Fifth Edition

Appleton & Lange's Review of
PEDIATRICS

Fifth Edition

Appleton & Lange's Review of
PEDIATRICS

Martin I. Lorin, MD
Professor of Clinical Pediatrics
Director of Medical Education
Department of Pediatrics
Baylor College of Medicine
Houston, Texas

Appleton & Lange Reviews/McGraw-Hill
Health Professions Division

New York   St. Louis   San Francisco   Auckland   Bogotá   Caracas   Lisbon   London
Madrid   Mexico City   Milan   Montreal   New Delhi   San Juan
Singapore   Sydney   Tokyo   Toronto

McGraw-Hill

A Division of The McGraw·Hill Companies

12 13 14 15 / 00

Library of Congress Cataloging-in-Publication Data

Lorin, Martin I.
    Appleton & Lange's review of pediatrics / Martin I. Lorin — 5th ed.
        p. cm.
    Includes bibliographical references and index.
    ISBN 0–8385–0057–9
    1. Pediatrics—Examinations, questions, etc. I. Title.
II. Title: Appleton & Lange's review of pediatrics. III. Title:
Review of pediatrics.
    [DNLM: 1. Pediatrics—examination questions.   WS 18 L872p 1993]
RJ48.2.L67   1993
618.92′00076—dc20
DNLM/DLC
for Library of Congress   93–57
                                                                 CIP

Acquisitions Editor: Jamie L. Mount
Production Editor: Sondra Greenfield
Designer: Penny Kindzierski

PRINTED IN THE UNITED STATES OF AMERICA

*This book is dedicated to my family, who made it possible,
and to my students and residents, who made it worthwhile.*

Contents

Preface ix

References xi

1. Warm-Up Questions and Exam-Taking Skills 1
Answers and Explanations 6

2. Growth and Development and Psychosocial Pediatrics 15
Answers and Explanations 24

3. The Newborn 35
Answers and Explanations 46

4. Feeding and Nutrition 59
Answers and Explanations 63

5. Accidents, Poisoning, and Drug Abuse 67
Answers and Explanations 72

6. Infectious and Communicable Diseases 79
Answers and Explanations 89

7. Metabolic Disorders (Including Fluid and Electrolytes) 101
Answers and Explanations 106

8. Therapeutics 113
Answers and Explanations 120

9. General Pediatrics 129
Answers and Explanations 139

10. Case Diagnosis—Management Problems 153
Answers and Explanations 167

11. Practice Test 181
Answers and Explanations 195
Practice Test Subspecialty List 211

Index 213
Practice Test Answer Grid 219

Preface

There are as many ways to acquire knowledge as there are to test it. This book addresses itself to the acquisition, as well as the testing, of knowledge and ability. It provides a means of comprehensive self-evaluation, which can direct your attention to areas of weakness in overall mastery of the subject material of pediatrics. The book also will enable you to become familiar with the types of questions used on most national examinations.

Chapter 1 is a warm-up practice examination that will also help you evaluate your test-taking skills. Chapters 2 through 9 are organized by topics and provide an opportunity to test your basic fund of pediatric knowledge. Chapter 10, Case Diagnosis—Management Problems, provides a chance to test your ability to apply that knowledge to a series of clinical problems. The Practice Test (Chapter 11) is a sample examination with questions drawn from all topic areas.

This book is meant to be a source of information and understanding. Each answer includes an explanation and one or more references. The latter will direct the reader to additional data and discussion as necessary. The reader should strive for understanding rather than memorization, although, undeniably, a substantial fund of knowledge must be committed to memory. Read all answers completely, even if you answered the question correctly. Many answers contain important and relevant information beyond that required simply to answer the question.

To make this book the best learning experience possible, there are some instances in which a series of questions deals with a single topic in a sequential or progressive manner. In this situation, a subsequent question may provide a clue to a previous question. Always answer one question at a time and refrain from looking ahead.

Occasionally, you will find a note in square brackets [Note: . . .] in the answer. Rather than medical information per se, these notes pertain to question construction and techniques for answering multiple-choice examination questions. Although there is no substitute for knowledge and understanding, it is recognized that exam-taking ability is a legitimate academic skill, and it is not inappropriate for you to strengthen your ability in this regard.

An index of questions is provided, primarily to help you locate questions that you answered and wish to review or check again.

It is hoped that you will learn as much from using this book as the author did by preparing it.

References

Following is a list of the textbooks used repeatedly as references for the answers in this book. This list has been kept as short as possible to facilitate your referencing task. It is recognized that most students and house officers do not have an extensive personal library and that a long list of reference texts would be inconvenient. On the other hand, no single source provides adequate, in-depth coverage of all topics that the author considers appropriate for this review book. In those situations in which the needed material could not be found in any of these core texts, reference was provided to material in other textbooks or journals.

It is hoped that the provision of direct references, without a number system, will eliminate page turning and save time. The name in parentheses below is the name used to refer to these references in the Answers and Explanations sections.

(Athreya) Athreya BH, Silverman BK: *Pediatric Physical Diagnosis.* Norwalk, CT, Appleton-Century-Crofts, 1985.

(Feigin) Feigin RD, Cherry JD: *Textbook of Pediatric Infectious Diseases,* 3rd ed. Philadelphia, Saunders, 1992.

(Hathaway) Hathaway WE, Groothius JR, Hay WW, et al: *Current Pediatric Diagnosis and Treatment,* 10th ed. Norwalk, CT, Appleton & Lange, 1991.

(Hoekelman) Hoekelman RA, Friedman SB, Nelson NM, et al: *Primary Pediatric Care,* 2nd ed. St. Louis, Mosby Year Book, 1992.

(Oski) Oski FA, DeAngelis CD, Feigin RD, et al: *Principles and Practice of Pediatrics.* Philadelphia, Lippincott, 1990.

(Rudolph) Rudolph AM, Hoffman JIE, Rudolph CD: *Pediatrics,* 19th ed. Norwalk, CT, Appleton & Lange, 1991.

(Schaffer) Schaffer R, Avery ME: *Schaffer and Avery's Diseases of the Newborn,* 6th ed. Philadelphia, Saunders, 1991.

CHAPTER 1

Warm-Up Questions and Exam-Taking Skills
Questions

In the remaining chapters of this book, and for some of the answers in this chapter, each explanation begins with a letter in boldface type indicating the correct answer choice. However, in this chapter, several of the questions and answers begin with a clue to help you analyze the question and your approach to answering it.

This chapter should be studied with no time constraints. Proceed at your own pace, taking as much time as you need for each question.

DIRECTIONS (Questions 1 through 29): Each of the numbered items or incomplete statements in this section is followed by answers or by completions of the statement. Select the ONE lettered answer or completion that is BEST in each case.

Clue: Questions 1 and 2 are simple and straightforward, with only one possible correct answer. For this type of question, try to answer the question before looking at the choices. Then read the choices to verify that your answer is there. Finally, review all the other choices just to be sure that none is better than the one you have selected.

1. The pattern of genetic transmission of cystic fibrosis is

    (A) autosomal dominant
    (B) autosomal recessive
    (C) X-linked recessive
    (D) X-linked dominant
    (E) autosomal recessive in some families and X-linked in others

2. The virus most commonly associated with the clinical picture of acute bronchiolitis in infants and young children is

    (A) adenovirus
    (B) respiratory syncytial virus
    (C) rhinovirus
    (D) coxsackievirus B
    (E) herpes virus type 2

Clue: Unlike the preceding two questions, the answer to Question 3 cannot be anticipated before viewing the list of suggested answers, because there are many possible completions to the question. Nevertheless, the question is simple and straightforward.

3. Minimal-change disease

    (A) is the most common cause of nephrotic syndrome in childhood
    (B) has a peak incidence in children between 10 and 15 years of age
    (C) usually results in end-stage renal disease in 3 to 5 years
    (D) is characterized by normal serum lipids and cholesterol
    (E) responds poorly to corticosteroids

Clue: Pay attention to key words when you read a question. Question 4 contains the key word "common."

4. Which of the following is a common side effect of phenytoin (Dilantin) therapy?

    (A) Raynaud's phenomenon
    (B) Lymphoma syndrome
    (C) Lupus erythematosus syndrome
    (D) Gingival hyperplasia
    (E) Optic atrophy

5. Infants born to mothers who have been using crack cocaine are at increased risk of

    (A) anemia
    (B) cerebral infarction
    (C) hypercalcemia
    (D) macrosomia
    (E) postmaturity

6. You examine an 18-year-old male college student with a 5-day history of fever, sore throat, and fatigue. Physical examination reveals an exudative tonsillitis and bilateral enlarged and slightly tender posterior cervical lymph nodes. The spleen is palpable 3 cm below the rib cage. The agent most likely responsible for this child's illness is

(A) group A beta-hemolytic *Streptococcus*
(B) adenovirus
(C) toxoplasmosis
(D) Epstein-Barr virus
(E) *C. diphtheriae*

Clue: The following question uses a negative qualifier, "all ... EXCEPT." You must be certain either that one of the features given is *not* associated with CMV or that four of the items *are* associated.

7. Intrauterine cytomegalovirus infection (CMV) has been associated with all of the following EXCEPT

(A) mental retardation
(B) deafness
(C) blindness
(D) jaundice
(E) intestinal obstruction

8. Clinical features associated with the 47,XXY karyotype include all of the following EXCEPT

(A) small, defective testes
(B) gynecomastia
(C) tall stature, with disproportionately long legs
(D) subnormal intelligence
(E) microcephaly

9. Meconium aspiration syndrome usually is associated with

(A) neonatal meningitis
(B) congenital heart disease
(C) cystic fibrosis
(D) fetal distress
(E) tracheoesophageal fistula

10. Which of the following statements regarding the use of NPH insulin in children is correct?

(A) The hypoglycemic effect peaks in 4 to 6 hours
(B) The hypoglycemic effect lasts about 12 hours
(C) It should not be mixed in the same syringe with regular insulin
(D) It is usually administered twice daily
(E) It should not be used in children less than 5 years old

11. A child in the preicteric phase of hepatitis A most likely will exhibit

(A) fever, rash, and diarrhea
(B) headache, hepatosplenomegaly, and clay-colored stools

(C) anorexia, fever, and vomiting
(D) fever, coma, and convulsions
(E) stiff neck and photophobia

12. Which of the following statements regarding immunization against *Hemophilus influenzae* type B (Hib) is correct?

(A) It is indicated for high-risk children only
(B) Currently available conjugated Hib vaccines can be administered effectively as early as 2 months of age
(C) Children who have had allergic reactions to egg should not be given the Hib vaccine
(D) It is recommended that the conjugated Hib vaccine not be administered to children with a history of reactions to DPT immunization
(E) The current recommendation is that the conjugated Hib vaccine be given as a single dose without a booster

13. It recently has been recommended that young infants should sleep in the supine rather than in the prone position. This is based on data suggesting that the prone position is associated with an increased incidence of

(A) delayed eruption of the first deciduous teeth
(B) gastroesophageal reflux and aspiration
(C) macrognathia
(D) strabismus
(E) sudden infant death

14. The feeding of honey to infants less than 6 months of age has been associated with

(A) hypoglycemia
(B) hypernatremia
(C) infantile botulism
(D) jaundice
(E) listeriosis

15. The mother of a healthy 6-month-old infant is planning to stop breast feeding within the next month and asks your advice about how she should proceed. The child had been fed on the breast only, without bottle supplementation and without solids. You should advise her that

(A) infant formula is an acceptable alternative for infants who are not being breast fed
(B) all infants should receive daily multivitamin (A, B complex, C, D) and mineral supplements to assure optimal nutrition
(C) after the introduction of cereals, food intolerances can be minimized by introducing solid foods in the following order: vegetables, fruits, meats, then eggs
(D) beginning at about the age of 6 months, an infant should be encouraged to consume solid foods at bedtime to facilitate sleeping through the night

(E) the infant should be started on milk by cup only, avoiding the use of a bottle

16. The term *small for gestational age* refers to an infant who weighs less than the

(A) 50th percentile for gestational age
(B) 25th percentile for gestational age
(C) 10th percentile for gestational age
(D) 5th percentile for gestational age
(E) 3rd percentile for gestational age

17. You have just examined a term, healthy, male newborn infant and found no abnormalities. In speaking to the mother, she asks you whether or not she should have the child circumcised. In your discussion with the mother, it would be most appropriate to explain that circumcision is associated with

(A) a decreased incidence of urinary tract infection in infancy and a decreased incidence of penile cancer in adulthood
(B) a decreased incidence of urinary tract infection in infancy and an increased incidence of penile cancer in adulthood
(C) an increased incidence of urinary tract infection during infancy and a decreased incidence of penile cancer in adulthood
(D) an increased incidence of urinary tract infection in childhood and an increased incidence of penile cancer in adulthood
(E) no change in the incidence of either urinary tract infection or penile cancer

18. The mother listens carefully and appears to consider the information you have given. She then asks whether you, personally, would recommend circumcision for her infant. You should reply that routine neonatal circumcision is

(A) medically indicated
(B) medically indicated, but parents must be aware of the risks, which include bleeding, infection, and scarring
(C) not medically indicated
(D) not medically indicated and associated with certain risks, but in the final analysis the decision should be made by the parents on the basis of personal preference
(E) not medically indicated, and you personally would advise against it

19. Which of the following is responsible for the greatest number of infants or children with failure to thrive?

(A) Renal disease
(B) Metabolic disorders
(C) Tuberculosis
(D) Endocrine disorders
(E) Nonorganic causes

20. A 2-year-old child is being evaluated because the mother notes that her right eye has been turning in. Physical examination documents strabismus with a right esotropia. Attempts to visualize the fundi are unsuccessful, but it is noted that the red reflex is replaced by a yellow-white pupillary reflex in the right eye. This child most likely has

(A) retinitis pigmentosa
(B) retinoblastoma
(C) rhabdomyosarcoma
(D) severe hyperopia
(E) severe myopia

21. A 2-year-old child is admitted because of weakness and coma. According to the parents he had been well until several hours prior to admission, when they noted diarrhea, cough, wheezing, and sweating. Physical examination reveals a comatose child with diffuse weakness and areflexia. Pupils are pinpoint and unresponsive. Examination of the chest reveals generalized wheezing. Oral secretions are copious. At this time you ought to administer a dose of

(A) adrenaline
(B) atropine
(C) cefotaxime
(D) methylprednisolone
(E) tensilon

22. A 3-week-old infant is admitted with vomiting of 5 days' duration. Physical examination reveals a rapid heart rate, evidence of dehydration, and ambiguous genitalia. Serum electrolytes are Na^+ 120 mEq/L, K^+ 7.5 mEq/L, HCO_3^- 12 mEq/L, BUN 20 mg/dL. In addition to intravenous fluid replacement with normal saline, administration of which of the following would be most important?

(A) Diuretics
(B) Potassium exchange resin
(C) Glucose and insulin
(D) Antibiotics
(E) Hydrocortisone

23. A previously well 12-year-old girl is admitted because of painful swellings on the front of the legs of about 3 days' duration. Examination reveals tender erythematous nodules, 1 to 2 cm in diameter, on the extensor surfaces of the lower legs. The remainder of the physical examination is unremarkable. Which of the following is most likely to confirm the cause of this condition?

(A) Stool smear and culture
(B) Urinalysis and BUN
(C) Throat culture and ASO titer
(D) Slit-lamp examination of the eye
(E) Echocardiogram

24. You have been asked to consult on an 8-year-old boy who has been followed elsewhere for several years because of microscopic hematuria. The child has been totally asymptomatic; medical history and family history are noncontributory; and the physical examination, including growth parameters, is entirely within normal limits. Repeated urine analyses have been normal except for microscopic hematuria. BUN, creatinine, and chest roentgenogram are normal. Which of the following would be LEAST useful at this time?

(A) Creatinine clearance
(B) ASO titer
(C) Urine calcium/creatinine ratio
(D) Renal ultrasound
(E) Analysis of a 24-hour urine specimen

25. A 12-year-old child is seen because of a rash and severe headache. The skin lesion began as a red macule on the thigh, which gradually expanded over 1 week to reach approximately 15 cm in diameter with red borders and central clearing. The lesion was slightly painful. A few days after the onset of the skin manifestation, the child developed severe headache, stiff neck, myalgias, arthralgias, malaise, fatigue, lethargy, and generalized lymphadenopathy. Low-grade fever was present. The mother recalls that the child was bitten by a tick about 1 week prior to the onset of symptoms. This patient's disorder is probably best treated with

(A) corticosteroids
(B) diphenhydramine
(C) methotrexate
(D) nonsteroidal anti-inflammatory drugs
(E) penicillin

26. An 8-year-old child is hospitalized because of paroxysms of severe colicky abdominal pain that do not radiate to the back or the groin. Physical examination is unremarkable except for generalized abdominal tenderness. The child is taken to the operating room, where exploratory laparotomy reveals an edematous intestine without specific lesions. The appendix appears normal but is removed. Postoperatively the abdominal pain persists, and melena develops. On the second postoperative day, tender swelling of both ankles and knees is noted. This child should be observed closely for the development of

(A) shock
(B) meningitis
(C) hepatitis
(D) a purpuric rash
(E) hemorrhagic pancreatitis

27. You are asked to evaluate a 10-year-old boy who has been having episodes of repetitive and semipurposeful movements of the face and shoulders. The parents believe that these movements are worse when the child is under emotional stress. They also volunteer that they have never noted the movements while the patient is asleep. The movements have been present for more than 6 months. The parents are now especially concerned because the child has developed repetitive episodes of throat clearing and snorting. Physical and neurological examination are entirely normal. During the examination you note that the child has some blinking of the right eye, twitching of the right face and grimacing. You ask him to stop these movements, and he is temporarily successful in doing so, but the movements recur. The home situation, social history, and child's development and social adjustment appear normal. Of the following, which would be the most appropriate next step?

(A) Order a CT of the head
(B) Prescribe carbamazepine
(C) Prescribe corticosteroids
(D) Prescribe haloperidol
(E) Refer the child to a psychiatrist

28. A 3-month-old infant is hospitalized because of recurrent right focal seizures that progress to generalization. Birth and perinatal history are unremarkable. There is a flat, purplish-red hemangioma on the left side of the face extending onto the forehead. The remainder of the examination (neurologic and physical) is within normal limits. The results of a lumbar puncture are within normal limits. You order a CT scan of the head and anticipate seeing

(A) agenesis of the corpus callosum
(B) a porencephalic cyst
(C) gyriform calcifications
(D) hydrocephalus
(E) normal findings

29. On routine examination of the children of a migrant farm worker, you notice that a 12-year-old child who has received little previous medical care is short and mentally retarded. Physical examination reveals that the liver is enlarged to 5 cm below the right rib cage, and the spleen is enlarged 6 cm below the left rib cage. Lumbodorsal kyphosis is prominent. The child has a peculiar facies with thick lips and a large tongue. Attempts to visualize the retina are unsuccessful because of clouding of the corneas. You expect that examination of this child's urine will reveal

(A) dermatan and heparan sulfate
(B) galactose
(C) mannose
(D) the odor of maple syrup
(E) the odor of sweaty feet

DIRECTIONS (30 through 36): Each set of matching questions in this section consists of a list of 4 to 26 lettered options followed by several numbered items. For each numbered item select the ONE lettered option with which it is most closely associated. Each lettered option may be selected once, more than once, or not at all.

Questions 30 through 33

- (A) Miliaria rubra
- (B) Verrucae vulgaris
- (C) Condyloma acuminatum
- (D) Molluscum contagiosum
- (E) Pityriasis rosea

30. Small (pinhead to 1 cm), pearly papules with translucent tops and waxy, whitish material inside, distributed on the face and anterior trunk. Some lesions are umbilicated.

31. Soft, flesh-colored papular or pedunculated lesions around the genitalia and rectum

32. Oval, maculopapular lesions oriented with the long axis along skin tension lines

33. Characteristically pruritic

Questions 34 through 36

- (A) ABO incompatibility
- (B) Alpha₁-antitrypsin deficiency
- (C) Biliary atresia
- (D) Breastfeeding jaundice
- (E) Breast milk jaundice
- (F) Choledochal cyst
- (G) Cholelithiasis
- (H) Crigler-Najjar syndrome
- (I) Cystic fibrosis
- (J) Dubin-Johnson syndrome
- (K) Erythroblastosis (Rh incompatibility)
- (L) Galactosemia
- (M) Glucose 6-phosphate dehydrogenase deficiency
- (N) Hepatitis
- (O) Hereditary spherocytosis
- (P) Hypothyroidism
- (Q) Physiologic hyperbilirubinemia
- (R) Sepsis

34. A 3-day-old term, healthy infant is noted to be jaundiced. Physical examination is otherwise normal. Laboratory values: Hb 16.8 g/dL; reticulocytes 1.0%; bilirubin unconjugated 8.5 mg/dL, conjugated 0.8 mg/dL.

35. A 5-week-old infant has been jaundiced for about 2 weeks. He has been asymptomatic and physical examination is otherwise normal. Laboratory values: Hb 14.2 g/dL; reticulocytes 1.2%; bilirubin unconjugated 4.5 mg/dL, conjugated 5.5 mg/dL; ALT 25 IU/L, AST 75 IU/L. Abdominal ultrasound examination reveals a normal-sized liver; a gallbladder is not visualized.

36. An otherwise well 4-week-old infant has remained jaundiced since day 3 of life despite two exchange transfusions and continuous phototherapy. Laboratory values: Hb 14 g/dL; reticulocytes 1.0%; bilirubin unconjugated 16 mg/dL, conjugated 0.2 mg/dL; ALT 15 IU/L, AST 40 IU/L. A Coombs test prior to the first exchange transfusion was negative. Ultrasound examination reveals a normal liver and gallbladder.

Answers and Explanations

For many of the questions below, the boldface letter indicating the correct answer appears within, or at the end of, the explanation rather than at the beginning. When this is the case, take care to not look ahead. Try to respond to the clues as you go along.

1. The correct answer is **(B)**. Cystic fibrosis (CF) is an autosomal recessive disorder with a disease incidence in Caucasians of about 1:1,500 and a corresponding carrier state of about 1:20. This is said to make CF the most common lethal genetic disease in the white population. The disease is much less common among blacks and Asians. *(Oski:1363; Rudolph:1526)*

2. Like question 1, this question has only one possible correct answer, and you should have been able to come up with that answer before looking at the list of choices. The answer is **(B)**, respiratory synctial virus (RSV), the most commonly identified cause of viral bronchiolitis. The choice here is especially easy because influenza and parainfluenza viruses, which are second behind RSV as causes of bronchiolitis, were not listed. *(Rudolph:1520; Oski:1332)*

3. The correct answer is **(A)**. This question is simple in that it deals with well-known and important clinical features of a common disease—minimal-change nephrotic syndrome (MCNS). It is straightforward in that not only is one of the listed choices clearly the best, but the other four choices all are clearly incorrect.

Minimal-change disease is clearly the most common cause of nephrotic syndrome in childhood, accounting for more than all other causes combined. The peak incidence is between 2 and 5 years of age. The prognosis is very favorable, and the process rarely progresses to end-stage renal disease. Serum lipids and cholesterol are elevated, as they are with other causes of nephrotic syndrome. Finally, the disease characteristically responds well to treatment with corticosteroids, with only a small minority of patients failing to remit.

If you answered this question incorrectly, try to determine why. Since the question is so straightforward, the most likely reason would be an incomplete fund of knowledge. *(Rudolph:1267–1271; Oski:1637–41)*

4. The correct answer is **(D)**. Optic atrophy is not a recognized complication of phenytoin (Dilantin) therapy. A lupus erythematosus-like syndrome, a lymphoma-like syndrome, and Raynaud's phenomenon all have been noted *rarely* with this drug. Gingival hyperplasia is a *common* and troublesome side effect, which often can be minimized by scrupulous dental hygiene.

If the examinee knew that lymphoma-like syndrome has been reported with phenytoin and focused in on that without carefully considering all other choices, he or she might have selected **(B)**. You could avoid this error by carefully reading the question and asking yourself, "What are the *common* side effects of this drug?," even before looking at the choices. Knowing that gingival hypertrophy is a very common side effect of phenytoin would be sufficient knowledge to answer the question correctly. *(Rudolph:966,982; Hathaway:674)*

5. This is another straightforward, completely factual question. Only one choice is correct. As a matter of fact, two answers are not only incorrect, they are exact opposites of what actually happens with cocaine, so it should be easy to be confident that they are incorrect. Infants born to women using cocaine, especially crack cocaine, have an increased incidence of *prematurity* (not postmaturity) and *low birth weight* (not macrosomia). The vasoconstrictive action of cocaine not only impairs uterine and placental blood flow but also may result in cerebral infarction in the fetus or neonate and probably is a key factor in the increased incidence of necrotizing enterocolitis seen in these infants. The correct answer is **(B)**. *(Schaffer:244–245)*

6. Although this question also is simple and straightforward, it is potentially more difficult than the preceding questions because several of the agents listed

could explain many of the features of this child's illness. If you read the instructions carefully, you noted that you were asked to select the one *best* answer, which does not imply that all other choices are totally without merit. Consider which of the above choices *best* fits the clinical scenario and which is *most likely* responsible for this illness.

The correct answer is (**D**). The agent most likely responsible for this child's illness is the Epstein-Barr (EB) virus. The clinical picture is strongly suggestive of mononucleosis. Although this child could be infected with group A *Streptococcus* or adenovirus, several features are much more characteristic of EB virus infection than either of these: the fact that the child is a college student, the presence of splenomegaly, and the fact that the adenopathy is posterior and only slightly tender. These findings also could be explained by toxoplasmosis, but this diagnosis is rarely confirmed as a cause of acute exudative tonsillitis and cervical adenitis in this country. Although it is appropriate to think of diphtheria in patients with acute exudative tonsillitis, there is nothing specific in this case to suggest that diagnosis. Infectious mononucleosis is certainly the *most likely* diagnosis.

If you missed this question, was it because you didn't know enough about EB virus or some of the other choices, or because you didn't make the right judgmental decision? *(Rudolph:649–650; Hathaway:832–833)*

7. It is generally easier to be sure that two items are associated than it is to be sure that they are not. If we know of the association, then it exists. If we don't know of an association, it may be because it doesn't exist or it may be *that we just don't know about it.* Recognized manifestations of cytomegaloviral infection in the neonate include deafness, blindness, jaundice, petechiae, fever, convulsions, and mental retardation. Intestinal obstruction has not been noted. Since congenital CMV infection is not uncommon, it is fortunate that most infections are asymptomatic.

Even if you knew nothing about congenital CMV infection, a careful reading of the choices would suggest a *best guess.* Answer (**E**) is different from all the other choices in the sense that neonatal intestinal obstruction usually is caused by a discrete congenital abnormality such as intestinal atresia, malrotation, or annular pancreas. The other manifestations listed generally result from diffuse tissue damage or inflammation. Even if you knew nothing about congenital CMV infection, a careful reading of the choices would suggest a *best guess.* Guessing, obviously, is a last resort, but almost always you should be able to make an *educated* rather than a *blind* guess. *(Feigin:979; Hathaway:84–85)*

8. Several factors make this question difficult, even though it deals with the most common human sex

chromosomal aberration, the 47,XXY karyotype. First, the name of the disorder (Klinefelter's syndrome or seminiferous tubule dysgenesis) is not provided in either the question or the answer. Second, the use of "all ... EXCEPT," as discussed above, adds to the complexity of the question.

Klinefelter's syndrome is associated with small, defective testes, azoospermia, and sterility. Gynecomastia and other signs of eunuchoidism occur in about half the patients. Patients usually are long-legged and tall. Although mental deficiency, often severe, is common, microcephaly is not a feature. Therefore, the correct answer is (**E**). *(Rudolph:1661–1662)*

9. (**D**) Meconium aspiration usually is associated with fetal distress. The mechanism involves the loss of sphincter tone, passage of meconium into the amniotic fluid, and aspiration by the distressed, gasping infant during the process of birth. The thick meconium obstructs the airways, causing tachypnea, retractions, and grunting.

This is the type of question in which a little knowledge can go a long way. If you knew that meconium aspiration was a relatively common problem in the delivery room, you could eliminate (**C**) cystic fibrosis (a relatively uncommon disease) as its cause. Meconium ileus, which is associated with cystic fibrosis, has nothing to do with meconium aspiration. If you realized that aspiration of meconium can only occur before or during delivery, you also could eliminate (**B**) congenital heart disease and (**A**) neonatal meningitis, as neither of these usually causes symptoms or distress during the delivery. Finally, you should be able to figure out that a tracheoesophageal fistula, with or without associated esophageal atresia, might lead to aspiration of saliva, milk, or gastric contents but would not predispose to aspiration of meconium. *(Rudolph:1493; Hathaway:74)*

10. You should try to answer this question by selecting the one best choice and then confirm it by verifying the alternate choices as incorrect. If you are not certain which answer is best, eliminate as many of the choices as possible and then make an intuitive guess among the remaining choices. Note that the question specifies *use in children.* Are there any differences in the effects of, or use of, NPH insulin in children as compared to adult? No, not really, except that in the case of children, one is almost always dealing with insulin-dependent diabetes.

The effect of NPH insulin peaks at 8 to 12 hours and lasts about 24 hours. It is usually administered together with regular insulin (in the same syringe) *twice a day*, before breakfast and before supper. NPH insulin is useful in the management of diabetic children of all ages. Therefore, the only correct statement is (**D**), that NPH insulin is usually administered twice a day. *(Rudolph:339,1981; Hathaway:812–813)*

11. (C) Although the material covered by this question is neither difficult nor complex, failure to pay attention to the precise wording of the question could be disastrous. The *preicteric* phase of viral hepatitis A is characterized by anorexia, fever, vomiting, and abdominal pain. Tender hepatomegaly (rather than hepatosplenomegaly) also is common. Rash is more frequent with hepatitis B than with hepatitis A. Clay-colored stools usually appear coincident with jaundice rather than during the preicteric phase. If you answered this question incorrectly, consider why. Inadequate attention to the words *preicteric phase* or *hepatitis A* might have led to the selection of choice **(B)**. *(Feigin:679–680)*

12. The majority of questions in national examinations deal with basic material that is covered in standard textbooks, and therefore, standard texts is where examinees should spend the majority of their reading time. A percentage of questions, however, deal with recent data, which although important and often well known, may not yet have been incorporated into standard texts. This is somewhat more likely to be the case for questions dealing with treatment than with manifestations or diagnosis of diseases. This question is an example of material that was incorporated into a question prior to its inclusion in standard textbooks. *Hemophilus influenzae* type B (Hib) infection is a major cause of morbidity and mortality in the young infant. The introduction of Hib immunization is relatively new. The Hib polysaccharide is not very immunogenic, and the first generation of vaccines were effective only when administered to children 2 years and older. Unfortunately, the greatest incidence of Hib meningitis is in the child less than 2 years. Just as information about the first vaccines was being incorporated into textbooks, a second generation of vaccines, which could be administered effectively at 18 months of age, was introduced into clinical use. Finally, in late 1990, conjugated vaccines were licensed. These vaccines are effective when administered as early as age 2 months.

The correct answer to this question, therefore, is **(B)**. It is now recommended that all infants be immunized with the conjugated Hib vaccine. Depending on the brand of vaccine used, infants should receive a series of two or three immunizations between 2 and 6 months of age, followed by a final booster dose at either 12 or 15 months of age. *(Pediatrics 88:169–172,1991)*

13. (E) This is another example of a question dealing with new material not yet in the standard texts. In this case, the information involved, although new, has received a great deal of national attention in the lay press as well as in the medical literature. Recent data have suggested an increased incidence of sudden infant death syndrome (SIDS) among infants sleeping prone as compared to those sleeping supine.

Although the prone sleeping position has been traditionally favored in the United States for many years, and although the data associating the prone position with SIDS is epidemiologic and not conclusive, the American Academy of Pediatrics and others now recommend that infants routinely be put to sleep in the supine position. However, since there appears to be less tendency to gastroesophageal reflux (GER) in the prone position, probably because the esophagus enters the stomach posteriorly, infants with GER are an exception and should be permitted to sleep in the prone position. Normal infants should sleep supine. *(Pediatrics 89:1120–1125,1992)*

14. This is a straightforward but difficult question because it involves information not so widely known as the material in most of the preceding questions. Can you recall reading or hearing about honey being associated with a specific infection or disease? If not, can you eliminate any of the choices to improve your chances of a correct guess? Isn't it unlikely that a complex carbohydrate such as honey would cause hypoglycemia? You may have heard that *Listeria* is often spread through contaminated milk and cheese, but you have not heard that it is spread by honey. Jaundice is a common problem in the neonate, but the question refers to infants less than 6 months of age, not specifically to neonates.

The answer is **(C)**. Infants are especially vulnerable to *infantile* botulism. This disorder differs from the adult form of the disease in that it is indolent rather than acute and is characterized by progressive muscle weakness. The infantile form of botulism results from ingestion of *C. botulinum* spores, in contrast to the adult form, which results from the ingestion of the preformed toxin in contaminated food. Honey has been incriminated as one source of *C. botulinum* spores, and, therefore, honey is not recommended for infants younger than 6 months of age. *(Rudolph:566; Hathaway:861)*

15. This question is very open ended, with many potentially correct completions. You must evaluate each choice, estimate its validity, and rank it against the other choices.
(A) Is infant formula an acceptable alternative to breast feeding? Common sense and experience suggest that it is. It may not be optimal or ideal, but it is widely used and, therefore, presumably acceptable.
(B) Should all infants be supplemented with multivitamins and minerals? The idea sounds reasonable, but is it necessary? Should *all* infants be supplemented?
(C) Does the exact order in which foods are introduced really matter?
(D) Is 6 months of age an appropriate time to introduce solids, and if so, why? Is it to get the infant to sleep through the night?
(E) When is a child developmentally ready to drink

from a cup? Clearly not at 6 months, so this answer can be eliminated.

So we have eliminated (**E**) and cast doubt on (**B, C, and D**). Therefore, the best answer is (**A**). Human milk is the preferred method of feeding throughout the first year of life. If breast feeding is discontinued, infant formula is an acceptable alternative. During the second 6 months of life, the normal infant fed iron- and vitamin-D-fortified formula and a diet that includes an adequate source of vitamin C does not require other vitamin or mineral supplementation. There is little basis for routine administration of additional vitamin or mineral preparations to normal children except for fluoride supplementation if there is insufficient fluoride in the drinking water.

Solid foods should be introduced one at a time, at intervals of a week or more, so that intolerances can be easily identified. The order of introduction is not critical, although a single-grain, iron-fortified infant cereal often is advised as the first solid food. Because allergy to egg is relatively common, introduction of this food is often delayed. Most authorities do recommend introducing solid foods at about 4 to 6 months, but at meal time rather than at bedtime. Misguided attempts to provide as many calories as possible at bedtime (to encourage infants to sleep) should be discouraged because such eating patterns established in infancy may contribute to overeating and obesity in later life. *(Rudolph:28–29; Hathaway:117–119)*

16. (**C**) Quantitative questions are intrinsically difficult in that they require very specific information rather than a concept. However, an understanding of the basic concept will often help narrow the choices. In this case, an understanding of the concept of *small for gestational age* would intuitively lead the examinee to eliminate choices (**A**) and (**B**) as including too many infants. To get beyond that point, other than by guessing, one has to know the data, in this case, a definition.

Most authors define the small-for-dates or small-for-gestational-age infant as one whose weight is less than the 10th percentile or more than two standard deviations below the mean for infants of that gestational age. Infants who are significantly small for gestational age require special care and observation. *(Rudolph:167)*

17. Although the topic of this question, circumcision, is a controversial and often emotional issue, this question is straightforward and deals only with facts. There are now several studies indicating a decreased incidence of urinary tract infection among circumcised as compared to noncircumcised males during infancy. This effect is restricted to the first few months of life, clearly not extending beyond the first birthday. If you were aware of these data, you would be able to exclude answers (**C**), (**D**), and (**E**), giving

yourself a 50% chance of guessing the correct answer. You may also know that data show a decreased incidence of penile cancer among circumcised males in late adulthood. Therefore, (**A**) is the correct answer. *(Pediatrics 84:388–390,1989; Rudolph:184)*

18. In contrast to the preceding question, this is a subjective question and therefore difficult and often frustrating for the examinee. The question looks not only for your fund of knowledge but also for how you would use that knowledge in dealing with parents. When faced with such questions, you should try to answer in accordance with what you know or believe to be closest to standard medical practice or the majority opinion, even if you personally disagree. Most authorities suggest that the brief decrease in prevalence of urinary tract infections and the decrease in penile cancer in late adulthood are not sufficient benefits to medically justify a routine recommendation for the surgical procedure of circumcision. In the final analysis, the decision must be made by the parents on the basis of personal preference. The correct answer, therefore, is (**D**), which is logical in regard to the available data and also is in accordance with the recommendations of the American Academy of Pediatrics. *(Pediatrics 78:96–99,1986; 84:388–390,1989; Am J Dis Child 134:484–486,1980)*

19. (**E**) Failure to thrive (FTT) is a common pediatric problem characterized by poor growth, especially in regard to weight gain. Today, in the United States, nonorganic causes of FTT account for 30% to more than 50% of the cases in most series and are responsible for more cases than any other etiology. Nonorganic causes encompass a diverse spectrum extending from poverty and lack of food, through poor parenting skills and misguided feeding to frank neglect or abuse. If you missed this question, why? Were you unaware of the importance and frequency of nonorganic causes of FTT? Did you think that one of the other choices was more common? If so, that reflects a lack of information rather than uncertainty between close items, because *none of the other choices listed accounts for more than 5% or 10% of cases.* If gastrointestinal problems had been a choice, the question would have been more difficult, because gastrointestinal disorders account for up to 25% of cases of FTT in most series. *(Oski:969)*

20. (**B**) Retinoblastoma is the most likely cause of this child's strabismus and white pupillary reflex (leukokoria, "cat's eye reflex"). Although rhabdomyosarcoma may involve the orbit, it is extrinsic to the globe and doesn't cause a white pupillary reflex. Other causes of leukokoria include visceral lava migrans (*Toxocara canis* infection) and retrolental fibroplasia. Although retinoblastoma is rare, the association with leukokoria is a classic and important pediatric entity with which all students as well as

pediatric house officers should be familiar. *(Rudolph: 1909; Oski:1597; Althreya:219)*

21. This format is common on national medical examinations. It makes the question difficult because, unlike all the previous questions, this format requires *recall* rather than *recognition*. The question asks you to identify a disease but does *not* provide a list of diseases from which to choose; instead, it provides a list of associated findings, in this case, treatments. To answer the question correctly, therefore, requires that you analyze the clinical findings and *recall* the disease rather than *selecting* it from a list.

The sudden onset of neurological signs or symptoms in a previously well toddler always ought to raise suspicion of a toxin or poisoning. Review the question. Can you think of any toxins that might explain the findings in this case?

The correct answer is **(B)**. This child is a victim of organophosphate poisoning. Organophosphate and carbamate insecticides are widely used throughout the United States and are an important cause of poisoning in children. These drugs produce both muscarinic effects (rhinorrhea, wheezing, pulmonary edema, salivation, vomiting, cramps, bradycardia, and pinpoint pupils) as well as nicotinic effects (twitching, weakness and paralysis, convulsions, coma, and respiratory failure). These children often ingest the toxic substance unobserved, and the diagnosis must be suspected on the basis of the clinical picture even when there is no history of ingestion or exposure. Atropine will reverse the muscarinic effects of these agents and is a useful part of treatment. *(Rudolph:814–815; Hathaway:945–946)*

22. **(E)** The child described probably has congenital adrenal hyperplasia (CAH), an inborn metabolic error of the adrenal cortex. The acidosis (HCO_3^- 12 mEq/L) helps to rule out pyloric stenosis as the cause of the emesis, as most infants with pyloric stenosis have a metabolic alkalosis. The enzyme deficiency in CAH results in decreased production of cortisol and other adrenal cortical hormones and secondary hypertrophy of the adrenal gland. Accumulation of androgen-like precursors of cortisol during fetal development leads to masculinization of the female fetus and ambiguous genitalia, which is the important clue in this case. The low serum sodium and high potassium levels are classic findings in this condition, reflecting the lack of mineralocorticoids. In addition to the use of saline, administration of a mineralocorticoid such as cortisone or hydrocortisone is critical. The elevated serum potassium level usually responds rapidly to administration of saline and steroids, and specific therapy with exchange resins or glucose and insulin usually is unnecessary.

As did the preceding question, this question tests the examinee's ability of recall rather than recognition, a more difficult but clinically more relevant skill. Instead of providing a list of diseases or syndromes as possible answers, it provides a list of additional features or findings, one of which is associated with the disorder in question. In this case, as in the preceding question, the feature to be selected is the appropriate therapy. The question tests more than the examinee's ability to recite the treatment of hyperkalemia. It tests his or her ability to analyze the clinical situation, make a correct diagnosis, set priorities, and tailor therapy to the specific pathophysiology involved. *(Rudolph:1596–1597; Hathaway: 802–803)*

23. Again, this question requires recall rather than recognition. The stem of the question gives no information except the age and sex of the patient and a description of the skin lesions—*tender* erythematous nodules on the *extensor* surfaces of the legs. On the basis of these data you must decide what disease the patient probably has. Which of the following best fits the skin lesions described: erythema nodosum, rheumatic nodules, subcutaneous fat necrosis, hematomas, septic emboli, or Henoch-Schöenlein purpura?

The correct answer is **(C)**. To answer this question you must not only identify the rash as erythema nodosum (an uncommon but not rare disease) but also know that group A beta-hemolytic streptococcal infection is a common cause. Erythema nodosum is a reactive phenomenon characterized by tender, erythematous nodules 1 to 2 cm in diameter. The lesions usually are on the extensor surfaces of the extremities and are more common on the legs. This rash is seen in a variety of infections including histoplasmosis, tuberculosis, coccidioidomycosis, and group A streptococcal infection. Today, the most common cause in an otherwise well child is said to be group A streptococcal infection. *(Rudolph:916; Hathaway:286)*.

24. Negative questions always are potentially more difficult than positive questions. At first glance, all of the choices listed seem plausible, but which test would be *least* useful? Examine each choice carefully. How likely is it that the test would be positive, and how important would a positive result be? How useful would a negative result be? Obviously, it would be important if the creatinine clearance were abnormal, and a 24-hour urine collection could quantitate the hematuria and any associated proteinuria. What would be the significance of an elevated urinary calcium/creatinine ratio? (Hypercalciuria is a common cause of hematuria.) What would you be looking for with a renal ultrasound? (It could reveal polycystic disease or small kidneys indicative of chronic nephritis.) What would be the significance of an elevated ASO titer in a patient with hematuria of several years' duration? (Probably none. The ASO titer is a reflection of *recent* group A streptococcal in-

fection and would not be helpful in this child with chronic hematuria.) Therefore, the correct answer is **(B)**. *(Rudolph:1241–1243; Hathaway:609)*

25. Here again, you are required to make a diagnosis but are not given a list of diseases from which to choose. You should analyze the data, identify the important features, and generate a list of most likely diagnoses. The major problems appear to be fever, a localized rash, and meningeal inflammation (headache and stiff neck). The malaise, fatigue, lethargy, generalized lymphadenopathy, and arthralgia are less specific. Of note is the fact that the child was bitten by a tick a week prior to the onset of the illness. If the tick bite is related to the illness, it would suggest an infectious etiology. The systemic findings, the central clearing of the rash, and the time course permit us to rule out a simple cellulitis. What are the common infections carried by ticks? Rocky Mountain spotted fever, Lyme disease, Q fever, tularemia, relapsing fever, and Colorado tick fever are all spread by ticks, but only Lyme disease fits with the localized rash described—erythema migrans chronicum. This disease is caused by the spirochete *Borrelia burgdorferi*. The organism is sensitive to a number of antibiotics, including penicillin, which generally is the treatment of choice and is the correct answer, **(E)**. *(Feigin:1063–1066; Hathaway:896–897)*

26. This question also challenges you to identify a disease without providing a list of diagnoses from which to choose. What disease do you believe this child most likely has: juvenile rheumatoid arthritis, inflammatory bowel disease, cystic fibrosis, Henoch-Schönlein purpura, *Salmonella* infection?

    The correct answer is **(D)**. This child has anaphylactoid purpura, also known as Henoch-Schönlein purpura (HSP). This is an important and not rare pediatric entity, well known to pediatric residents but not so well known by students. The question is difficult because the scenario given is infrequent although well recognized in this disorder. The most characteristic feature of the disease, a purpuric rash limited to the area below the waist, is not present in this case, and the purpuric rash listed as a possible answer is not specified as to location or distribution. If you missed this question, was it because you weren't familiar with HSP or because you didn't recognize it from this uncommon presentation? *(Rudolph:color plate 13,490–491,1158; Hathaway:504–505)*

27. What disorder do you believe this child probably has: psychomotor seizures, Tourette's syndrome, drug abuse, brain tumor, or psychological disorder?

    The child most likely has Tourette's syndrome, a disorder characterized by blinking, twitching, grimacing, and jerking movements that often have a repetitive and semipurposeful character. Like simple habit tics, the movements usually can be voluntarily suppressed momentarily, disappear during sleep, and are made worse by emotional tension. These features could mislead the examinee to assume a psychological etiology. Ultimately, the muscles of respiration and swallowing become involved so that throat clearing, coughing, snorting, hiccups, and other noises are common. Coprolalia, echolalia, and spitting are classic features but are not always present.

    The correct answer is **(D)**. Haloperidol is the drug of choice for Tourette's syndrome, although not all patients require therapy. *(Oski:1385,1937–1938; Hathaway:702)*

28. This question deals with a rare but dramatic pediatric syndrome. What is the significance of the hemangioma on one side of the face? If you can identify the disease, can you then anticipate the findings on CT scan?

    Suppose the question had read: "... The most likely diagnosis is"

    (A) congenital toxoplasmosis
    (B) holoprosencephaly
    (C) Sturge-Weber syndrome
    (D) subdural effusions
    (E) porencephalic cyst

    Providing a list of diagnoses would change the question from one of recall to one of recognition.

    The correct answer to the question above is **(C)**, Sturge-Weber syndrome. The association of a unilateral facial hemangioma, particularly in the distribution of the trigeminal nerve, and focal seizures suggests Sturge-Weber syndrome (also referred to as Sturge-Weber-Dmitri syndrome and encephalotrigeminal angiomatosis). This syndrome is characterized by a port-wine capillary nevus on the face (classically in the distribution of the first division of the trigeminal nerve), focal seizures on the contralateral side, and intracranial calcifications on the ipsilateral side. Therefore, the correct answer to question 28 is **(C)**, gyriform calcifications. The intracranial pathology is caused by hemangiomatous changes of the meninges. This is a congenital disorder, probably of nongenetic basis. The seizures often are very difficult to control. Other frequent features include mental deficiency and a contralateral hemiparesis.

    Pay attention to all information. When analyzing such a question, you need to consider the potential significance of each piece of data, such as the hemangioma, although there is always the possibility that some incidental information, unrelated to the diagnosis, has been included.

    If you were able to make the correct diagnosis only after seeing the list of diseases above, it would suggest that your fund of knowledge in this area is adequate but that your ability to recall what you know needs strengthening. If you were unable to identify the correct answer even with the list above, you are unfamiliar with this syndrome. This question is very difficult because the subject matter (Sturge-Weber syndrome) is rare and because the question requires recall rather than recognition, a double dose of difficulty. *(Rudolph:915; Hathaway:695–696)*

29. This question is exceedingly difficult, so don't be discouraged. Do you know what disease or condition this child has, and if so, what would be found in the urine? Your first task is to establish a probable diagnosis. If you were not able to deduce the diagnosis from the question, how about from the list of answers? Do you know for what condition each finding is suggestive or diagnostic? Think about *each* one.

Urinary finding	Disease
Dermatan and heparan sulfate	Hurler syndrome
Galactose	Galactosemia
Mannose	Mannosidosis
Odor of maple syrup	Branched-chain aminoacidemia
Odor of sweaty feet	Isovaleryl CoA dehydrogenase deficiency

The correct answer is **(A)**. The child described has Hurler syndrome (a form of mucopolysaccharidosis). This rare autosomal recessive disorder is characterized by growth retardation that generally starts after the first year of life. Classically, facial features become coarse and eventually appear gargoyle-like. Hepatosplenomegaly results from the accumulation of mucopolysaccharide and often is striking. Bone and joint involvement with kyphosis and joint contractures is frequent. Corneal clouding results from the deposition of mucopolysaccharide in that organ. The accumulation of the mucopolysaccharide within the brain leads to mental retardation.

If you were not familiar with Hurler syndrome and did not know that it is characterized by dermatan and heparan sulfate in the urine, you would not be able to answer the question. On the other hand, you might know that information and still not be able to answer the question if you could not successfully recall the disease. Exploring each potential answer and trying to recall the conditions with which it is associated could help. *(Rudolph:377–378,1859; Hathaway:1013)*

30. **(D)** In a matching question with six or fewer choices it is practical to read and analyze each choice before attempting to answer the question. However, read the questions before analyzing the list of potential answers, otherwise you may waste time on unnecessary analysis. For example, if you read or analyze the list of conditions given here (**A** through **E**), you may waste time thinking about etiology when the question addresses only the *appearance* of the rash or lesion. Know the question before attempting to analyze the answers.

The lesions of molluscum contagiosum are typically quite small, from pinhead size to 5 or 10 mm in diameter. Larger lesions do occur but are infrequent. The lesions usually have an easily recognized appearance: round, dome-shaped papules with a translucent top and a waxy, whitish material inside. Umbilication is common, especially of larger lesions. The condition is caused by a DNA pox virus and is spread by direct contact with an infected individual. Lesions may occur anywhere but are most common on the arms and trunk. *(Rudolph:931; Oski:831)*

31. **(C)** Condyloma accuminatum are soft, fleshy, papular or pedunculated lesions occurring around the genitalia and/or rectum. Although these lesions are caused by the human papillomavirus and are sexually transmitted in adolescents and older children, it is now believed that the majority of cases in infants and very young children are not sexually acquired but rather are acquired during passage through the birth canal. *(Rudolph:931; Oski:831)*

32. **(E)** The typical lesion of pityriasis rosea is an ovoid, pink papule or plaque with fine scales. Lesions typically follow tension lines on the skin, giving the appearance of the branches of a pine tree or a Christmas tree on the patient's back. A single lesion appearing a week or two before other lesions is a common occurrence and is referred to as a herald patch. *(Oski:831–832)*

33. **(E)** Of the five conditions listed, only pityriasis rosea is typically pruritic. Itching in this condition is often intense and prolonged. *(Oski:831–832)*

34. In this type of matching question, up to 26 options are presented for each item. When the list of options is long (more than six), it becomes inefficient and time consuming to evaluate each possible choice for each item. However, it is helpful to scan or preview the list of options. Then, for each numbered item, decide what the best answer would be and look for it in the list of possible choices.

It is clear that the 3-day-old term infant in this question has *unconjugated* hyperbilirubinemia but is otherwise well and has no evidence of hemolysis. The most likely cause of these findings would be physiologic jaundice, a generally benign condition of neonates associated with hepatic immaturity and a peak bilirubin level of less than 13 mg/dL on day of life 3 or 4 for a term infant and 15 mg/dL or less on day 5 to 7 for a preterm infant. Since physiologic jaundice is one of the options listed **(Q)**, the examinee need look no further. Although it is true that some of the other conditions listed, such as breastfeeding jaundice or Crigler-Najjar syndrome, could cause similar findings, we are not told that the infant is being breast fed, and Crigler-Najjar syndrome is exceedingly rare. Physiologic jaundice is clearly the *most likely cause* and therefore the *best* choice. *(Hathaway:78–81)*

35. **(C)** This 5-week-old infant has persistent *mixed* hyperbilirubinemia, suggesting a hepatic disorder. The normal liver enzymes indicate an obstructive rather than an inflammatory condition. Finally, the inability to visualize a gallbladder on ultrasound examination makes biliary atresia **(C)** the most likely diagnosis. *(Hathaway:576–580,589)*

36. This infant has had severe, *persistent unconjugated* hyperbilirubinemia for 4 weeks but is otherwise well. The normal serum levels of conjugated bilirubin and hepatic enzymes rule out most forms of liver disease (obstructive or inflammatory), yet there is no evidence of hemolysis. The Coombs test was negative, and the hyperbilirubinemia is too severe and prolonged for either a blood group incompatibility or breast-milk jaundice. Such a course for neonatal jaundice is very rare, and therefore one must consider rare causes. Crigler-Najjar syndrome (answer **H**), a congenital deficiency of hepatic enzymes involved in conjugation of bilirubin, is the only disorder that could explain this patient's findings. If the examinee were unable to recall the entity of Crigler-Najjar syndrome, a quick scan of the list might "ring a bell." If this fails, make the best guess possible and return to the question, if time permits, after completing the test booklet to evaluate each option for the best fit. *(Hathaway:581)*

BIBLIOGRAPHY

AAP, Committee on Infectious Diseases. Haemophilus influenzae Type b conjugate vaccines: recommendations for immunization of infants and children 2 months of age and older: update. *Pediatrics.* 1991;88:169–172.

AAP Task Force on Circumcision. Report of the Task Force on Circumcision. *Pediatrics.* 1989;84:388–390.

AAP Task Force on Infant Positioning and SIDS. Positioning and SIDS. *Pediatrics.* 1992;89:1120–1125.

Athreya BH, Silverman BK. *Pediatric Physical Diagnosis.* Norwalk, Conn: Appleton-Century-Crofts; 1985.

Feigin RD, Cherry JD. *Textbook of Pediatric Infectious Diseases.* 3rd ed. Philadelphia, Pa: Saunders; 1992.

Hathaway WE, Groothius JR, Hay WW, et al. *Current Pediatric Diagnosis & Treatment.* 10th ed. Norwalk, Conn: Appleton & Lange; 1991.

Kochen M, McCurdy S. Circumcision and the risk of cancer of the penis. *Am J Dis Child.* 1980;134:484–486.

Oski FA, DeAngelis CD, Feigin RD, et al. *Principles & Practice of Pediatrics.* Philadelphia, Pa: JB Lippincott; 1990.

Rudolph AM, Hoffman JIE, Rudolph CD. *Pediatrics.* 19th ed. Norwalk, Conn: Appleton & Lange; 1991.

Schaffer R, Avery, ME. *Schaffer and Avery's Diseases of the Newborn.* 6th ed. Philadelphia, Pa: Saunders; 1991.

Wiswell TE, Roscelli JD. Corroborative evidence for the decreased incidence of urinary tract infections in circumcised male infants. *Pediatrics.* 1986;78:96–99.

CHAPTER 2

Growth and Development and Psychosocial Pediatrics
Questions

The area of growth and development occupies an important and unique position in the field of pediatrics. Both national general medical examinations and pediatric specialty examinations devote a significant percentage of questions to growth and development. Although this is a topic rich in concepts, it is also an area where memorization is important. The age at which a specific function or ability appears, or at which a child normally masters a certain skill, is called a developmental *landmark*. Unfortunately, a number of these landmarks must be committed to memory, either by study or by examining a sufficient number of children at different ages. Observing the behavior and abilities of normal children in *nonmedical* settings can be a helpful and enjoyable way to learn about landmarks and other aspects of child development, and the student should make the most of every opportunity to do so. The student also must commit to memory a number of normal values relating growth and physiologic parameters (such as weight, head circumference, blood pressure) to age. Finally, although some national examinations provide a list of normal *laboratory* values with the examination booklet, they usually provide adult norms only rather than age-related norms. Many laboratory values (for example, hemoglobin and serum alkaline phosphatase) are very age dependent, and the examinee will need to know these norms. Don't be discouraged by the amount of such numerical information asked for in this chapter. There also is a great deal of conceptual material about growth and development.

Psychosocial pediatrics, including child psychiatry, child psychology, and behavioral pediatrics as well as socioeconomic issues, is an important part of pediatrics and has been referred to as the new frontier in pediatrics. The implication is that now that many childhood killers have been essentially eliminated (eg, smallpox, diphtheria), others rendered much less common (eg, measles), and others relatively easily treated (eg, bacterial infections), the focus for further improvement of child health needs to be on psychosocial issues, including the prevention of trauma. The topic of psychosocial pediatrics is addressed in every general pediatric textbook and is included in all national examinations.

DIRECTIONS (Questions 1 through 74): Each of the numbered items or incomplete statements in this section is followed by answers or by completions of the statement. Select the ONE lettered answer or completion that is BEST in each case.

1. In the normal infant and child, neuromotor development progresses

   (A) in a cephalocaudal and proximodistal manner
   (B) in a cephalocaudal and distoproximal manner
   (C) in a caudocephalal and proximodistal manner
   (D) in a caudocephalal and distoproximal manner
   (E) in a random manner

2. A 4-week-old infant normally

   (A) is unresponsive
   (B) is oblivious to surroundings
   (C) is aware of noise and discomfort only
   (D) will regard the human face
   (E) can distinguish mother from other people

3. Which of the following is a criterion for the diagnosis of learning disorder?

(A) Above average intelligence
(B) Reversal of letters in writing
(C) Absence of emotional, behavioral, or motivational problems
(D) Discrepancy between intelligence and achievement in one or more areas
(E) Evidence of visual or auditory perceptual defects

4. A 4-month-old infant can

(A) hold her head reasonably steady in the sitting position
(B) sit alone without support
(C) say "mama" and "dada," but indiscriminately
(D) say "mama" and "dada" appropriately
(E) point to objects that she wants

5. A 6-month-old infant differs from a 3-month-old in regard to his or her ability to

(A) control bowel and bladder
(B) crawl
(C) sit, or almost sit, without assistance
(D) smile socially
(E) walk holding on to furniture

6. The most advanced language function a 14-month-old child usually can perform is to

(A) babble
(B) speak several recognizable words
(C) combine two different words
(D) speak in complete sentences
(E) use the past tense

7. A newborn infant is noted to have the stigmata of Down's syndrome. In regard to telling the parents the presumed diagnosis, which of the following would be most appropriate?

(A) Delay any discussion with either parent until the diagnosis is confirmed by chromosomal analysis
(B) Permit the mother to bond to the infant (1 to 5 days) before discussing the diagnosis
(C) Explain the diagnosis to the father and have him tell the mother, either privately or with a physician present, as he prefers
(D) Inform both parents of the presumed diagnosis as soon as possible
(E) Explain the diagnosis to the father at once, but delay discussion with the mother for 48 to 72 hours

8. Temper tantrums are least likely to indicate a significant behavioral or emotional problem in

(A) an 18-month-old child
(B) a 5-year-old child
(C) a child whose parents are separated

(D) a child with a chronic physical disease
(E) a firstborn child

9. Which of the following laboratory values is normally higher in childhood than in adulthood?

(A) Hemoglobin concentration
(B) Serum alkaline phosphatase
(C) Serum bicarbonate
(D) Serum cholesterol
(E) Serum sodium

10. The developmental thrust of the toddler is best expressed by the phrase

(A) "me do it"
(B) "show me how"
(C) "that can't be right"
(D) "why?"
(E) "you do it"

11. Which of the following statements regarding total body water (TBW) expressed as a percentage of body weight is most correct?

(A) The percentage of TBW is less in the infant than in the older child
(B) The percentage of TBW is greater in the infant than in the older child
(C) The percentage of TBW is the same in the infant as in the older child
(D) The percentage of TBW is less in the male infant than in the older male, but the same in the female infant as in the older female
(E) The percentage of TBW is more in the female infant than in the older female, but the same in the male infant as in the older male

12. In the male, body fat expressed as a *percentage* of total body weight is at its maximum at

(A) birth
(B) about 1 year
(C) about 5 years
(D) preadolescence
(E) adolescence

13. A child who can walk downstairs alternating his or her feet, do a broad jump, and throw a ball overhand, also would be expected to

(A) add five and five
(B) identify three or four coins
(C) name two or three colors
(D) multiply three times three
(E) write his or her name

14. A toddler who resists going to bed at the appropriate time probably is

(A) emotionally deprived and eager for human contact
(B) being intentionally negative to get attention

(C) preoccupied with current activities
(D) physically ill
(E) depressed

15. A child who can correctly count 10 objects, name four colors as well as a penny, nickel, and dime, but cannot add, subtract, or correctly copy a diamond, is probably

(A) a normal 5-year-old
(B) a normal 8-year-old
(C) a normal 10-year-old
(D) emotionally disturbed
(E) brain damaged

16. A child who can skip with alternate feet, stand on one foot for ten seconds, and tie his own shoelaces has reached a developmental motor level of

(A) 2 years
(B) 4 years
(C) 6 years
(D) 8 years
(E) 10 years

17. Which of the following would indicate Tanner stage 3 sexual development in a female child?

(A) Acne
(B) Breast and papilla elevated as a small mound
(C) Darkly pigmented, slightly curly pubic hair
(D) Fine hair on upper lip
(E) Menstruation

18. In the normal infant, the grasp reflex has been replaced by voluntary grasp activity by

(A) 2 months
(B) 4 months
(C) 6 months
(D) 8 months
(E) 12 months

19. The ability to copy forms develops in a regular order. Which of the following is the correct sequence?

(A) Copy a square, a cross, a circle
(B) Copy a square, a circle, a cross
(C) Copy a cross, a circle, a square
(D) Copy a circle, a square, a cross
(E) Copy a circle, a cross, a square

20. In the term newborn, which of the following statements regarding fetal hemoglobin is correct?

(A) Essentially all the hemoglobin is fetal hemoglobin
(B) Fetal hemoglobin binds oxygen less tightly than adult hemoglobin
(C) Oxygenated fetal hemoglobin is blue rather than red
(D) Fetal hemoglobin prevents sickling of sickle cells

(E) Fetal hemoglobin hemolyses easily and is a major cause of neonatal jaundice

21. The normal respiratory rate of a 1-year-old child is

(A) over 80/min
(B) between 60 and 80/min
(C) between 35 and 50/min
(D) between 20 and 30/min
(E) between 10 and 15/min

22. As compared to older children and adults, the electrocardiogram (ECG) of an infant normally shows

(A) a shorter RR and shorter PR interval
(B) a shorter RR and longer PR interval
(C) a longer RR and shorter PR interval
(D) a longer RR and shorter PR interval
(E) an equal RR and PR interval

23. The average blood pressure at 2 years of age is

(A) 50/30
(B) 60/30
(C) 75/50
(D) 95/60
(E) 120/80

24. The concentration of protein in the cerebrospinal fluid of infants during the first few weeks of life normally may be as high as

(A) 20 mg/dL
(B) 45 mg/dL
(C) 125 mg/dL
(D) 500 mg/dL
(E) 1,000 mg/dL

25. The first deciduous tooth usually erupts

(A) before 5 months
(B) between 5 and 9 months
(C) between 9 and 12 months
(D) between 12 and 18 months
(E) whenever nipple feedings are discontinued

26. By 1 year, most children have

(A) one to two deciduous teeth
(B) two to four deciduous teeth
(C) six to eight deciduous teeth
(D) two to four deciduous teeth and two permanent teeth
(E) six to eight deciduous teeth and two permanent teeth

27. The first permanent teeth to erupt are usually the

(A) central incisors
(B) lateral incisors
(C) first molars
(D) second molars
(E) premolars

28. By 4 years of age one would expect a child's conversation to be

(A) fully understandable, although mispronunciations and grammatical errors are common
(B) fully understandable, with few if any mispronunciations and grammatical errors
(C) fully understandable to the parent but not necessarily to others
(D) somewhat understandable although garbled and indistinct
(E) somewhat understandable, with mostly correct use of nouns and mostly incorrect use of verbs

29. The interaction between a normal mother and her normal 1-month-old infant is best described as

(A) purely physical
(B) mutually responsive and social
(C) mutually affectionate
(D) purely physical for the infant but highly social for the mother
(E) affectionate for the mother but neutral or unresponsive for the infant

30. A mother is concerned that her 30-month-old son occasionally repeats words spoken to him. Physical and neurologic examinations are entirely normal, and the child's developmental landmarks are within normal limits. This child probably

(A) is displaying precocious verbal behavior
(B) has a subtle neurologic abnormality
(C) has poor language development
(D) has infantile autism
(E) is normal

31. A child with an intelligence quotient (IQ) of 65 would be classified as

(A) at the lower limits of normal
(B) mildly retarded and educable
(C) moderately retarded and trainable
(D) moderately retarded and untrainable
(E) severely retarded and untrainable

32. The most important reason for advocating immediate physical contact between a mother and her newborn infant is that such contact

(A) stimulates uterine contraction and lessens postpartum bleeding
(B) facilitates transfer of maternal respiratory flora to the infant
(C) improves the infant's muscle tone and respiration
(D) encourages maternal-infant bonding
(E) stimulates expulsion of the placenta

33. The skeletal age, or bone age, of a child is judged by the

(A) presence or absence of specific ossification centers as compared to known standards
(B) radiodensity of the long bones as compared to known standards
(C) width-length ratios of certain bones as compared to known standards
(D) relative lengths of specific long bones as compared to the width of the skull
(E) relative lengths of specific long bones as compared to the width of the vertebral bodies

34. At birth, the skull (cranium)

(A) is larger than the face
(B) is smaller than the face
(C) and face are equal in size
(D) may be larger or smaller than the face
(E) is usually flattened anteriorly

35. Most infants lose weight immediately after birth. Normal, term infants generally regain their birth weight by

(A) 24 hours
(B) 48 hours
(C) 72 hours
(D) 3 to 5 days
(E) 7 to 10 days

36. Compared with the adult in terms of body proportions, the young infant has

(A) a larger head and trunk
(B) a larger head and neck
(C) a smaller neck and trunk
(D) a smaller trunk and legs
(E) longer arms and legs

37. A weight gain of about 1.2 kg (2½ lb) during the first 3 months of life is

(A) about average
(B) above average but within normal limits
(C) below average but within normal limits
(D) below average and probably abnormal
(E) above average and probably abnormal

38. Development of the skeleton is by progression from connective tissue to cartilage to bone. At birth, the anterior fontanel is

(A) bone
(B) cartilage
(C) connective tissue
(D) a combination of cartilage and bone
(E) a combination of connective tissue and cartilage

39. The anterior fontanel usually feels closed on physical examination (palpation)

(A) by 3 months
(B) between 3 and 9 months
(C) between 9 and 18 months
(D) between 18 and 24 months
(E) between 24 and 36 months

40. In explaining the normal pattern of physical growth to a parent, the most appropriate statement would be that growth is

(A) rapid during infancy and childhood, then slows
(B) rapid in early infancy, then gradually slows to a steady pace from about 5 years until just before puberty, when it speeds up again moderately
(C) slow at first, then accelerates until the completion of puberty, when it slows down again
(D) steady during early infancy and childhood, then progressively more rapid through later childhood and early puberty, finally slowing in later puberty
(E) so individualized that a so-called normal pattern really does not exist

41. In regard to puberty, maximal growth in muscle mass

(A) occurs just before the onset of puberty
(B) precedes the maximal growth in height
(C) parallels the maximal growth in height
(D) follows the maximal growth in height
(E) is sporadic and unpredictable

42. The growth curve shown in Figure 2–1 is most compatible with a diagnosis of

(A) androgen excess
(B) constitutional growth delay
(C) craniopharyngioma
(D) normal variant
(E) thyroid dysgenesis

43. Children with isolated growth hormone (GH) deficiency usually

(A) have a normal bone age
(B) have associated mild hypothyroidism
(C) grow parallel to, but below, the normal growth curve
(D) have an associated ("compensating") hyperthyroidism
(E) show deceleration of growth velocity and fall away from the normal growth curve

44. Children with delayed puberty (without endocrine abnormality) generally can expect to be ultimately

(A) very short and obese
(B) short but of proportionate weight
(C) of normal height and weight
(D) very tall but of proportionate weight
(E) very tall and obese

45. A 14-year-old boy is brought to clinic because of tenderness of the right breast. Examination reveals a small, firm nodule, which feels like hypertrophied breast tissue, beneath the areola. The most likely explanation for this finding is

(A) hermaphrodism
(B) pseudohermaphrodism
(C) physiologic gynecomastia
(D) an estrogen-secreting adrenal tumor
(E) an androgen-secreting adrenal tumor

46. It is estimated that the average school-age American child watches television for about

(A) 1 to 2 hours a week
(B) 3 to 4 hours a week
(C) 5 to 10 hours a week
(D) 30 to 40 hours a week
(E) 70 to 100 hours a week

47. Which of the following would be most important in preventing or reducing the psychic trauma of hospitalization for a 9-month-old infant?

(A) Encouraging the mother to room in or to visit as much as possible
(B) Keeping a television set turned on during the waking hours
(C) Liberal use of sedation for frightening procedures
(D) Minimizing the number of different nurses and doctors involved in the care of the patient
(E) Providing a familiar blanket or stuffed animal

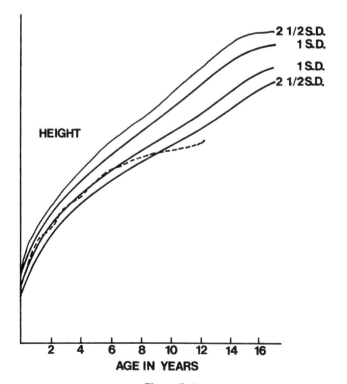

Figure 2–1

48. A 2½-year-old child is hospitalized. For the first 3 days the mother visits during the day, and the child appears frightened and cries for her when she leaves. For the next 3 days the mother does not visit, and the child cries and calls for her. On the seventh day, although the mother does not visit, the child is noted to be very quiet. It would be best to

(A) tell the mother that her visits seem to upset the child and he or she will adjust better if she does not visit for a few days
(B) explain to the mother that if she cannot room in with the child, it would be best for her not to visit at all
(C) encourage the mother to visit more often and for longer periods
(D) prescribe a tranquilizer or sedative for the child
(E) leave things as they are

49. A mild lumbar lordosis and a protuberant abdomen are most characteristic of the

(A) infant
(B) toddler
(C) preschooler
(D) school-age child
(E) adolescent

50. Adolescence is best defined as the period

(A) immediately before, during, and after puberty
(B) of maximal physical growth
(C) of maximal sexual development
(D) of physiologic adjustment to maturity
(E) of psychosocial transition from childhood to adulthood

51. Declining scholastic grades, refusal to participate in family activities, and unwillingness to communicate with either parent in an adolescent usually indicate

(A) a normal stage of development
(B) a normal response to peer pressure
(C) a normal reaction to overprotective parents
(D) a transient phase of ambivalence
(E) an emotional or psychiatric problem

52. Ovulation usually

(A) precedes menarche by 12 to 24 months
(B) precedes menarche by 1 to 2 months
(C) occurs at the same time as menarche
(D) follows menarche by 1 to 2 months
(E) follows menarche by 12 to 24 months

53. The normal (average) hemoglobin concentration at 1 year of age is about

(A) 17 g/dL
(B) 15 g/dL
(C) 12 g/dL
(D) 10 g/dL
(E) 8 g/dL

54. Compared with the adult, lymphoid swelling and hyperplasia in response to infection in the child are

(A) more pronounced
(B) equal
(C) less pronounced
(D) equal in magnitude but delayed
(E) equal in magnitude but briefer

55. The number of alveoli present in the term infant lung is

(A) equal to that of the adult
(B) twice that of the adult
(C) five to ten times that of the adult
(D) one-half that of the adult
(E) $\frac{1}{10}$ to $\frac{1}{5}$ that of the adult

56. The number of glomeruli in the kidney of a term infant is

(A) equal to that of the adult
(B) twice that of the adult
(C) five times that of the adult
(D) one-half that of the adult
(E) one-fifth that of the adult

57. Which of the following statements about renal function of the infant, as compared to that of the adult, is true?

(A) The bicarbonate threshold is lower
(B) The phosphate threshold is lower
(C) The threshold for acid excretion is lower
(D) The ability to concentrate the urine is greater

58. During the first year of life, an infant who weighed 7.5 lb (3.4 kg) at birth ordinarily would gain about

(A) 5 lb (2.3 kg)
(B) 10 lb (4.5 kg)
(C) 15 lb (6.8 kg)
(D) 20 lb (9 kg)
(E) 25 lb (11.4 kg)

59. During the second year of life, the average weight gain is about

(A) 1.5 kg
(B) 3 kg
(C) 5 kg
(D) 8 kg
(E) 12 kg

60. During the first year of life, the average gain in body length is about

(A) 5 inches (12.7 cm)
(B) 10 inches (25 cm)
(C) 15 inches (38 cm)
(D) 20 inches (51 cm)
(E) 25 inches (64 cm)

61. During the second year of life, the average child grows about

(A) 12 to 15 cm
(B) 20 to 25 cm
(C) 30 to 40 cm
(D) 40 to 50 cm
(E) over 50 cm

62. During the school-age years, the average child grows about how much per year?

(A) Less than 5 cm
(B) 5 to 8 cm
(C) 10 to 15 cm
(D) 15 to 20 cm
(E) More than 20 cm

63. The average head circumference of a term infant at birth is about

(A) 25 cm
(B) 30 cm
(C) 35 cm
(D) 40 cm
(E) 50 cm

64. During the first month of life, head circumference grows about

(A) 0.5 cm
(B) 1.25 cm
(C) 2.5 cm
(D) 5 cm
(E) 7.5 cm

65. The average growth in head circumference during the first year of life is about

(A) 4 cm
(B) 12 cm
(C) 25 cm
(D) 37 cm
(E) 50 cm

66. The ratio of upper to lower body segments (the distance from crown to symphysis pubis, to the distance from the symphysis to the sole of the foot) is about

(A) 2.0 at birth and 1.5 at adolescence
(B) 1.7 at birth and 1.0 by adolescence
(C) 1.2 at birth and 0.8 by adolescence
(D) 2.0 at birth and unchanged thereafter
(E) 1.0 at birth and unchanged thereafter

67. As part of a routine 18-month check-up, your nurse administers the Denver Developmental Screening Test (DDST) to the child. She reports to you that the child appeared to function at about a 15- to 18-month level, but he was noncompliant and difficult to test. You tell her that the child probably is developmentally

(A) advanced and was stressed by the test
(B) delayed and psychologically disturbed
(C) delayed and was stressed by the test
(D) normal, and noncompliance is common at this age
(E) normal but psychologically disturbed

68. Which of the following statements regarding menarche in the adolescent girl is most correct?

(A) It precedes the spurt in linear growth
(B) It occurs simultaneously with Tanner stage 2 breast development
(C) It generally occurs when Tanner stage 3 breast and pubic hair development have been achieved
(D) It occurs simultaneously with Tanner stages 4 to 5 pubic hair and breast development
(E) It generally occurs a year or more after Tanner stage 5 breast and pubic hair development have been achieved

Please note the use of a negative qualifier such as EXCEPT, UNLIKELY, or NOT in each of the following questions (Questions 69 through 74).

69. All of the following statements about familial short stature are true EXCEPT

(A) growth retardation is present from early childhood
(B) ultimate height is below average
(C) the bone age is usually markedly retarded
(D) the onset of puberty usually occurs at the normal time
(E) the shape of the growth curve is normal

70. Developmental screening or assessment of the infant or young child generally is divided into four (Denver Developmental Screening Test) or five (Gesell Developmental Screening Inventory) categories. Which of the following is NOT one of these categories?

(A) Fine motor
(B) Gross motor
(C) Language
(D) Intellectual
(E) Personal-social

71. A normal 3-month-old infant is UNLIKELY to

(A) produce vocal sounds other than crying
(B) be able to lift his chest off the mattress when prone
(C) smile in response to a human face
(D) cry at the presence of a stranger
(E) cry when hungry

72. Which of the following statements regarding the attainment of bladder control is NOT correct?

   (A) Bowel control (day and night) usually occurs at an earlier age than bladder control (day and night)
   (B) Females generally achieve bladder control at an earlier age than males
   (C) Fewer than 5% of children will have achieved nocturnal bladder control by 2½ years of age
   (D) More than 50% of children will have achieved nocturnal bladder control by 4 years of age
   (E) At least 2% of children have not achieved nocturnal bladder control by 10 years of age

73. A 1-year-old child would be expected to do all of the following EXCEPT

   (A) build a tower of three cubes
   (B) grasp a pellet
   (C) reach for an object
   (D) stand alone
   (E) transfer an object from hand to hand

74. A 6-year-old child would NOT be expected to be able to

   (A) identify correctly the longer of two lines
   (B) draw a recognizable picture of a man with six parts
   (C) identify colors and body parts
   (D) identify his or her right and left arms
   (E) define abstract terms such as justice and honesty

DIRECTIONS (75 through 85): Each set of matching questions in this section consists of a list of 4 to 26 lettered options followed by several numbered items. For each numbered item select the ONE lettered option with which it is most closely associated. Each lettered option may be selected once, more than once, or not at all.

Questions 75 through 78

   (A) 0 to 2 years
   (B) 3 to 6 years
   (C) 6 to 12 years
   (D) 12 to 14 years
   (E) 14 to 19 years

75. Suicidal behavior

76. Gender identity

77. Oedipal years

78. Latency

Questions 79 through 82

   (A) Clinical neurologic examination
   (B) Electroencephalogram

   (C) Gesell schedules
   (D) Thematic apperception test
   (E) Wechsler Intelligence Scale (WISC) test

79. Measure development of a 1-year-old

80. Measure intelligence of a 10-year-old

81. Detection of hemiparesis in a 3-month-old

82. Detection of blindness or deafness in a 2-month-old

Questions 83 through 85

   (A) Normal 1-year-old infant
   (B) Normal 2-year-old child
   (C) Normal 3-year-old child
   (D) Normal 4-year-old child
   (E) Normal 5-year-old child
   (F) Normal 7-year-old child
   (G) Normal 10-year-old child

83. Can build a tower of 8 to 10 cubes and imitate a bridge built of cubes; can copy a circle but not a cross; can ride a tricycle but cannot catch a ball; can partly dress self but cannot button or unbutton clothes.

84. Can walk backwards and hop on one foot but cannot use alternate feet when climbing stairs; can refer to self as I, use multiword phrases, and give first and last name but cannot count to five or recite the days of the week.

85. Can catch a ball, skip with alternate feet, copy a circle and a cross, tell his age, identify his right and left hands, count to 10 or beyond, dress himself. Cannot define words, tie his shoelaces, identify the day of the week, do simple addition and subtraction, or count backwards.

DIRECTIONS (Questions 86 through 96): Each group of items in this section consists of lettered headings followed by a set of numbered words or phrases. For each numbered word or phrase, select

   A if the item is associated with (A) *only*,
   B if the item is associated with (B) *only*,
   C if the item is associated with *both* (A) *and* (B),
   D if the item is associated with *neither* (A) *nor* (B).

Questions 86 through 93

   (A) 7-month-old child
   (B) 14-month-old child
   (C) Both
   (D) Neither

86. Social smile

87. Social laugh

88. Sit without assistance

89. Walk unassisted

90. Release an object into a mug or an offered hand

91. Walk up steps

92. Regard and reach for a pellet or raisin

93. Tonic neck reflex

Questions 94 through 96

    (A) Tall during childhood
    (B) Tall ultimate adult height
    (C) Both
    (D) Neither

94. Untreated congenital adrenal hyperplasia

95. Marfan's syndrome

96. Cushing's syndrome

Answers and Explanations

1. **(A)** Normal neuromotor development progresses in a cephalocaudal and proximodistal order. Control of the eyes and head precedes control of the arms and legs. Control of the arms precedes control of the hands, which precedes control of the fingers. Although the rate of development varies considerably, even among normal infants, the pattern and sequence of acquisition of neuromotor control is relatively constant. *(Hathaway:8–22)*

2. **(D)** Although the psychosocial responses of 4-week-old infants are limited, these infants are far from oblivious to their surroundings. They are responsive to noise, albeit producing a subtle and often difficult to demonstrate response. They clearly react to pain or discomfort by movements and by crying. However, the 4-week-old also is capable of responding to the human face and establishing eye contact. In fact, it can be shown that the newborn infant is more responsive to a human face than to a similar-size neutral stimulus. Although some investigators have suggested that by as early as 3 days an infant will turn preferentially to the sound of its mother's voice, it will take many more months before the infant reliably demonstrates the ability to distinguish mother from others. [*Note*: Despite the fact that such data could be interpreted as indicating that choice **(E)** also is correct, choice **(D)** clearly is the best answer. Remember that the directions call for the best answer and do not stipulate that this answer be perfect or that all other choices be totally incorrect.] *(Hathaway:8–9; Pediatrics 56:544,1975)*

3. **(D)** The key criterion to the diagnosis of learning disorder is a significant discrepancy between the child's estimated intelligence and his or her achievement in one or more learning areas. Although reversal of letters is common in these children, it is not present in all patients and is not a criterion for diagnosis. Furthermore, some reversal of letters may occur in normal children as they begin to learn to write. Children with learning disorders are usually of average or above average intelligence, but above average intelligence is not a criterion for diagnosis. Similarly, visual or auditory perceptual defects are frequently seen in

these patients but are not criteria for diagnosis. Many of these patients do have emotional, behavioral, or motivational problems in addition to, or in reaction to, their learning disorder. *(Hathaway:38–40)*

4. **(A)** A 4-month-old infant cannot sit alone, but, if supported in the sitting position, she will be able to hold her head reasonably steady. The vocal efforts of the 4-month-old infant are restricted to laughs and squeals and do not yet include the use of words, either appropriately or indiscriminately. The 4-month-old is many months away from being able to indicate her wants by pointing. *(Rudolph:19; Hathaway:22–25)*

5. **(C)** Most infants are able to sit without assistance by 6 to 7 months. The social smile is present by 10 to 12 weeks. Creeping and crawling are achieved by 8 to 10 months, walking while holding on to furniture at 9 to 10 months, and bowel and bladder control not until well after the first year. Of the developmental milestones listed, only the ability to sit or almost sit without assistance discriminates between the normal 6-month-old and the normal 3-month-old. *(Rudolph:19; Hathaway:22–25)*

6. **(B)** At 1 year, most (but not all) children have a vocabulary of several recognizable words. During the second year of life, they will begin to combine words into simple phrases, with 50% doing so by 20 months. The most advanced language function a 14-month-old usually performs is to speak a few recognizable words. *(Rudolph:19; Hathaway:20–25)*

7. **(D)** Studies have shown that the majority of parents prefer to be informed of Down's syndrome and other causes of impairment or mental retardation in their baby as soon as possible. Delay only makes the shock greater. The diagnosis should be presented to both parents together, gently and compassionately, preferably by a physician with whom they are familiar. It is not necessary to delay informing the parents while awaiting the results of chromosomal analysis or other tests. Most parents will accept the fact that the diagnosis is less than 100% certain while confir-

mation is pending. Often, the small ray of hope that this permits eases the acceptance of reality. *(Rudolph:296;* Pediatr Clin North Am *22:561,1975)*

8. **(A)** Temper tantrums in an 18-month-old generally represent the child's primitive dealing with a growing sense of independence and the conflict for self-control. As such, these outbursts, if brief and temporary, may be considered normal. In an older child, however, they would be a developmentally inappropriate response and indicate an underlying problem. Children whose parents are separated and children with chronic physical disease are at increased risk of behavioral and emotional problems. The fact that a child is first born would be irrelevant to the significance of tantrums. [*Note:* The word "least" was intentionally not capitalized, and the question was not grouped with the other negative questions. The student must remain alert and always read the entire question carefully.] *(Levine ML, et al:* Developmental-Behavioral Pediatrics. *Philadelphia, Saunders, 1983, p 84; Rudolph:30; Hathaway:672)*

9. **(B)** Serum concentration of alkaline phosphatase is consistently higher throughout childhood than in adulthood. It is very high at birth. Although it falls during childhood, it still remains considerably above adult values and then peaks again during adolescence. Hemoglobin concentration at birth is higher than normal adult values, falls to a physiologic nadir of 10 to 12 g/dL at 2 to 4 months, and then rises, remaining at or below adult values for the rest of childhood. Serum bicarbonate and cholesterol concentrations are slightly low in infancy but then reach levels that are about equal to adult values. Serum sodium concentration is not different in children than in adults. [*Note:* The question specifies that the value normally be higher in *childhood.* Hemoglobin values are normally higher than adult values in *early infancy* only. It is especially important in reading pediatric questions to pay careful attention to any indication of age or stage of childhood.] *(Hathaway:1099)*

10. **(A)** Toddlerhood is the period of developing autonomy, when the child normally is seeking to establish his or her own identity and to prove his or her own ability. Toddlers want to control and do everything by themselves. They are too impatient and immature to seek or accept explanations. The toddler's slogan is "me do it." *(Rudolph:26; Hathaway:19)*

11. **(B)** Total body water (TBW), as a percent of total body weight, is greater in the infant than in the child or adult. The percentage of TBW is highest at birth and decreases steadily from infancy to late childhood, averaging almost 70% of body weight in early infancy and only 60% in late childhood. Age-related changes in body composition and water content have clinical significance. Daily fluid needs in relation to body weight are greatest in the young infant. The in-

fant who is moderately to severely dehydrated will have lost 10% to 15% of his body weight as water, whereas the corresponding figure for the older child or adult is only 6 to 9%. *(Rudolph:226; Hathaway:1065)*

12. **(B)** Body fat comprises about 16% of body weight at birth, increases to about 22% at about a year of age, and then gradually declines. At adolescence there is a second marked increase in body fat in females but not in males. In the normal male, percentage of body fat is at its relative highest at about 1 year of age. *(Rudolph:132–133)*

13. **(C)** The gross motor tasks described (walking downstairs with alternate feet, throwing overhand, broad jump) are accomplished at 3 to 4 years of age. A child of this age also should be able to identify two or three colors. The other abilities listed generally come at, or after, 5 years of age. [*Note:* This format is common in pediatric examination questions about development. The student should recognize that often, as is the case in this question, the correct answer can be surmised even if the reader cannot identify the age of the child described in the body of the question. Logically, in this case, the correct choice must be the one corresponding to the youngest age. The ability to name colors precedes all the other items listed and therefore must be the correct answer. Knowing the sequence of development without knowing the corresponding ages would be sufficient to answer this question.] *(Hathaway:22–25; Rudolph:19)*

14. **(C)** Resistance to going to bed is a common pattern of normal maturation in the young child. The toddler is preoccupied with current activities and unaware of tomorrow and the need for sleep. Consequently, he frequently is unwilling to suspend his present activity. At this age, resistance to going to bed (unless extreme) is unlikely to represent an emotional problem, although it may present a management problem for the parents. (Pediatrics *50:312–324,1972; Rudolph:29).*

15. **(A)** The average 5-year-old child can count 10 objects and identify colors and coins but usually cannot yet add and subtract or correctly copy a diamond. An 8- or 10-year-old would be able to do all of these tasks. The child described most likely is a normal 5-year-old. *(Rudolph:19; Hathaway:22–23)*

16. **(C)** The ability to skip with alternate feet and the ability to stand on one foot for 10 seconds are gross motor milestones usually achieved by 5 or 6 years. Tying shoelaces is a complex, fine motor task that, also is usually achieved by children at about 5 or 6 years. (J Pediatr *71:181,1967; Rudolph:19; Hathaway:22–24)*

17. **(C)** Tanner staging of female children is based on the physical appearances of pubic hair and breasts. A small mound of breast tissue is considered stage 2.

Stage 3 is characterized by enlargement of the breast and areola beyond a simple mound and the progression from light, straight to dark, curly pubic hair. Although facial hair, acne, and menstruation are related to the development and function of sexual organs, these features are not utilized in the Tanner staging system. *(Oski:712–713; Hathaway:224–226)*

18. (B) The primitive grasp *reflex* disappears between 2 and 3 months, and *voluntary* grasping actions begin to appear between 3 and 4 months. The grasp reflex gradually is replaced by active grasp activity between 2 and 4 months. By 4 months of age, almost 90% of normal infants will grasp a rattle. *(J Pediatr 71:181,1967; Rudolph:19; Hathaway:19–22)*

19. (E) The ability to copy certain printed forms is considered a fine motor-adaptive characteristic and develops in a regular order. The ability to copy a vertical line appears first, at about 2 to 3 years. The following abilities then appear in sequence: a circle at 2½ to 3½ years, a cross at 3½ to 4½ years, and finally, a square at 5 to 6 years. *(J Pediatr 71:181,1967; Rudolph:19; Hathaway:22–25)*

20. (D) At term birth (40 weeks' gestation), the percentage of fetal hemoglobin varies greatly from infant to infant but usually is between 60% and 90%. Fetal hemoglobin binds more tightly to oxygen than does adult hemoglobin, giving the newborn infant a relative advantage in picking up oxygen in the lung but a disadvantage in releasing oxygen to the tissues. The presence of significant amounts of fetal hemoglobin (which protects the sickle erythrocyte against sickling) is the major reason that young infants with sickle cell disease rarely are symptomatic. Oxygenated fetal hemoglobin is red, just like adult hemoglobin. Fetal hemoglobin does not predispose the red cell to hemolysis. *(Rudolph:1093; Hathaway:1102)*

21. (D) Both heart rate and respiratory rate are greater in infants and young children than in adults, reflecting the relatively larger surface area and higher metabolic rate of the youngsters. The respiratory rate of most normal 1-year-old children is between 20 and 30 times a minute. This is slower than a neonate and faster than an older child or adult. *(Rudolph:1463)*

22. (A) For the reasons explained in answer 21 above, the infant normally has a more rapid heart rate than an adult. Rates of up to 180 beats per minute can be normal in the first year of life. This increased rate is associated with both a shorter RR and a shorter PR interval on the electrocardiogram. *(Hathaway:415–419)*

23. (D) The blood pressure of a normal 2-year-old child averages about 95/60. There is almost no change in normal blood pressure values between 2 and 6 years,

but after 6 years there is a gradual increase to an average of 120/75 at 16 years. It is generally recommended that *routine* measurement of blood pressure in children commence at 2 to 3 years of age; however, blood pressure should be measured in younger children, including neonates, whenever clinically indicated. *(Hathaway:624)*

24. (C) The cerebrospinal fluid concentration of protein in the immediate newborn period normally may be as high as 125 mg/dL; some series have suggested normal values up to 200 mg/dL. The concentration gradually falls to "normal values" of less than 45 mg/dL by 6 to 8 weeks. *(Hathaway:655)*

25. (B) The first deciduous teeth to erupt are usually the central incisors, appearing between 5 and 9 months of age, the lower erupting before the upper. As is the case with most developmental milestones, there is much variation in timing but relatively little variation in sequence. Eruption of the first "baby" teeth is a good time to instruct parents about dental hygiene. Children who are permitted to go to sleep with a bottle of milk or juice in the mouth may develop rampant decay of all teeth, especially the upper incisors (the tongue provides relative protection for the lower incisors). This has been referred to as the "bottle caries syndrome." *(Rudolph:973,979; Hathaway:315)*

26. (C) By 1 year, most children have six to eight deciduous teeth and no permanent teeth. Early eruption of teeth generally is of no significance except possibly for discomfort to the mother during breast feeding. Delayed eruption usually is a normal variation but may be indicative of hypothyroidism or a metabolic disturbance such as rickets. *(Rudolph:972–978; Hathaway:314–315; Hoekelman:87)*

27. (C) The first *permanent* teeth to erupt are the molars, usually at about 6 to 7 years. It is important that these molars be maintained in good health. They not only provide a major chewing surface but also maintain the dental arch in place when the primary (deciduous) molars are lost. *(Rudolph:972–975; Hathaway:315; Hoekelman:87–89)*

28. (A) The physician needs to distinguish speech (pronunciation, articulation, and fluency) from language (content, meaning, vocabulary, and grammar) and to evaluate each separately. Normally, both speech and language are sufficiently developed by 4 years so that the child's verbal communications are fully understandable, even by strangers. Mispronunciations and grammatical errors, however, remain common until about 4½ years or even 5 years. *(Hathaway:20–21; Pediatrics 82:447,1988; Hoekelman:655–656)*

29. (B) Although the young infant has a limited repertoire of social responses, it is clear (experimentally) that by 2 or 3 weeks the infant prefers the mother's voice and body odor and reacts more positively to these than to the voice and smell of other women. For her part, the mother quickly learns what soothes or comforts her own infant. In other ways also (e.g., eye contact), the relationship between the normal mother and infant is highly social and mutually responsive. It would be presumptuous, however, to call the infant's preferential behavior at this age "affection." "Attachment" would be a more biologic, less judgmental term. *(Hoekelman:473–476; Levine MD: Developmental–Behavioral Pediatrics. Philadelphia, Saunders, 1983, p 81; Oski:280)*

30. **(E)** Some echolalia (echoing back of spoken words) during toddlerhood is common and usually of no concern. When severe or persistent beyond toddlerhood, echolalia may be a sign of disturbed language development, mental retardation, or neurologic disease. Although echolalia is common in infantile autism, most toddlers who display word repetition are not autistic. [*Note:* The question did not ask whether autism should be considered (it should) but whether the child probably has autism (he probably does not).] *(Hathaway:20–21; Rudolph:90–91)*

31. **(B)** An IQ between 50 and 70 or 75 (depending on the test employed) usually indicates mild mental retardation. Such children generally are educable if given appropriate support and opportunity. An IQ between 30 and 50 is considered moderate retardation; less than 30 is considered severe and profound retardation. *(Rudolph:125–126; Hathaway:43–45)*

32. **(D)** There is evidence that early (the first hours and days after delivery) visual and physical contact between mother and infant promotes maternal-infant bonding and psychological attachment by the mother. Although there is considerable controversy about the long-range effects of such early contact, it is generally accepted that this represents an important period in establishing harmonious relations between the mother and her infant. The biologic effects, if any, of early contact are less certain. It is recognized that in the nursing mother, sight or sound of the infant stimulates the milk letdown reflex. *(Am J Dis Child 136:251–257,1982; Pediatrics 72:79,1983; Oski:280; Hathaway:58–59; Hoekelman:473–474)*

33. **(A)** The order in which ossification begins in different growth centers of the bones is very regular and predictable. Standards have been compiled for various age groups, indicating which centers should be ossified (and therefore visible on roentgenograms) at any given age. Comparison of the patient with these norms permits an estimate of his or her degree of skeletal maturation, or "bone age." This can be helpful in evaluating short stature, monitoring the treatment of certain endocrine disorders, and predicting remaining growth potential and ultimate height. *(Rudolph:133–135)*

34. **(A)** At birth, the skull (cranium) normally is considerably larger than the face. This proportion can be noted on physical examination and on roentgenograms. The high cranium-to-face ratio is both absolute and relative to the later relationship of these two structures. An exaggerated cranium-to-face ratio may indicate hydrocephalus, and a diminished ratio may indicate microcephaly. *(Hathaway:17–18,690–693)*

35. **(E)** Infants lose weight during the first few days of life, partly because of a loss of body water and partly because initial caloric intake is substantially below requirement. Premature infants lose relatively more weight and take a longer time to regain birth weight. Term infants generally return to birth weight by 7 to 10 days of life; bottle-fed infants regain weight more rapidly than breast-fed infants. *(Rudolph:183)*

36. **(A)** Compared with the adult, the infant has a larger head, a smaller neck, a larger trunk, and shorter legs. Seemingly, the infant is all head and trunk. These differences are, of course, physiologic. The infant has relatively little use for arms or legs yet does need a functioning central nervous system as well as a large liver and gastrointestinal tract to handle his relatively high caloric intake. *(Hathaway:18)*

37. **(D)** During the first 3 months of life, the normal infant gains an average of about 1 kg (or 2 lb) a month for a total of 3 kg (or about 6 to 6½ lb). A weight gain of only 1.2 kg for the first 3 months is far less than average and quite abnormal. If the infant had weighed 3.6 kg (8 lb) at birth, he or she would now weigh only 4.8 kg (10½ lb). This corresponds to a drop from the 50th to below the 3rd percentile for weight. Poor weight gain (failure to thrive) is a common and important pediatric problem. Psychosocial problems, including frank neglect, improper feeding techniques, and systemic diseases are some of the more frequent causes. [*Note:* National medical examinations generally use the metric system exclusively. The student would do well to learn the conversions or, better yet, learn to think in both systems. One pound equals 0.45 kg, and 1 kg equals 2.2 lb.] *(Rudolph:1958–1959; Hathaway:13–14)*

38. **(C)** At birth, the anterior fontanel, which is the junction of the coronal and saggital sutures in the region between the frontal and parietal bones, is composed of connective tissue, which is why it feels like a hole or soft spot. It will be replaced gradually by bone. Examination of the anterior fontanel during infancy can provide information about intracranial pressure. A full or bulging fontanel may indicate meningitis or intracranial hemorrhage. A sunken fontanel can be seen in dehydrated infants. *(Rudolph:137,171; Althreya:93)*

39. (C) Despite wide variations in size and rate of closure, it is generally accepted that the anterior fontanel closes some time between 9 and 18 months. That is, by this time, it is composed of cartilage and bone and no longer is palpable as a soft spot. Early closure may be indicative of a disorder such as premature cranial synostosis. Late closure may be seen in conditions such as hypothyroidism, rickets, hypophosphatasia, hydrocephalus, or trisomy-18 syndrome. *(Athreya:93; Rudolph:137)*

40. (B) Despite great individual variations in rate of growth and ultimate size, the overall pattern of growth is fairly predictable for all normal children. Growth is rapid at first (infancy), then slow and steady (preschool and school age), then rapid again (before and during puberty). Figure 2–2, which plots growth *velocity* (rather than height) against age, makes the point very graphically. [*Note*: Although response (**A**) is technically a true statement, it is a poor choice by virtue of being incomplete. Choice (**B**) is the *best* choice.] *(Rudolph:17–18,1959)*

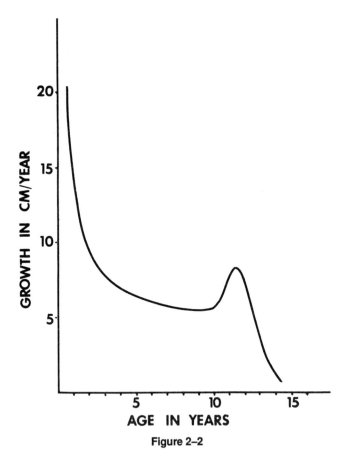

Figure 2–2

41. (D) Growth in muscle mass is a relatively late event of puberty. Maximal growth of muscle follows maximal growth in height. First the adolescent grows taller; then he or she fills out. Knowledge of this normal pattern can help the adolescent and his or her parent deal with aspirations and expectations regarding physical appearance and performance. *(Rudolph:138)*

42. (C) Craniopharyngioma often is associated with hypothalamic and pituitary destruction, which may present as growth failure any time during later childhood or adolescence. A rather sudden arrest of previously normal linear growth should make one consider this diagnosis. Thyroid dysgenesis would cause growth failure from early infancy. The growth impairment shown is too severe to be considered either a normal variation or constitutional growth delay. Although androgen excess can lead to ultimate short stature because it stimulates closure of the skeletal growth centers, it also stimulates linear growth, so the child initially is tall for his age. *(Rudolph:1572,1743)*

43. (E) About 50% of patients with isolated GH deficiency grow normally during the first year of life. Growth then decelerates, and both height and weight fall further and further away from the normal curves. Bone age generally is delayed. By definition, in *isolated* growth hormone deficiency other endocrine functions are normal; there is no associated disturbance of thyroid function. Before concluding that a child has isolated growth hormone deficiency, however, it is necessary to rule out physical destruction of the pituitary gland (as for example, by a craniopharyngioma), or an associated pituitary abnormality such as ACTH deficiency. Isolated growth hormone deficiency can be sporadic or genetic. [*Note*: The astute student will realize that it is very unlikely that statements (**C**) and (**E**) are *both* incorrect and will concentrate on these, even if uncertain about the remaining choices.] *(Rudolph:1570–1574; Oski:1806–1807; Hathaway:770–772)*

44. (C) Children with delayed puberty not associated with an endocrine abnormality are initially short but have a longer than normal period of growth and a later than normal adolescent growth spurt. *Ultimate* height, therefore, generally is normal, and *ultimate* weight is normal and proportionate to height. *(Rudolph:1572; Oski:1805)*

45. (C) Physiologic gynecomastia, mild hypertrophy of breast tissue in boys, is a common and completely normal occurrence in the early pubescent period. This hypertrophy usually presents as a firm nodule, which often is tender. In the majority of cases, the nodule disappears at the end of puberty or shortly thereafter. Such hypertrophy is unilateral in a significant proportion of cases. *(Oski:1802; Hathaway:245)*

46. (D) Remarkable as it seems, American children spend an average of 30 to 40 hours a week in front of the television set, whereas, in general, they spend only 25 to 30 hours a week in school. Television has a major influence on children's knowledge, attitude, and behavior. The nature and quality of the program material is, of course, as much a problem as the volume. There are considerable concern and some data that such excessive viewing adversely affects children's attitudes towards violence, gender roles, concepts of racial stereotypes, and commercialism. *(Am J Dis Child 140:78–79,1986;* Pediatrics *75:233,1985)*

47. (A) At the age of 9 months, a child's world is centered about his or her primary caregiver, usually the mother. It is not possible to use language, familiar items such as blankets or toys, or anything else to reassure an infant in the parent's absence, although such measures can be helpful for the toddler and preschool child. Rooming in is the single *most important* and most effective way to reduce the emotional trauma of hospitalization for an infant and should be encouraged. Appropriate use of sedation for painful or frightening procedures can be helpful and is appropriate but is not a substitute for rooming in. *(Oski:525–526;* Pediatr Clin North Am *22:583,1975)*

48. (C) The toddler and preschooler react initially to hospitalization and separation by fear, crying, and searching for the parent. This is normal. If the separation continues, however, the child may become anxious, withdrawn, and apathetic. This reaction of emotional despair is a serious signal that may be misinterpreted as quiet adjustment. The parents should be encouraged to *increase* visits, and the staff should step up its "tender loving care." Sedative drugs have no role in the management of this problem. *(Oski:525–526;* Pediatr Clin North Am *22:583,1975)*

49. (B) A relatively large abdomen is common throughout infancy and early childhood, reflecting a relatively large liver and considerable gas in the small bowel. This is most noticeable during toddlerhood, from 1 to 3 years. It is also during this period of early ambulation that a lumbar lordosis is common. The lordosis exaggerates the large and protuberant abdomen, resulting in the typical "pot-bellied" appearance of the toddler. This normal pot-bellied appearance may be one reason that abdominal tumors (Wilms's tumor or neuroblastoma) at this age are often diagnosed late. *(Athreya:155–156; Oski:1746)*

50. (E) Adolescence is the period of psychosocial transition from childhood to adulthood. Puberty is a physiologic event. Adolescence is a psychosocial phenomenon, albeit strongly influenced by the child's reaction to the physical and physiologic changes of puberty. Adolescence cannot be defined by a fixed temporal relation to puberty. Often, adolescence appears to occur some time after the onset of puberty. *(Rudolph:40–42,137–138)*

51. (E) Although adolescence is characteristically a difficult period of psychosocial and emotional growth, change, and adjustment, current understanding of this period indicates that emotional turmoil, disruptive behavior, and family crises are not the norm and, when present, represent significant pathology. Declining scholastic grades are always worrisome. Such behavior warrants investigation and intervention rather than acceptance and reassurance. The differential diagnosis includes emotional problems, maladjustment, psychosis, drug abuse, and, rarely, organic disease. *(Rudolph:40–42,86,97–98)*

52. (E) The first menstrual cycles following menarche generally are anovulatory. Most but not all girls do not begin to ovulate for 12 to 24 months following menarche. Anovulatory cycles tend to be irregular and are painless. The onset of ovulation a year or more after menarche can be associated with surprise pregnancy in the girl who had been sexually active while using no type of contraception. *(Oski:722)*

53. (C) The average hemoglobin value at birth is about 17 g/dL. It then falls rapidly over the next 2 to 3 months to a low of about 11 g/dL in the term infant. Hemoglobin values then gradually rise, although remaining below adult values until the early teen years. The mean value at 1 year of age is about 12 g/dL. *(Hathaway:471)*

54. (A) A marked lymphoid response to infection is characteristic of the infant and child. Swelling and hyperplasia of lymphoid tissue are frequent and often persistent. "Hypertrophy" of tonsils, adenoids, and cervical lymph nodes in young children provides common examples of this age-related phenomenon. A predominant lymphocytosis of the peripheral white blood cell count also is characteristic of infancy and early childhood. *(Hathaway:11,471)*

55. (E) The number of alveoli present at birth is only about $\frac{1}{10}$ to $\frac{1}{5}$ that of the adult. As the child grows, new terminal bronchioles and alveoli will form from the distal airways. Clinically, this is an important factor that permits the infant eventually to recover from pulmonary diseases such as bronchopulmonary dysplasia, a protracted postinflammatory state following respiratory distress syndrome (hyaline membrane disease). *(Rudolph:1462)*

56. (A) At term, the formation of nephrons in the kidney is complete, and generally no new units are formed after birth. Recovery from destroyed glomeruli, therefore, is minimal. In cases of premature infants, however, it is believed that some new nephrons are formed postnatally. *(Rudolph:1223)*

57. (A) Infants have a lower bicarbonate threshold than do older children or adults. This is why they normally have a lower serum bicarbonate (17 to 22 mEq/L) than older individuals. They also have *impairment* of phosphate excretion (higher threshold) and a relative *inability to increase* acid excretion in response to an acid load. This adds to their risk for metabolic acidosis at times of stress. Infants also have an impaired ability to excrete a sodium load and a relative *inability to concentrate* the urine maximally. *(J Pediatr 86:485,1975)*

58. **(C)** Although there is great variation within the normal range, the average infant roughly triples his or her birth weight by the first birthday. This means an increase from an average of 7.5 lb (3.4 kg) at birth to 22 lb (10 kg) at 1 year. Thus, the weight gain during the first year of life is about 15 lb (6 kg). *(Hathaway:12–17; Rudolph:129–137)*

59. **(B)** Average weight gain during the second year of life is considerably less than during the first year, averaging only about 3 kg (6 or 7 lb). This reflects the general principle that growth is most rapid early in life and then slows down, until a slight jump at about puberty. Failure to recognize this pattern as normal causes many parents undue concern about their child's growth and eating habits. [*Note*: As explained earlier, many examinations use *only* the metric system.] *(Hathaway:12–17; Rudolph:129–137)*

60. **(B)** During the first year of life, linear growth is rapid, and the average infant grows from about 20 inches (51 cm) at birth to about 30 inches (75 cm) at the first birthday. This is an increase of approximately 10 inches (25 cm) in length. *(Hathaway:12–17; Rudolph:129–137)*

61. **(A)** As with weight gain, gain in height during the second year of life is considerably less than during the first year. During the first year, the child grows about 25 cm (10 inches). Between the first and second birthdays, the youngster grows an average of only 13 cm (about 5 inches), about half that of the first year. [*Note*: Again, only the metric value is provided in this question.] *(Hathaway:12–17; Rudolph:129–137)*

62. **(B)** Growth is slower during toddlerhood than during infancy. During the school years growth is slower still, averaging only 5 to 8 cm gain in height per year. [*Note*: One centimeter equals 0.39 inch; 5 to 8 cm equals about 2 to 3 inches.] *(Hathaway:12–17; Rudolph:129–137)*

63. **(C)** The average head circumference of a term infant at birth is 35 cm (14 inches). A low-birth-weight infant, whether or not preterm, will have a smaller head. A larger than normal head at birth may indicate hydrocephalus or an intracranial hemorrhage. A smaller than normal head may indicate microcephaly. *(Hathaway:12–17; Rudolph:129–137)*

64. **(C)** Head circumference increases relatively rapidly after birth, growing about 2.5 cm (1 inch) the first month. Of course, this is related to the rapid growth of the brain that occurs during infancy. A greater than normal increase in head circumference may indicate subdural effusions or hydrocephalus. Less than normal growth may reflect brain injury, for example, from intrauterine infection, or microcephaly. *(Hathaway:12–17; Rudolph:129–137)*

65. **(B)** During the first year of life, the average total increase in head circumference is about 12 cm (5 inches): 6 cm (2½ inches) during the first 3 months; 3 cm (1¼ inches) from 3 to 6 months; and another 3 cm from 6 to 12 months. A convenient rule to remember is that growth in head circumference averages 2 cm per month during the first 3 months (equals 6 cm), 1 cm per month during the next 3 months (equals 3 cm), and ½ cm per month for the last 6 months of the year (equals 3 cm). This totals (6 + 3 + 3) 12 cm for the year. *(Hathaway:12–17; Rudolph:129–137)*

66. **(B)** The ratio of upper (crown to pubis) to lower (pubis to heels) body segments is about 1.7 at birth and falls to about 1.0 by 10 years. It remains at about that value (1.0) thereafter. In children being evaluated for short stature, persistence of infantile proportions can be a clue to diseases such as hypothyroidism or short-limbed dwarfism. [*Note*: To answer this question correctly, the student need only know that the upper/lower ratio in adolescents and adults is approximately 1.0 and that it is significantly higher at birth.] *(Rudolph:137)*

67. **(D)** About half of normal children during the second year of life are noncompliant when faced with a task such as the DDST. This is itself a developmental phenomenon, reflecting the child's movement toward independence and his new-found ability to resist control and do things himself. The range of normal on screening tests such as the DDST is broad, and a score in the 15- to 18-month range for an 18-month-old child is not bothersome. Usually, more formal and complete evaluation is indicated for the child who is functioning *more than one-third* below his chronologic age. *(Hoekelman:236–239)*

68. **(D)** Menarche usually occurs as, or shortly after, breast and pubic hair development reach Tanner stage 4. Menarche generally follows rather than precedes the adolescent growth spurt. In fact, for most girls, menarche heralds the end of the adolescent growth spurt, and there is little further increase in height following menarche. *(Rudolph:137–138; Hathaway:226)*

69. **(C)** In patients with familial short stature, the bone age usually is normal or only slightly delayed. In these children, slow linear growth is apparent in early childhood. The growth curve is of normal shape, paralleling but remaining below the bottom of the normal curve (3rd or 5th percentile or 2½ standard deviations). Because the bone age tends to parallel the chronological age rather than the height, ultimate height for these patients is below average. *(Oski:1804–1805)*

70. **(D)** The four categories of development assessed by the Denver Developmental Screening Test are fine motor-adaptive, gross motor, language, and personal-social. The Gesell Developmental Screening Inventory uses the same scheme, except that fine motor and adaptive are examined separately, giving a total of five rather than four categories. "Intellectual" is not a category in either instrument and is difficult to define or assess in the young infant. It is important to keep these categories distinct when evaluating an infant or child. For example, delay in gross motor achievement only may indicate a myopathy or other peripheral neurologic disorder. Impairment of only fine motor abilities may indicate mild cerebral palsy. Delayed language may be the result of deafness, and delayed personal-social development may be a clue to a poor social environment. Global delay (all categories) can result from a variety of problems such as severe birth asphyxia, Down's syndrome, or an inborn error of metabolism. *(J Pediatr 71:181–191,1967; Hathaway:22)*

71. **(D)** Normal 3-month-old infants are unlikely to cry at the presence of a stranger. Infants at this age have a social, although nondiscriminating, smile and do not yet recognize strangers as being "strange." They will smile at a human face but will not cry at the sight of a stranger. They lift their chests off the mattress when prone and make social vocal noises. Crying with hunger is a basic response throughout early infancy. *(J Pediatr 71:181–191,1967; Rudolph:19)*

72. **(C)** In the United States, a very substantial percentage of children, probably more than 50%, will have achieved bladder control by 2½ years of age. The child usually learns to control his stooling functions before achieving control of urinary function, especially at night. Lack of bladder control (enuresis) is a much more prevalent problem than lack of bowel control (encopresis). The diagnosis of enuresis generally refers to children 4 years or older. Studies suggest that about 15% of children are still enuretic at 5 years of age and that a smaller but significant percentage persist into adolescence. *(Pediatrics 42:614, 1968; Rudolph:110–111; Hathaway:757–758)*

73. **(A)** A 1-year-old child would try to build a tower of two cubes but probably would not succeed (only 25% of 1-year-old children can do so). He or she certainly would not be able to build a tower of three blocks. He or she should be able to reach for an object (4-month achievement), transfer an object (6 months), grasp a pellet (10

months), and stand alone (11 months). [*Note:* Although a certain percentage of normal children will not be able to stand without support at 1 year of age, almost none can build a tower of three cubes at that age. Choice **(A)** is, therefore, the *better* answer.] *(J Pediatr 71:181,1967; Rudolph:19; Hathaway:22–25)*

74. **(E)** The ability to define highly abstract terms such as justice and honesty develops at about 10 or 11 years and would not be expected in a 6-year-old. The other tasks listed all would be expected of a 6-year-old: correctly identify the longer of two lines (3 to 4 years), draw a man with 6 parts (5 years), identify colors and body parts (3 to 4 years), and identify right and left arms (5 to 6 years). [*Note:* Although the 6-year-old child certainly might have some *understanding* of words such as honesty, he would not be able to *define* them. The question specifies that he "define" abstract terms.] *(J Pediatr 71:181,1967; Hathaway:20–25)*

75. **(E)** Suicide is the third (males) or fourth (females) leading cause of death during adolescence. Although suicide is seen during childhood and preadolescence (12 to 14 years), it is decidedly uncommon before adolescence. *(Oski:664–665; Hathaway:231;* Pediatr Clin North Am *22:595,1975)*

76. **(A)** Current studies indicate that gender identity is well established by 2 years of age. The major determinant of gender identity appears to be the parents' attitudes, behavior, and expectations rather than genetic or biologic factors. *(Rudolph:1664;* Pediatr Clin North Am *22:643,1975; Hoekelman:539)*

77. **(B)** According to classic psychodevelopmental theory, some time around 3 years children become aware of the anatomic differences between the sexes. The child develops erotic feelings toward the parent of the opposite sex and feelings of rivalry toward the parent of the same sex. This stage in psychosocial development has been labeled the Oedipal period and is characterized by a great deal of curiosity about the genitalia (self and others) and a strengthening or reaffirmation of gender identity. *(Pediatr Clin North Am 22:643,1975; Hoekelman:532–533)*

78. **(C)** The term *latency*, which may be a misnomer, refers to the period between the Oedipal stage and adolescence (that is, from 6 to 12 years). During this period, genital and sexual curiosity are less overt than before or after but, nevertheless, are present. During latency, sexual feelings and curiosity can be recognized in sexual references in games and in the well-recognized propensity of young children to repeat "dirty words." *(Rudolph:91;* Pediatr Clin North Am *22:643,1975; Hoekelman:533)*

79. **(C)** The Gesell schedules are designed to evaluate the developmental achievements of infants and chil-

dren less than 5 years of age. *(Rudolph:669,68;* Pediatr Clin North Am *29:359,1982)*

80. **(E)** The Wechsler Intelligence Scale (WISC) is designed to measure the intelligence of children from 5 to 15 years of age. The WISC and the Gesell are different in what they measure as well as in the age groups for which they are designed. The thematic apperception test (TAT) assesses the personality and adjustment patterns of the subject (4 years to adult). *(Rudolph:669,68;* Pediatr Clin North Am *29:359,1982)*

81. **(A)** Neurologic defects such as a hemiparesis are best detected by a thorough neurologic examination. Neither the Gesell nor the WISC is designed to detect visual, auditory, or focal motor impairment, although, of course, such impairment could result in a diminished performance. *(Rudolph:669,68;* Pediatr Clin North Am *29:359,1982)*

82. **(A)** Blindness or deafness is best detected by the routine neurologic examination. Confirmation may require specific testing such as measurement of visual or auditory evoked brain potentials. *(Rudolph:669,68;* Pediatr Clin North Am *29:359,1982)*

83. **(C)** These are difficult questions because of the relatively wide range for normal developmental milestones. Nevertheless, it should be apparent that the child described here is more advanced than a 2-year-old (who could only build a tower of seven cubes, could not imitate a bridge built of cubes, and could not ride a tricycle) and not yet at the 4-year-old level (catch a ball and begin to button and unbutton clothes). The description, therefore, best fits a 3-year-old. *(Hathaway:21–25; Rudolph:19)*

84. **(C)** The child described here also is closer to 3 than to 2 or 4 years of age. He can walk backwards (30 months) and hop on one foot (3 to 4 years) but cannot use alternate feet walking up stairs (3 to 4 years). He refers to himself as I (30 months), uses multiword phrases (3 years), and gives his first and last name (3 years) but cannot count to 5 (4 to 5 years) or recite the days of the week (4 to 5 years). *(Hathaway:21–24; Rudolph:19)*

85. **(E)** This youngster is 5 years old. He can catch a ball (5 to 6 years), copy a circle (3 years) and a cross (5 years), skip with alternate feet (5 years), and identifies right and left (5 to 6 years). He cannot yet define words (6 to 7 years) or do 6- to 8-year tasks such as tie his shoelaces, tell the day of the week, or perform simple addition and subtraction. *(Hathaway:21–25; Rudolph:19)*

86. **(C)** Smiling is a very early and important social tool for the infant. The smile response of the infant helps bond the mother to the infant. Over 90% of infants are capable of smiling in response to a human face or

voice by as early as 2 months. A social smile is therefore appropriately matched to both a 7- and a 14-month-old. *(Rudolph:19; Hathaway:24–25;* J Pediatr *71:181–191,1967)*

87. **(C)** A social laugh appears a little later than the social smile. About 50% of infants exhibit some laughing behavior by 2 months, and almost 90% by 3 months. Thus, both a 7-month-old and a 14-month-old are capable of social laughter. *(Rudolph:19; Hathaway:24–25;* J Pediatr *71:181–191,1967)*

88. **(C)** About 50% of normal children can sit without assistance by 6 months, and almost 90% can do so by 7 months. The ability to sit without assistance, therefore, is properly matched to both the 7- and the 14-month-old. *(Rudolph:19; Hathaway:24–25;* J Pediatr *71:181–191,1967)*

89. **(B)** Unassisted bipedal ambulation (unassisted walking) is achieved between 10 and 14 months. A very few 7-month-old children can walk assisted or holding on to furniture, but essentially none can walk unassisted or alone. In contrast, approximately 90% of youngsters can walk without assistance by 14 months. *(Rudolph:19; Hathaway:24–25;* J Pediatr *71:181–191,1967)*

90. **(B)** The ability to release an object when desired and in a controlled manner is more advanced and is achieved at an older age than the ability to reach for or grasp an object. Most children can purposely release an object such as a cube into a mug or into an offered hand by 1 year or shortly thereafter. *(Rudolph:19; Hathaway:24–25;* J Pediatr *71:181–191,1967)*

91. **(D)** Very few children can walk up steps by 14 or 15 months. About 50% can do so by 18 months, and most can do so by 2 years. The ability to walk up steps is properly associated with neither the 7-month-old nor the 14-month-old. *(Rudolph:19; Hathaway:24–25;* J Pediatr *71:181–191,1967)*

92. **(C)** Both the 7-month-old and the 14-month-old will notice and regard a small object such as a raisin or pellet; about 90% of normal infants can do so by 5 months. Both the 7- and the 14-month-old can reach for a small object, although the 7-month-old will do so crudely, with an attempted palmar grasp, whereas the 14-month-old child will use a neat pincer grasp. The former will rake in the pellet or raisin, whereas the latter will pick it up and probably put it in his mouth. [*Note:* The question was phrased "regard and reach for." This does not require that the infant successfully pick up the object.] *(Rudolph:19; Hathaway:24–25;* J Pediatr *71:181–191,1967)*

93. **(D)** The tonic neck reflex is a primitive reflex that appears within a few weeks of birth and normally disappears by 4 to 6 months. Persistence of the tonic

neck reflex beyond 5 or 6 months is abnormal and would be suggestive of a central nervous system problem involving the motor system: cerebral palsy is one example. *(Athreya:248; Hathaway:18; Oski:609–610; Rudolph:176–177)*

94. (A) Excessive growth in height during childhood is one of the signs of virilization and may be seen in children with untreated congenital adrenal hyperplasia. These children, however, will ultimately be short because while androgens stimulate linear growth, they also speed up epiphyseal closure, and therefore, growth stops early. *(Hathaway:635,803–804)*

95. (C) Patients with Marfan's syndrome are characteristically tall as children and as adults. *(Hathaway: 635,803–804)*

96. (D) Cushing's syndrome, as in other situations of glucocorticoid excess, is associated with excessive gain in weight but *retardation of linear growth* (height). Children with Cushing's syndrome, therefore, are short. *(Hathaway:635,803–804)*

BIBLIOGRAPHY

Anders TF, Weinstein P. Sleep and its disorders in infants and children: a review. *Pediatrics.* 1972;50:312–324.

Athreya BH, Silverman BK. *Pediatric Physical Diagnosis.* Norwalk, Conn: Appleton-Century-Crofts; 1985.

Coplan J, Gleason JR. Unclear speech: recognition and significance of unintelligible speech in preschool children. *Pediatrics.* 1988;82:447–452.

Frankenburg WK, Dodds JB. The Denver Developmental Screening Test. *J Pediatr.* 1967;71:181–191.

Gayton WF. Management problems of mentally retarded children and their families. *Pediatr Clin North Am.* 1975;22:561–570.

Goren CC, Sarty M, Wu PYK. Visual following and pattern discrimination of face-like stimuli by newborn infants. *Pediatrics.* 1975;56:544.

Hathaway WE, Groothius JR, Hay WW, et al. *Current Pediatric Diagnosis & Treatment.* 10th ed. Norwalk, Conn: Appleton & Lange; 1991.

Hoekelman RA, Friedman SB, Nelson NM, et al. *Primary Pediatric Care.* 2nd ed. St. Louis, Mo: Mosby Year Book; 1992.

Horowitz FD. Child development for the pediatrician. *Pediatric Clin North Am.* 1982;29:359–375.

Kenny TJ. The hospitalized child. *Pediatr Clin North Am.* 1975;22:583–593.

Levine M, Carey WB, Crocker AC, et al. *Developmental-Behaviorial Pediatrics.* Philadelphia, Pa: Saunders; 1983.

Loggie JHM, Kleiman LI, Van-Maanen EF. Renal function and diuretic therapy in infants and children. *J Pediatr.* 1975;86:485–496.

McAnarney ER. Suicidal behavior of children and youth. *Pediatric Clin North Am.* 1975;22:595–604.

Oppel WC, Harper PA, Rider RV. The age of attaining bladder control. *Pediatrics.* 1968;42:614–626.

Oski FA, DeAngelis CD, Feigin RD, et al. *Principles & Practice of Pediatrics.* Philadelphia, Pa: JB Lippincott; 1990.

Rudolph AM, Hoffman JIE, Rudolph CD. *Pediatrics.* 19th ed. Norwalk, Conn: Appleton & Lange; 1991.

Satterfield S. Common sexual problems of children and adolescents. *Pediatric Clin North Am.* 1975;22:643–652.

Siegel E: Early and extended maternal-infant contact: a critical review. *Am J Dis Child.* 1982;136:251–257.

Smith RD, Fosarelli PD, Palumbo F, et al. The impact of television on children. *Am J Dis Child.* 1986;140:78–79.

Zuckerman DM, Zuckerman BS. Television's impact on children. *Pediatrics.* 1985;75:233–240.

CHAPTER 3

The Newborn
Questions

Neonatology, the study of the newborn infant, is a major part of pediatrics, much more than just a subspecialty. Most youngsters go through childhood without ever having a cardiac, neurologic, or renal problem, but all children are originally neonates. Neonatology is associated with major morbidity and mortality, severe organic disease, unique physiology and pathophysiology, and intensive technology. The examinee will be expected to understand this unique physiology and pathophysiology as well as to have a knowledge of the diseases and management technology associated with this period of life. The examinee will also be expected to know that the norms for many laboratory values (eg, Hb, CSF protein) are quite different for the neonate than for the older infant or child. Most children are hospitalized because of diseases unrelated to their age (eg, ashma, sickle cell disease, trauma, osteomyelitis). The newborn, in contrast, is almost always sick as the result of a problem directly related to his age—respiratory distress syndrome, pneumonia, meningitis and sepsis, intestinal obstruction, congenital malformations, etc.

The neonatal period is formally defined as the first 30 days of life. However, very premature, small, or sick newborns may remain in the neonatal intensive care unit for several months. The fact that a 15-day-old infant has been *previously well* does not have the same significance as a previously well 15-month-old or 15-year-old. For the neonate, congenital malformations, congenital diseases, and genetic diseases should always be considered, even for what appears to be new and acute symptoms. Finally, the student must always remember that the *normal* neonate is *not* immunologically normal and is vulnerable to severe infection by "unusual" organisms.

DIRECTIONS (Questions 1 through 105): Each of the numbered items or incomplete statements in this section is followed by answers or by completions of the statement. Select the ONE lettered answer or completion that is BEST in each case.

1. The organism most commonly recovered from a breast abscess in a newborn is

   (A) *Escherichia coli*
   (B) *Staphylococcus aureus*
   (C) *Listeria monocytogenes*
   (D) an anaerobic organism
   (E) group B *Streptococcus*

2. A premature infant is delivered precipitously and appears asphyxiated. The infant is cyanotic, there are no respiratory efforts, and the heart rate is 80 per minute. The infant is meconium stained, and thick, particulate meconium is noted in the amniotic fluid and in the infant's mouth. At this point you should

   (A) pass an umbilical artery catheter to measure pH and PO_2
   (B) start bag-and-mask ventilation with 100% oxygen
   (C) suction the oropharynx and trachea with an endotracheal tube to remove the meconium
   (D) intubate the trachea and begin ventilation with 100% oxygen
   (E) establish monitoring with ECG and pulse oximeter

3. At birth, most newborn infants with congenital cytomegalovirus infection are

   (A) asphyxiated
   (B) asymptomatic
   (C) preterm
   (D) small for gestational age
   (E) stillborn

4. The most common permanent complications of congenital cytomegalovirus infection involve the

(A) central nervous system
(B) heart
(C) hematopoietic system
(D) immune system
(E) liver

5. The prognosis of bacterial meningitis in the neonate is

(A) excellent, with over 90% surviving and very few suffering permanent neurologic damage
(B) excellent for survival, with a less than 10% mortality, but with a high incidence of permanent neurologic damage
(C) poor for survival, with a mortality greater than 50%, but with few cases of neurologic damage among the survivors
(D) guarded, with a mortality of 20% or greater and a significant incidence of permanent neurologic abnormalities in survivors
(E) dismal, with a 90% mortality rate

6. Late-onset neonatal infection with *Listeria monocytogenes* generally is manifested by

(A) meningitis
(B) osteomyelitis
(C) pneumonia
(D) renal infection
(E) sepsis

7. A presumptive diagnosis of gonococcal ophthalmia neonatorum

(A) can be ruled out by a history of silver nitrate prophylaxis
(B) can be made on the basis of a Gram's stain of exudate from the eye
(C) can be made on the basis of injection of the palpebral conjunctiva
(D) can be made on the basis of a history of vaginal discharge in the mother
(E) is never warranted

8. A 1-week-old infant is noted to have several pustules with erythematous margins in the diaper area. The largest lesion is about 6 mm in diameter. The child is afebrile, appears well, and is eating normally. The remainder of the physical examination is within normal limits. Culture of a lesion probably will reveal

(A) group B *Streptococcus*
(B) *Staphylococcus*
(C) herpes simplex virus
(D) *E. coli*
(E) no organism

9. A 28-year-old woman in her 38th week of pregnancy develops fever and the rash of varicella. Two days later she goes into labor. You anticipate that the infant will be

(A) stillborn
(B) normal at birth but will develop disseminated varicella
(C) normal at birth but will develop mild varicella
(D) normal at birth and will not develop varicella
(E) normal at birth but will die in 5 to 10 days without any clinical signs of varicella

10. Which of the following statements is most accurate?

(A) Most newborn infants are immune to pertussis
(B) Infants are immune to pertussis only if their mothers received diphtheria-pertussis-tetanus (DPT) immunizations
(C) Infants are immune to pertussis only if their mothers actually had pertussis
(D) Infants are immune to pertussis if their mothers either received DPT immunization or had pertussis
(E) Most newborn infants are susceptible to pertussis

11. Oral candidiasis (thrush) in a 1-week-old term newborn infant usually

(A) responds well to topical therapy with mycostatin
(B) requires systemic therapy with amphotericin B
(C) requires both topical (mycostatin) and systemic (amphotericin) therapy
(D) requires investigation to rule out DiGeorge's syndrome

12. In the United States today, neonatal tetanus occurs

(A) commonly in infants born to nonimmunized mothers
(B) commonly in infants born to intravenous drug-using mothers
(C) commonly in infants with immunodeficiency
(D) commonly in hypocalcemic infants
(E) rarely

13. The major route for excretion of bilirubin in the fetus in utero is

(A) via the kidney
(B) transplacental passage
(C) degradation to biliverdin
(D) reincorporation into hemoglobin
(E) hepatic secretion and storage in the intestinal lumen

14. The breakdown of 1 g of hemoglobin yields about

(A) 0.035 mg of bilirubin
(B) 0.35 mg of bilirubin
(C) 3.5 mg of bilirubin
(D) 35 mg of bilirubin
(E) 350 mg of bilirubin

15. Which of the following might be an indication for intrauterine transfusion of the fetus?

(A) Erythroblastosis fetalis
(B) Sickle cell anemia
(C) Spherocytosis
(D) Fetal distress and bradycardia

16. The most common complication of intrauterine transfusion is

(A) a transfusion reaction (mismatch)
(B) graft-versus-host reaction
(C) premature onset of labor
(D) acquired immunodeficiency syndrome (AIDS)
(E) renal failure

17. Kernicterus is most closely related to the serum level of

(A) total bilirubin
(B) conjugated bilirubin
(C) unconjugated bilirubin
(D) haptoglobin
(E) hemoglobin

18. Early signs of kernicterus include

(A) bradycardia
(B) diarrhea
(C) lethargy and poor sucking
(D) seizures and opisthotonos
(E) weakness and paralysis

19. In most cases of ABO isoimmune hemolytic disease of the newborn, the mother is

(A) type A and the infant is type B
(B) type A and the infant is type AB
(C) type O and the infant is type A
(D) type O and the infant is type AB
(E) type O and the infant is type B

20. The earliest and most consistent finding in mild hemolytic disease of the newborn usually is

(A) pallor
(B) jaundice
(C) tachycardia
(D) bilirubinuria
(E) light-colored stools

21. Small amounts of unconjugated bilirubin in the plasma generally do not enter the brain because

(A) unconjugated bilirubin is not lipid soluble
(B) unconjugated bilirubin is tightly bound to albumin
(C) unconjugated bilirubin is tightly bound to hemoglobin
(D) the blood-brain barrier is impermeable to unconjugated bilirubin
(E) unconjugated bilirubin is rapidly metabolized by cerebrospinal fluid

22. Mortality during the neonatal period (the first 28 days of life)

(A) is the lowest of any period during infancy and childhood
(B) is the highest of any period during infancy and childhood
(C) is the highest of any period during the first year of life but is lower than during adolescence
(D) has increased over the past two decades
(E) has not changed significantly since 1950

23. Among infants of comparable weight and gestational age

(A) there is no difference in mortality between males and females and blacks and whites
(B) males have a higher mortality than females, and blacks have a higher mortality than whites
(C) males have a lower mortality than females, and blacks have a lower mortality than whites
(D) males have a higher mortality than females, and blacks have a lower mortality than whites
(E) males have a lower mortality than females, and blacks have a higher mortality than whites

24. Infants weighing less than 2,500 g at birth are

(A) always premature
(B) usually, but not always, premature
(C) rarely premature
(D) indistinguishable from premature infants
(E) premature by definition

25. Of the following infants, all weighing 1,500 g at birth, which would have the greatest chance of survival?

(A) One born at 38 weeks
(B) One born at 34 weeks
(C) One born at 28 weeks
(D) One born at 24 weeks
(E) One born at 20 weeks

26. Of the following group of infants, which has the highest anticipated mortality rate?

(A) Term and large for gestational age
(B) Term and normal size for gestational age
(C) Postterm and large for gestational age
(D) Postterm and small for gestational age
(E) Postterm and normal size for gestational age

27. The average 28-week fetus weighs about

(A) 500 g
(B) 1,000 g
(C) 1,500 g
(D) 2,000 g
(E) 2,500 g

28. Of the following physical findings in a newborn, which would indicate most reliably that the infant was mature (40 weeks gestation)?

    (A) Presence of a 2-mm breast nodule
    (B) Presence of ear cartilage
    (C) Sole of foot covered with creases
    (D) Head circumference over 34 cm
    (E) Thick and silky scalp hair

29. An infant weighing 1,100 g at birth, without signs of specific disease or distress, probably would

    (A) feed adequately by bottle or breast
    (B) feed adequately by bottle (with a soft nipple) but not from the breast
    (C) feed adequately from the breast but not from a bottle
    (D) require and tolerate nasogastric or orogastric tube feedings
    (E) be unable to tolerate any feedings and require intravenous nutrition

30. The usual position of the hand in the term newborn infant is

    (A) open, with fingers spread apart
    (B) open, with fingers flexed but apart
    (C) open, with fingers flexed and touching each other
    (D) closed, with thumb inside the fingers
    (E) closed, with thumb outside the fingers

31. Erythema toxicum is

    (A) more common among term than premature infants
    (B) usually associated with fever and a general toxic state
    (C) uncommon before the fifth day of life
    (D) usually associated with an elevated peripheral white blood cell count
    (E) manifested by a papulovesicular rash

32. The lecithin-sphingomyelin ratio of amniotic fluid is a useful indicator of the maturity of the fetal

    (A) central nervous system
    (B) lungs
    (C) liver
    (D) kidneys
    (E) immunologic system

33. Bronchopulmonary dysplasia is the result of

    (A) an inflammatory insult to the lungs late in fetal development
    (B) failure of development of pulmonary arterioles during early fetal life
    (C) failure of development of the bronchial buds during early fetal life
    (D) intrauterine viral infection
    (E) the use of oxygen and positive-pressure breathing in the treatment of respiratory distress syndrome

34. Infants with untreated severe respiratory distress syndrome usually develop

    (A) isolated respiratory alkalosis
    (B) isolated metabolic acidosis
    (C) respiratory acidosis and metabolic acidosis
    (D) respiratory acidosis and metabolic alkalosis
    (E) respiratory alkalosis and metabolic acidosis

35. The most important factor predisposing to infantile respiratory distress syndrome is

    (A) cold stress
    (B) hypocalcemia
    (C) hypoglycemia
    (D) precipitous delivery
    (E) prematurity

36. Clinical signs of respiratory distress syndrome generally first appear

    (A) in the first 6 hours of life
    (B) between 6 and 24 hours of life
    (C) between 24 and 48 hours of life
    (D) after 72 hours of life
    (E) when the infant is first fed

37. The characteristic roentgenographic findings of infantile respiratory distress syndrome are

    (A) lobar atelectasis and interstitial edema
    (B) bilateral patchy densities and pneumothorax
    (C) diffuse reticulogranular changes and air bronchograms
    (D) diffuse hyperaeration and cardiomegaly
    (E) cardiomegaly and interstitial edema

38. The major goal of continuous positive airway pressure in the treatment of infants with respiratory distress syndrome is to

    (A) prevent infection
    (B) prevent pneumothorax
    (C) improve cardiac output
    (D) raise arterial PO_2
    (E) lower arterial PCO_2

39. The major danger associated with an arterial PO_2 greater than 100 mm Hg in a premature infant receiving oxygen for respiratory distress syndrome is

    (A) alveolar proteinosis
    (B) atelectasis
    (C) fire or explosion
    (D) kernicterus
    (E) retinopathy of prematurity (retrolental fibroplasia)

40. The pathophysiology of infantile respiratory distress syndrome in the premature infant appears to involve

    (A) increased production of pulmonary surfactant
    (B) decreased production of pulmonary surfactant
    (C) increased metabolism of pulmonary surfactant

(D) decreased metabolism of pulmonary surfactant
(E) rerouting of pulmonary surfactant to the systemic circulation

41. A low arterial PO_2 (below 50) in an infant with respiratory distress syndrome receiving 100% oxygen generally indicates

(A) congestive heart failure
(B) intrapulmonary hemorrhage
(C) pulmonary fibrosis
(D) secondary bacterial pneumonia
(E) shunting of blood past atelectatic alveoli

42. On routine examination, a newborn infant is found to have epiphora, photophobia, blepharospasm, and enlarged and cloudy corneas. The infant probably has

(A) congenital cataracts
(B) congenital glaucoma
(C) galactosemia
(D) intraocular hemorrhage
(E) retrolental fibroplasia

43. The highest incidence of intraventricular hemorrhage at autopsy is found in infants who

(A) are stillborn
(B) die in the first 24 hours of life
(C) die between 1 and 3 days of life
(D) die between 10 and 30 days of life
(E) die after 30 days of life

44. A well-appearing newborn infant is noted to have cyanosis limited to the extremities. Except for the cyanosis, physical examination is entirely normal. The most likely cause of this finding is

(A) cyanotic congenital heart disease
(B) respiratory distress syndrome
(C) a patent ductus arteriosus
(D) methemoglobinemia
(E) poor vasomotor control

45. A newborn infant is noted to be cyanotic and tachypneic. He is placed in 50% oxygen, and the cyanosis clears completely. This infant most likely has

(A) cyanotic congenital heart disease
(B) lung disease
(C) central nervous system disease
(D) liver disease
(E) methemoglobinemia

46. An infant with low-set ears, hypocalcemia, absence of a thymic shadow on chest roentgenogram, and persistent candidiasis probably has

(A) autoimmune disease
(B) DiGeorge's syndrome
(C) idiopathic hypoparathyroidism
(D) renal failure
(E) severe combined immunodeficiency

47. A 3-week-old infant is noted to have microcephaly, cerebral calcifications on skull roentgenogram, and blindness. Which of the following is the most likely cause of these findings?

(A) Bilateral subdural hemorrhages
(B) Cerebral agenesis
(C) Cytomegalovirus infection
(D) Erythroblastosis
(E) Primary microcephaly

48. A 5-day-old infant with white, cheesy patches on the tongue and buccal mucosa, with mild inflammation of the mucosa, probably is infected with

(A) *Candida albicans*
(B) *Listeria monocytogenes*
(C) *Escherichia coli*
(D) group A *Streptococcus*
(E) group B *Streptococcus*

49. The Wilson-Mikity syndrome is best diagnosed by the typical clinical picture plus the findings on

(A) cerebral arteriogram
(B) chest roentgenogram
(C) computerized tomographic (CT) scan of the head
(D) electrocardiogram
(E) renal biopsy

50. A newborn infant has signs of congestive heart failure. Physical examination does not reveal a significant cardiac murmur. Auscultation of the head reveals a loud cranial bruit. The most likely diagnosis is

(A) polycythemia
(B) hyperthyroidism
(C) ruptured cerebral aneurysm
(D) transposition of the great vessels
(E) arteriovenous malformation of the great vein of Galen

51. Excessive sweating in a young infant may be a manifestation of

(A) cystic fibrosis
(B) heart failure
(C) polycythemia
(D) phenylketonuria
(E) pneumonia

52. A 24-hour-old infant weighing 1,700 g is noted to have irritability, apnea, cardiac arrhythmias, and, finally, seizures. Of the following metabolic derangements, which would be the most likely to cause these symptoms?

(A) Hypercalcemia
(B) Hypocalcemia
(C) Hyperglycemia
(D) Hypoglycemia
(E) Hyponatremia

53. A 3,600-g term infant with a brachial plexus palsy develops cyanosis and respiratory distress at the age of 72 hours. Which of the following is most likely?

(A) Infantile respiratory distress syndrome (RDS)
(B) Diaphragmatic paralysis
(C) Pulmonary hemorrhage
(D) Pneumothorax
(E) Cystic adenomatoid malformation of the lung

54. Which of the following tracheoesophageal anomalies is most common?

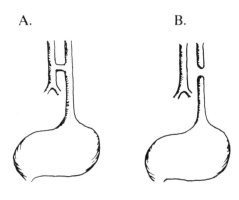

A.   B.

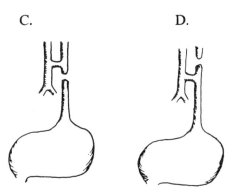

C.   D.

Figure 3–1

55. A cephalhematoma is best differentiated from caput succedaneum by

(A) absence of a history of prolonged or difficult labor
(B) limitation of swelling to the area over one bone
(C) a normal neurologic examination
(D) a prolonged prothrombin time
(E) a normal lumbar puncture

56. Genetic disorders of organic acid metabolism are most likely to present in the first week of life with

(A) acute renal failure
(B) signs of intestinal obstruction

(C) vomiting, coma, and acidosis
(D) cardiac arrhythmias
(E) poor growth

57. An infant born to a mother with adult-onset myasthenia gravis

(A) would not have any special problems
(B) might be apneic at birth but, after proper resuscitation, would have no further problems
(C) might develop muscle weakness lasting several weeks
(D) might develop muscle weakness lasting several years
(E) might develop permanent muscle weakness

58. Hypoglycemia in a term infant less than 48 hours old usually is defined as a blood glucose level below

(A) 10 mg/dL
(B) 20 mg/dL
(C) 40 mg/dL
(D) 60 mg/dL
(E) 80 mg/dL

59. The most common type of congenital clubfoot deformity is

(A) calcaneovalgus
(B) talipes varus
(C) metatarsus varus
(D) talipes equinovarus

60. The most urgent problem in infants with the Pierre Robin syndrome is

(A) heart failure
(B) seizures
(C) intestinal obstruction
(D) metabolic acidosis
(E) upper airway obstruction

61. Which of the following problems in a newborn infant might respond to a pharmacologic dose of pyridoxine?

(A) Blindness
(B) Convulsions
(C) Jaundice
(D) Rash
(E) Urinary retention

62. Premature synostosis of the sagittal suture usually is associated with

(A) scaphocephaly
(B) increased intracranial pressure
(C) microcephaly
(D) hydrocephalus
(E) subdural effusions

63. Of the following, which correlates best with subsequent neurologic abnormalities?

(A) Fetal bradycardia
(B) Failure to breathe at birth
(C) A low 1-minute Apgar score
(D) A low 5-minute Apgar score
(E) Seizures in the first 36 hours of life

64. An 8-day-old infant develops papules, pustules, and comedones on the forehead, nose, and malar areas of the face. The child is otherwise well, and the remainder of the physical examination is normal. The most likely diagnosis is

(A) congenital syphilis
(B) impetigo
(C) neonatal acne
(D) staphylococcal pustulosis
(E) tuberous sclerosis

65. Within a few hours after birth, the entire skin of the normal infant often becomes

(A) dry and scaly
(B) edematous
(C) hemorrhagic (petechiae and purpura)
(D) pale and cyanotic
(E) red

66. The decline in frequency of late-onset neonatal tetany in the United States is related to

(A) better prenatal care
(B) decreased frequency of breast feeding
(C) increased use of prepared formulas simulating breast milk
(D) use of prophylactic penicillin for all infants born outside of a hospital
(E) use of vitamin-D-fortified cow milk

67. A 1,700-g infant was asphyxiated at birth and, after successful resuscitation, had numerous apneic episodes. On the third day of life, the infant began to vomit, and abdominal distention and bloody stools were noted. The most likely diagnosis is

(A) aganglionosis
(B) intussusception
(C) necrotizing enterocolitis
(D) *Shigella* enteritis
(E) volvulus

68. The natural history of the elevated capillary or cavernous hemangioma is best described by which of the following statements?

(A) No significant change in size after birth
(B) An increase in size during the first few years after birth and then regression
(C) An increase in size during the first decade of life and then no further change

(D) A slow but progressive increase in size throughout life
(E) A slow but progressive decrease in size starting shortly after birth

69. Scalded skin syndrome (toxic epidermal necrolysis) of the newborn is associated with

(A) maternal diabetes
(B) staphylococcal infection or colonization
(C) thiamine deficiency
(D) an immunologic defect or deficiency
(E) excessive vitamin K administration

70. A Wright's stain of the contents from a lesion of erythema toxicum usually will reveal

(A) basophils
(B) eosinophils
(C) lymphocytes
(D) immature lymphocytes
(E) polymorphonuclear leukocytes

71. An infant born to a mother with hyperparathyroidism is likely to develop

(A) hypercalcemia
(B) hypocalcemia
(C) parathyroid carcinoma
(D) hyperthyroidism
(E) hyperparathyroidism

72. A newborn infant is noted to have a peculiar face with low-set ears and folded helices. The chin is small, and the nose is turned down at the tip. Examination of the placental membranes reveals amnion nodosum. One should suspect the possibility of

(A) bilateral renal agenesis
(B) congenital toxoplasmosis
(C) esophageal atresia
(D) group B streptococcal infection
(E) transposition of the great vessels

73. An infant with ambiguous genitalia and salt-losing congenital adrenal hyperplasia is found to be 46,XY. The enzymatic defect is probably

(A) complete 21-hydroxylase
(B) partial 21-hydroxylase
(C) 3β-hydroxysteroid dehydrogenase
(D) 11-hydroxylase
(E) 17-hydroxylase

74. Thyrotoxicosis in the first day of life is most likely to occur in an infant born to a mother

(A) with untreated hypothyroidism
(B) with untreated Graves's disease
(C) with Graves's disease being treated with antithyroid medications
(D) with euthyroid goiter
(E) receiving iodides as therapy for chronic bronchitis

75. Which of the following roentgenographic findings in a newborn infant would be most suggestive of hypothyroidism?

(A) Epiphyseal dysgenesis
(B) Absence of ossification of the hamate bone
(C) Prominent thymic shadow
(D) Osteoporosis
(E) Cardiomegaly

76. A difference between infants born to heroin-abusing mothers and infants born to phenobarbital-abusing mothers is that infants in the latter group

(A) do not have withdrawal symptoms
(B) have withdrawal symptoms appearing earlier than heroin withdrawal
(C) do not develop tremors
(D) have a high incidence of jaundice
(E) are usually term and full size

77. Which of the following organisms is the most frequent cause of neonatal meningitis?

(A) Group B streptococci
(B) *Escherichia coli*
(C) *Listeria monocytogenes*
(D) *Hemophilus influenzae*
(E) *Streptococcus pneumoniae*

78. One should be concerned about a term infant who has not passed a meconium stool

(A) during the process of birth
(B) within a few minutes of birth
(C) by 1 to 2 hours of life
(D) by 6 to 12 hours of life
(E) by 24 hours of life

79. On the fifth day of life, an infant is noted to have a violaceous, circumscribed, subcutaneous nodule immediately beneath fading forceps marks on one cheek. The most likely diagnosis is

(A) an abscess
(B) a hemangioma
(C) a pericytoma
(D) periorbital cellulitis caused by *Hemophilus influenzae*
(E) subcutaneous fat necrosis

80. The initial lesions of incontinentia pigmenti are

(A) deeply pigmented
(B) scaly
(C) waxy papules
(D) inflammatory bullae
(E) small vesicles

81. Which of the following infants is at greatest risk of developing an early iron deficiency anemia?

(A) A premature infant
(B) An infant with ABO incompatibility

(C) An infant with physiologic hyperbilirubinemia
(D) A postmature infant
(E) An infant with polycythemia

82. Fetal hemoglobin has an increased affinity for oxygen as compared with adult hemoglobin. This difference results from

(A) an increased mass of fetal hemoglobin
(B) thinness of the red cell membrane in the fetus
(C) the presence of unconjugated bilirubin in the red cell
(D) decreased binding with 2,3-diphosphoglycerate (2,3-DPG)
(E) intracellular alkalosis

83. The mass shown below is most likely a

(A) scalp abscess
(B) posterior hydrocephalus
(C) encephalocele
(D) diastematomyelia
(E) hydrocele

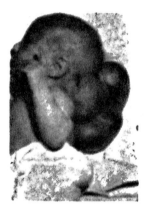

Figure 3–2

84. The roentgenogram shown below is that of an asymptomatic 3-week-old infant with a cardiac murmur. The radiodensity in the right upper chest probably represents

(A) pneumonia
(B) a right aortic arch
(C) a normal thymus
(D) lobar emphysema
(E) a lung abscess

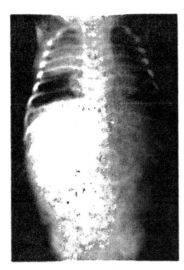

Figure 3–3

85. An infant born with malformed forearms is noted to develop severe hemorrhagic manifestations. A roentgenogram of the arm is shown below. Which of the following would be the most likely cause of the bleeding problem?

(A) Leukemia
(B) Hypoprothrombinemia
(C) Thrombocytopenia
(D) Hypersplenism
(E) Hemophilia

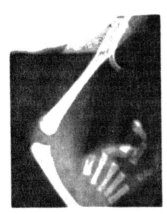

Figure 3–4

86. Which of the following statements about urinary tract infections in the neonatal period is correct?

(A) The most common organism is *E. coli*
(B) Anatomic obstructive lesions are present in most cases
(C) Renal vein thrombosis is a frequent complication

(D) A bag urine specimen for culture is generally the best method of establishing the diagnosis
(E) The BUN is elevated in the majority of patients

87. Which of the following is most suggestive of early congenital syphilis?

(A) Bilateral cataracts
(B) Bullous lesions of the palms and soles
(C) Hepatitis
(D) Myocarditis
(E) Pneumonia

88. "Physiologic jaundice" of the newborn

(A) is an unconjugated hyperbilirubinemia
(B) usually appears within the first 12 hours of life
(C) is more common in term than in preterm infants
(D) is generally associated with moderate anemia and reticulocytosis
(E) is uncommon in black infants

89. An infant born at 39 weeks of gestation and weighing 2,000 g should be classified as

(A) low birth weight
(B) premature
(C) small for gestational age
(D) low birth weight and small for gestational age
(E) premature and small for gestational age

90. Which of the following is more common among term rather than premature infants?

(A) Intraventricular hemorrhage
(B) Hemorrhagic disease of the newborn
(C) Sepsis
(D) Subdural hemorrhage
(E) Congenital infection

Please note the use of a negative qualifier such as EXCEPT, LEAST, or NOT in each of the following questions (Questions 91 through 105).

91. Which of the following serum values would be most UNUSUAL for an infant in the first 24 hours of life?

(A) Sodium 145 mEq/L
(B) Potassium 3.0 mEq/L
(C) Urea 20 mg/dL
(D) Glucose 55 mg/dL
(E) Chloride 105 mEq/L

92. Which of the following is NOT a common finding in respiratory distress syndrome (hyaline membrane disease)?

(A) Tachypnea
(B) Grunting
(C) Cyanosis
(D) Wheezing
(E) Retractions

93. A high-risk labor is being followed by electronic fetal heart rate monitoring (EFM). Which of the following would be LEAST ominous?

(A) Heart rate below 80/minute
(B) Accelerations of the heart rate
(C) Decelerations of the heart rate
(D) Decreased beat-to-beat variability in heart rate
(E) Fixed heart rate

94. Which of the following has NOT been associated with renal vein thrombosis in the newborn period?

(A) Infants born to diabetic mothers
(B) Polycythemia
(C) Dehydration
(D) Intraventricular hemorrhage
(E) Anoxia and shock

95. Which of the following is NOT a feature of extrahepatic biliary atresia?

(A) Jaundice appearing during the second or third week of life
(B) Elevated serum alkaline phosphatase levels
(C) Eventual occurrence of ascites and esophageal varices
(D) Cholelithiasis and cholecystitis
(E) Development of hepatosplenomegaly

96. Of the following, which is the LEAST likely cause of anemia in a newborn infant?

(A) Abruptio placentae
(B) Fetal-maternal transfusion
(C) Iron deficiency anemia
(D) Maternal-infant blood group incompatibility
(E) Twin-to-twin transfusion

97. Which of the following is LEAST likely as a cause of vomiting in the first day of life?

(A) Annular pancreas
(B) Duodenal atresia
(C) Hypertrophic pyloric stenosis
(D) Meconium ileus
(E) Volvulus

98. Which of the following is NOT associated with cyanosis?

(A) Polycythemia
(B) Methemoglobinemia
(C) Fetal hemoglobin
(D) Shock
(E) Apnea

99. Which of the following statements regarding polycythemia in the newborn infant is NOT correct?

(A) Chronic intrauterine hypoxemia is a cause
(B) Twin-to-twin transfusion and maternal-to-fetal transfusion are causes
(C) Ischemia of brain, kidneys, and other organs is a pathophysiologic consequence

(D) Persistent pulmonary hypertension is a complication
(E) Manifestations occur at the time of delivery

100. Which of the following findings has NOT been associated with congenital rubella infection?

(A) Eye defects such as cataracts or glaucoma
(B) Cardiac defects such as patent ductus arteriosus or ventricular septal defect
(C) Deafness
(D) Renal agenesis or hypoplasia
(E) Neonatal thrombocytopenic purpura

101. Factors that appear to lower the threshold for neurologic damage and kernicterus from unconjugated hyperbilirubinemia include all of the following EXCEPT

(A) acidosis
(B) asphyxia
(C) sepsis
(D) postmaturity
(E) hypothermia

102. Infants who are term but small for their gestational age have a high risk of all of the following EXCEPT

(A) hypoglycemia
(B) polycythemia
(C) convulsions
(D) respiratory distress syndrome
(E) pulmonary hemorrhage

103. Infants born to diabetic mothers are at risk for all of the following EXCEPT

(A) polycythemia
(B) hyperglycemic dehydration
(C) hypocalcemia
(D) congenital malformations
(E) cardiomyopathy

104. Which of the following statements about tremors in the neonate is NOT true?

(A) Movements may be either coarse or fine
(B) Movements may be elicited by stimulation of the infant
(C) Tremors usually progress to convulsions
(D) Movements can be stopped by holding the infant or the affected limb
(E) Differential diagnosis includes hypocalcemia and withdrawal from maternal narcotic abuse

105. Which of the following is NOT a contributing factor to physiologic hyperbilirubinemia of the newborn?

(A) Increased portal blood flow
(B) Decreased hepatic conjugation of bilirubin
(C) Increased enterohepatic circulation of bilirubin
(D) Increased bilirubin production
(E) Relative polycythemia of the newborn

DIRECTIONS (106 through 110): Each set of matching questions in this section consists of a list of 4 to 26 lettered options followed by several numbered items. For each numbered item select the ONE lettered option with which it is most closely associated. Each lettered option may be selected once, more than once, or not at all.

Questions 106 through 110

    (A) trisomy 13 (Patau's syndrome)
    (B) trisomy 18 (Edwards's syndrome)
    (C) 5p deletion (cri du chat syndrome)
    (D) trisomy 21 (Down's syndrome)
    (E) 45,X or XO (Turner's syndrome)

106. Low-set ears, nail hypoplasia, "rocker-bottom" feet, growth retardation, severe mental retardation

107. Holoprosencephaly, microphthalmia or arophthalmia, cleft lip and palate, polydactyly, severe mental retardation

108. Hypotonia and hyperextensible joints, clinodactyly, Brushfield's spots, duodenal atresia, flattening of the occiput

109. Microcephaly, mental retardation, hypertelorism and antimongoloid slant, cat-like (mewing) cry in infancy

110. Redundant skin at nape of neck, low posterior hairline, edema of dorsum of feet in newborn period, cardiac and renal anomalies

DIRECTIONS (Questions 111 through 119): Each group of items in this section consists of lettered headings followed by a set of numbered words or phrases. For each numbered word or phrase, select

    A if the item is associated with (A) <u>only</u>,
    B if the item is associated with (B) <u>only</u>,
    C if the item is associated with <u>both</u> (A) <u>and</u> (B),
    D if the item is associated with <u>neither</u> (A) <u>nor</u> (B).

Questions 111 through 116

    (A) Indication for exchange transfusion
    (B) Indication for phototherapy
    (C) Both
    (D) Neither

111. Serum level of unconjugated bilirubin of 20 mg/dL at the age of 14 hours

112. Serum level of unconjugated bilirubin of 5 mg/dL at the age of 3 days

113. Serum level of unconjugated bilirubin of 25 mg/dL at the age of 4 days

114. Serum level of unconjugated bilirubin of 15 mg/dL at the age of 2 days

115. Serum level of unconjugated bilirubin of 10 mg/dL at 12 days of life

116. 24-hour-old infant, blood type A; mother is type O; Coombs's test positive on cord blood; serum bilirubin 2 mg/dL

Questions 117 through 119

    (A) Normal term infant at birth
    (B) Normal term infant at the age of 10 days
    (C) Both
    (D) Neither

117. Platelet count of 50,000/mm^3

118. Reticulocyte count of 1% or less

119. Nucleated red blood cells in peripheral blood smear

Answers and Explanations

1. (B) Breast hypertrophy and engorgement, resulting from transplacental maternal hormones, is not uncommon during the first few weeks of life. Infection and abscess formation occasionally occur in the engorged breast. *Staphylococcus aureus* is the most frequent organism to be recovered from such abscesses in infants, accounting for over 90% of these infections in the newborn and young infant. Empiric antibiotic therapy, before the results of culture, should include effective coverage for staphylococci as well as adequate coverage for group B *Streptococcus* and gram-negative enteric organisms, even though these are less common. *(Rudolph:173; Oski:485;* Am J Dis Child *129:1031–1034,1975)*

2. (C) More than half of infants born with meconium staining have meconium below the vocal cords. If it is not removed before the first breath, the meconium will be aspirated with dire pulmonary complications. Especially if the meconium is thick or particulate ("pea soup"), removal by tracheal intubation and suctioning directly through the endotracheal tube should be accomplished *before* initiating ventilation. This is the first and most important step in resuscitation of such an infant. *(Rudolph:195–196)*

3. (B) Most neonates with congenital cytomegalovirus infection are asymptomatic *at birth*. Although the infection can be fatal, it usually is not. There is a tendency for *severely* affected fetuses to be growth retarded and small for dates, but most are within normal limits for size and for dates. *(Feigin:935; Hathaway:84)*

4. (A) Although the majority of newborn infants infected with cytomegalovirus are asymptomatic at birth, up to 20% eventually demonstrate central nervous system abnormalities. More than 75% of those infants *who are symptomatic at birth* are left with permanent neurologic sequelae, including deafness and mental retardation. The liver frequently is involved, but permanent hepatic damage is rare. *(Feigin:930–932; Hathaway:84)*

5. (D) Despite advances in diagnosis and therapy, the prognosis of bacterial meningitis in the newborn infant remains poor. In different series, mortality ranges from 20% to 50%. Many of the survivors are left with significant permanent neurologic damage. The outlook is especially poor for premature infants and for those infected with coliform organisms. *(Feigin:908; Hathaway:83;* Pediatrics *77:217,1986)*

6. (A) Neonatal infection with *Listeria monocytogenes* may be early onset or late onset. The former is usually associated with sepsis and pneumonia, whereas the latter generally presents as meningitis. *Listeria* rarely causes renal infection or osteomyelitis. *(Feigin: 899–900; Hathaway:884)*

7. (B) Gram's stain of the exudate is the most useful tool to establish a presumptive diagnosis of gonococcal ophthalmolitis. Conjunctival injection is not specific. A history of vaginal discharge in the mother is important but also is obtained frequently in cases of neonatal chlamydial conjunctivitis. Cases of gonococcal conjunctivitis continue to occur despite the use of appropriate prophylactic measures in the delivery room. In some cases, the prophylactic agent was improperly applied. In other cases, the infection was acquired postnatally, possibly via the mother's contaminated fingers. *(Feigin:546)*

8. (B) The lesions described are classic for superficial pustular staphylococcal disease (impetigo neonatorum). This infection tends to remain localized and usually responds well to topical measures, including antibacterial ointment. Lesions of herpes virus usually are vesicular rather than pustular and have no special predilection for the diaper area. *(Feigin:915–916)*

9. (B) Although varicella is usually a mild and relatively benign disorder, it can be very severe in the neonate as well as in the immunosuppressed patient (eg, leukemia). The timing of neonatal infection is a critical factor in determining outcome. If the mother's infection begins more than 5 days prior to delivery, apparently there is time for maternal antibody to cross the placenta, and disease in the neonate will be mild. However, if maternal infection occurs 4 days or less prior to delivery, infection in the infant will be severe and disseminated, with about 30% mortality. *(Feigin:950–951)*

10. **(E)** Newborn infants generally are susceptible to pertussis infection. Immunity secondary to immunization in infancy usually has waned by adulthood. Even if the mother is immune, there appears to be little transplacental protection against pertussis. This is probably because most bactericidal antibodies against the pertussis organism reside in the IgM class of immunoglobulins, which do not cross the placenta. *(Feigin:918;* Pediatr Clin North Am *19:387–412, 1972)*

11. **(A)** Oral candidiasis is a common and usually not serious problem. It is seen frequently in the first few weeks of life, sometimes resulting from poor cleaning of nipples and bottles. As an isolated finding in an otherwise asymptomatic neonate, it requires no immunologic investigation and usually responds rapidly to topical therapy with mycostatin suspension. Cases that fail to respond to therapy or that recur should make one think of immunodeficiency diseases such as DiGeorge's syndrome. In the sick, premature infant, especially those with central lines or other invasive devices, oral thrush is more serious and may herald systemic infection. *(Hathaway:349)*

12. **(E)** Neonatal tetanus is rare in developed countries such as the United States, occurring only in infants born outside of a hospital, under nonsterile conditions, to unimmunized mothers, a combination of conditions sometimes seen among migrant farm workers and illegal immigrants. Mothers who have completed their childhood immunizations but have not had a tetanus booster in more than 20 years may be "unimmunized." Unimmunized intravenous drug users may develop tetanus from contaminated needles, yet their offspring are safe if born in a hospital under sterile conditions; the same is true for infants born to other unimmunized women. Hypocalcemia causes the symptom tetany, which is unrelated to the disease tetanus. *(Oski:558,1059–1060,1077; Hathaway:862)*

13. **(B)** Unconjugated bilirubin passes easily across the placenta, and this is the major mechanism for fetal elimination of bilirubin. Intestinal degradation of bilirubin to biliverdin is accomplished primarily by the intestinal bacterial flora, which obviously are not present in utero. The inability of the fetus to conjugate bilirubin, therefore, is clearly advantageous during intrauterine life. *(Oski:400; Schaffer:749–752)*

14. **(D)** Breakdown and metabolism of 1 g of hemoglobin yields about 35 mg of bilirubin. This is important because it explains why very little hemolysis is required for the development of hyperbilirubinemia in the presence of impaired hepatic ability to conjugate or excrete bilirubin, such as occurs in the newborn (and especially the premature) infant. [*Note:* The exact number is unimportant to the clinician and the average reader. The individual values listed as choices, however, are sufficiently spread out so that answering the question really only requires knowledge of the concept that in the newborn a little bit of hemoglobin goes a long way toward hyperbilirubinemia.] *(*Pediatr Clin North Am *9:575–603, 1962; Rudolph: 1054; Schaffer:749)*

15. **(A)** Erythroblastosis fetalis, usually a result of Rh incompatibility, is the major indication for intrauterine transfusion. The transfusion is accomplished by injection of donor blood (packed red cells) into the fetal abdominal cavity or the vessels of the umbilical cord under ultrasound guidance. The technique is reasonably safe but highly specialized and generally is available only in high-risk obstetric centers. Were a fetus with erythroblastosis to develop signs of distress and bradycardia, it would be too late for transfusion, and delivery would be the only way likely to save the infant. Neither spherocytosis nor sickle cell disease causes serious intrauterine problems, although spherocytosis can cause neonatal jaundice. *(Schaffer:807–808)*

16. **(C)** Current technology, including the use of ultrasound monitoring during the procedure, has made intrauterine transfusion relatively safe. Premature onset of labor is the major complication. Graft-versus-host reaction has been reported but is rare. Testing of donor blood for human immunodeficiency virus (HIV) antibody is routine and usually will prevent transfusion transmission of AIDS, although blood from a recently infected individual may contain virus but not antibody. Transfusion reactions have not been a problem. *(*Clin Obstet Gynecol *18:1–23, 1975;* Br J Hosp Med *34:141,1985; Schaffer:807–808)*

17. **(C)** Kernicterus is a condition of neurologic damage that is the direct result of the toxic effects of bilirubin on the central nervous system. Since unconjugated bilirubin crosses the blood–brain barrier, whereas conjugated bilirubin does not, the risk of kernicterus is most closely related to the serum level of unconjugated bilirubin. *(Rudolph:1056; Oski:402; Hathaway:78–79)*

18. **(C)** Early signs of kernicterus include hypotonia, lethargy, and poor sucking. Fever, seizures, and opisthotonos are *late* findings. Paralysis, bradycardia, and diarrhea are not part of the clinical picture of kernicterus. [*Note:* The examinee must pay close attention to qualifying terms such as early, late, mild, or severe and not focus prematurely on an obvious relationship. Certainly, seizures and opisthotonos are *classic* signs of kernicterus. But these are late signs and, fortunately, today are seen only infrequently.] *(Rudolph:1056; Oski:402; Hathaway:78–79)*

19. (C) Blood type A appears to be the most antigenic blood group. In most cases of ABO isoimmune hemolytic disease of the newborn, the mother is type O and the infant is type A. Anti-A antibodies produced by the mother cross the placenta and cause hemolysis of fetal erythrocytes. *(Oski:406; Hathaway:80)*

20. (B) The most constant finding in *mild* hemolytic disease of the newborn is hyperbilirubinemia. The inability of the immature liver to conjugate bilirubin leads to a prompt rise in unconjugated bilirubin, even before there is significant anemia. Light-colored stools and bilirubinuria usually are associated with hepatic obstruction rather than hemolysis. Only in cases of severe hemolytic disease in utero will the infant be severely anemic at birth although only slightly jaundiced because of transplacental clearing of bilirubin. [*Note*: As indicated in Question 19, the student must pay close attention to terms such as mild, early, often, and serious.] *(Oski:403–406; Hathaway:80)*

21. (B) Unconjugated bilirubin in the serum is tightly bound to albumin. The unconjugated bilirubin molecule is lipid soluble, and that which is not bound to albumin enters the brain readily. This is why kernicterus usually occurs only at serum levels of unconjugated bilirubin exceeding 20 mg/dL (the approximate limit of albumin binding). Factors that are associated with low serum albumin levels (e.g., prematurity) and factors that impair bilirubin binding to albumin (eg, acidosis) can result in kernicterus at lower serum bilirubin levels. *(Rudolph:1054–1055; Oski:402–403)*

22. (B) Although neonatal mortality has declined more than 50% since 1950, the neonatal period remains the single period of highest mortality during all of infancy and childhood. The death rate during the first 28 days of life is almost 10 per 1,000 live births. *(Rudolph:5,165–166)*

23. (D) Males have a higher neonatal mortality rate than females, both overall and when corrected for weight and gestational age. Blacks have a higher rate of prematurity and low birth weight and therefore have an *overall* higher neonatal mortality than whites. Among infants of *comparable* weight and gestational age, however, black infants have a lower mortality than do white infants. *(Rudolph:165–166; Schaffer:4–6)*

24. (B) Prematurity is defined on the basis of gestational age, not body weight. About two-thirds of infants weighing less than 2,500 g at birth are premature; one-third are *not* premature; that is, they have a gestational age of greater than 38 weeks. These infants are small for gestational age but are not premature. Although survival decreases with decreasing birth weight, it is only at around a birth weight

of 1,000 g that the mortality rate begins to increase steeply. [*Note*: The student might be confused about interpretation of the word "usually." Is it meant to imply almost always, more than 90%, more than 80%, or just more than half of the time? Careful consideration will reveal that, in this case, the exact distinction is immaterial. "Usually, but not always, premature" clearly is the best choice because all the other answers are patently incorrect. Regardless of which of the above definitions is applied, response **(B)** is still more correct than any of the other statements.] *(Oski:297; Hathaway:50–51)*

25. (A) For any given birth weight, the older or more mature the fetus, the greater is the likelihood of survival. A 1,500-g, 38-week-old infant would be small for gestational age and would have a lower risk of death than a 1,500-g infant born at 28 to 32 weeks, whose weight would be appropriate for gestational age but who would be premature. *(Hathaway:50–51; Rudolph:165–166)*

26. (D) The postterm, small-for-gestational-age infant usually is a victim of placental insufficiency and has a significantly higher mortality rate than the other groups listed. For example, infants born at 44 weeks of gestation have a 1% mortality rate if they weigh over 4,500 g but a 6% mortality rate if they weigh less than 2,000 g. *(Hathaway:50–51; Rudolph:165–166)*

27. (B) The 28-week fetus weighs between 800 and 1,400 g, averaging about 1,100 g. These parameters (28 weeks and approximately 1,000 g) are convenient to remember, because survival begins to decline rapidly at less than 28 weeks or less than 1,000 g. *(Hathaway:51)*

28. (C) The breast nodule and ear cartilage appear at about 36 weeks of gestation. Sole creases appear at about the same time, but only on the anterior portion of the foot; creases do not cover the entire foot until 40 weeks of gestation. Head circumference is a poor indicator of fetal age and may reach 34 cm by 35 weeks. Scalp hair becomes thick and silky at about 37 weeks. *(Rudolph:167–168; Hathaway:54)*

29. (D) Low-birth-weight infants usually tolerate tube feedings without difficulty. This may be accomplished by passing a tube at each feeding (gavage) or by leaving a nasogastric tube in place. In the latter case, feeding may be by bolus or by continuous drip. It is doubtful that an infant of 1,100 g would be strong enough to take sufficient calories by sucking. Additionally, the immature sucking and swallowing reflexes would pose the threat of aspiration, making attempts at oral feeding by either bottle or breast hazardous. *(Rudolph:191)*

30. (D) The usual position of the newborn's hand is as a closed fist, with thumb inside the fingers. This is the so-called cortical thumb position (palmar grasp reflex), which would be abnormal in an older child but is the normal finding in the neonate, reflects the relatively primitive state of the infant's central nervous system. Even in the newborn, however, this position is not obligatory; that is, periodically the infant will open his hand. *(Schaffer:396–397)*

31. **(A)** Erythema toxicum is a benign condition seen in 30 to 70% of normal, term infants. It is much less common among premature infants. The skin lesions usually appear within the first 2 days of life and are not associated with any systemic signs or symptoms. Infants are afebrile, and the peripheral white blood cell counts are normal. The rash consists of blotchy erythematous macules 2–3 cm in diameter. *(Rudolph:170,879–880; Hathaway:270–271)*

32. **(B)** The lecithin-sphingomyelin (L/S) ratio of amniotic fluid reflects the composition of fetal lung fluid and is a useful indicator of the maturity of the fetal lung in regard to surfactant production and the risk of neonatal respiratory distress syndrome (RDS), also referred to as hyaline membrane disease (HMD). This disorder also has been called infantile respiratory distress syndrome (IRDS) to distinguish it from adult respiratory distress syndrome (ARDS). An immature L/S ratio indicates a high risk of RDS if the infant is delivered at that time. Conversely, a mature ratio suggests that there is little risk of RDS. *(Schaffer:501–502; Rudolph:158)*

33. **(E)** Some infants with severe respiratory distress syndrome who require therapy with positive-pressure respirators and high concentrations of oxygen develop chronic pulmonary changes known as bronchopulmonary dysplasia (BPD). It is believed that oxygen and barotrauma (positive pressure), superimposed on an inflamed lung, are the major pathogenic factors in the development of BPD. *(Schaffer:519–521; Hathaway:380–381)*

34. **(C)** Infants with severe respiratory distress syndrome commonly develop hypercapnia and respiratory acidosis. If untreated, they frequently develop metabolic acidosis secondary to hypoxemia. [*Note*: The key to correct interpretation of this question is attention to the words *severe* and *untreated*.] *(Rudolph:1487)*

35. **(E)** Prematurity is the single most important predetermining factor in the neonatal respiratory distress syndrome. Respiratory distress syndrome is rare in term infants. Cold stress occasionally may be an associated etiologic factor but is not the most important determinant. Precipitous delivery, hypoglycemia, and hypocalcemia do not, by themselves, cause or predispose to RDS. *(Rudolph:1485,1490; Hathaway: 74)*

36. **(A)** The signs of infantile respiratory distress syndrome (tachypnea, cyanosis, retractions) generally appear within the first few hours of birth. Infants who develop symptoms of respiratory distress after the first 12 hours of life are more likely to have pneumonia, heart disease, or other problems rather than RDS. *(Rudolph:1486–1487)*

37. **(C)** The characteristic roentgenographic findings in infants with respiratory distress syndrome are a diffuse reticulogranular pattern and air bronchograms. These changes are presumed to represent diffuse alveolar atelectasis. Lobar densities are infrequent, and lung volume usually is diminished rather than increased. Pneumothorax does occur, but generally as a complication of treatment rather than as a feature of the disease itself. *(Rudolph:1488; Hathaway:74)*

38. **(D)** The purpose of continuous positive airway pressure is to prevent alveolar collapse and thereby improve oxygenation. Such therapy usually does not improve arterial PCO_2 or cardiac output; in fact, these parameters may worsen. Pneumothorax actually is one of the complications of treatment with continuous positive airway pressure. There is no evidence that continuous positive airway pressure prevents infection. To the contrary, the invasive technology (eg, endotracheal tube) often required can predispose to infection. *(Rudolph:1491–1492)*

39. **(E)** Retrolental fibroplasia (retinopathy of prematurity) is the major danger of hyperoxemia and is the reason that the arterial PO_2 should not be permitted to exceed 100 mm Hg for any period of time in the premature infant. Oxygen therapy in the premature infant is an example of a situation in which too much of a good thing is not better. Premature infants appear to be uniquely sensitive to retinal damage from oxygen. *(Rudolph:1908; Hathaway:309–310)*

40. **(B)** A decrease in production of pulmonary surfactant by alveolar cells has been demonstrated in the lungs of infants and experimental animals with respiratory distress syndrome. The biologic function of surfactant is to lower the surface tension of the alveolar lining and thereby stabilize the alveoli. Absence of surfactant leads to alveolar collapse (atelectasis), which in turn causes the pathophysiologic, clinical, and roentgenographic changes characteristic of this disorder. *(Rudolph:1488–1489; Hathaway:74)*

41. **(E)** A low arterial PO_2 unresponsive to high concentrations of inspired oxygen in infants with RDS generally is the result of blood shunting past atelectatic alveoli; as such, it reflects the severity of pulmonary involvement. Although secondary bacterial pneumonia and intrapulmonary hemorrhage are seen occasionally in infants with RDS, one need not invoke their presence to explain why hypoxemia is unresponsive to 100% oxygen. Occasionally, the low PO_2

reflects a right-to-left shunt through a ductus arteriosus that has remained patent because of hypoxia. *(Rudolph:1486–1488)*

42. **(B)** The findings of enlarged and cloudy corneas leaves little doubt but that the infant has congenital glaucoma. Cataracts alone do not cause megalocornea, nor do they cause blepharospasm or other signs of inflammation. The same is true of retrolental fibroplasia. *(Rudolph: 171,1902–1903; Hathaway:300)*

43. **(C)** The incidence of intraventricular hemorrhage at autopsy is least in stillborns, greater for those dying in the first 24 hours, and greatest for those dying between 1 and 3 days. The incidence then decreases rapidly. These findings are compatible with the hypothesis that such hemorrhages are related to hypoxia, acidosis, and blood pressure changes, all of which are common in the first days of life of the premature infant. *(Pediatr Clin North Am 36:47,1989; Rudolph:1705–1706)*

44. **(E)** Peripheral cyanosis (acrocyanosis) is a common finding in the neonate, presumably a result of poor vasomotor control. The cyanosis generally clears if the infant is warmed. In infants with cyanotic heart disease or methemoglobinemia, the cyanosis is generalized rather than limited to the extremities. It is very unlikely that the cyanosis is caused by pulmonary disease in the absence of rales, retractions, or other respiratory findings. A patent ductus arteriosus usually is associated with a left-to-right shunt and tachypnea rather than cyanosis. *(Arthreya:280; Rudolph:1395–1396)*

45. **(B)** The excellent response to oxygen makes both a right-to-left cardiac shunt (cyanotic congenital heart disease) and methemoglobinemia unlikely, since neither of these conditions is easily corrected by increased ambient oxygen. Patients who are cyanotic because of central nervous system disease breathe slowly or shallowly, and the infant in the question is tachypneic. Although cyanosis associated with liver disease has been reported, it is exceedingly rare, especially in the newborn period. The infant described most likely has lung disease; most such infants improve with increased ambient oxygen. *(Pediatr Clin North Am 20:296,1973; Rudolph:1395–1396)*

46. **(B)** DiGeorge's syndrome is an abnormality of development of the structures arising from the third and fourth pharyngeal pouches. There is absence of the thymus and parathyroid glands, with resultant immunodeficiency and hypocalcemia. Chronic infection with bacterial, viral, and fungal organisms is the rule. Infants with severe combined immunodeficiency have neither ear abnormalities nor hypocalcemia. Infants with renal failure, idiopathic hypoparathyroidism, or autoimmune disease (which is very rare in the neonate) would not be expected to have

an absent thymic image on chest roentgenogram, although chronic stress can lead to involution of the thymus. *(Oski:191–192; Hathaway: 523–524)*

47. **(C)** The combination of microcephaly, cerebral calcifications, and blindness is typical of the damage caused to neural tissues by intrauterine infection with either cytomegalovirus or toxoplasmosis. Subdural bleeding causes enlargement of the head, cerebral agenesis is not associated with calcifications, and erythroblastosis would not explain any of the findings listed. Primary microcephaly is not associated with either cerebral calcifications or blindness. *(Rudolph:435–436,644–645; Hathaway:84–85)*

48. **(A)** The findings described are typical of thrush (oral infection with *Candida albicans*), which is common in young infants. Although *E. coli*, *Listeria monocytogenes*, and group B *Streptococcus* all are important pathogens in the neonatal period, they are not associated with pharyngeal infection or oral exudate. Group A *Streptococcus* is a common cause of exudative tonsillitis in the older child but is an extremely rare pathogen in the newborn infant. Additionally, the exudate noted with group A streptococcal infection would be in the area of the tonsils rather than on the buccal mucosa. *(Oski:792,1252–1253; Hathaway:349,922)*

49. **(B)** The Wilson-Mikity syndrome is a type of respiratory distress seen primarily in premature infants and associated with progressive dyspnea, tachypnea, and cyanosis. The syndrome involves a characteristic progression of radiographic findings from diffuse reticulonodular and bubbly changes to coarse streaks and hyperaeration. In most cases, the roentgenographic findings revert to normal after many months. The cause is unknown, and the syndrome appears to have become less common in the past decade. *(Schaffer:524; Oski:348)*

50. **(E)** Congestive heart failure is a common complication of large intracranial arteriovenous fistulas, and a cranial bruit usually is readily audible in these patients. The great vein of Galen is a frequent location for such arteriovenous malformations. Hyperthyroidism and polycythemia cause congestive heart failure only rarely; transposition of the great vessels usually is associated with a cardiac murmur and not with a cranial bruit. Ruptured cerebral aneurysms are exceedingly rare in the newborn period and present with neurologic findings rather than heart failure or cranial bruits. *(Rudolph:1753)*

51. **(B)** Excessive sweating has been noted as a sign of heart failure, especially in infants. The mechanism is believed to involve catecholamine release. None of the other items listed, including cystic fibrosis, are associated with excessive sweating. *(Rudolph:1319; Hathaway:425)*

52. (B) Hypocalcemia may cause lethargy, irritability, apnea, cardiac arrhythmias, seizures, and vomiting. Hypoglycemia and hyponatremia could explain some of these findings. Cardiac arrhythmias, however, are not part of the clinical symptomatology of either hypoglycemia or hyponatremia. *(Schaffer:931; Hathaway: 95)*

53. (B) Brachial plexus injury frequently is associated with phrenic nerve injury on the same side because of the proximity of the involved spinal nerve roots. The phrenic injury results in diaphragmatic paralysis, which can lead to progressive respiratory difficulty. The fact that this is a large infant strengthens the supposition of brachial plexus injury during birth. Respiratory distress syndrome is uncommon in term infants and almost always presents initially in the first 24 hours of life. Pulmonary hemorrhage, pneumothorax, and cystic adenomatoid malformation can cause cyanosis and respiratory distress but have no association with brachial plexus injury. *(Rudolph:181,1765)*

54. (D) The most common congenital defect of the esophagus is atresia of the proximal segment with a fistula between the distal segment and the trachea. The clinical significance of this configuration is that attempts to feed the infant will result in massive aspiration and that even prior to feeding, aspiration of gastric secretion may occur through the distal fistula. It is important to diagnose this condition as quickly as possible to prevent the development of aspiration pneumonia. *(Rudolph:995–997; Hathaway:88)*

55. (B) Both cephalhematoma and caput are associated with prolonged and difficult labors, and both are associated with a normal neurologic examination unless there has been concomitant intracranial trauma. Caput, however, is diffuse and poorly demarcated edema, whereas a cephalhematoma is a subperiosteal collection of blood and therefore is sharply demarcated and limited to a single bone. Cephalhematomas may be bilateral, but each is separate and sharply demarcated. Lumbar puncture is not indicated in the evaluation of either condition but, if done, would be normal in both cases. Coagulation parameters are normal in both. [*Note:* The student might wish to argue that response **(B)** is incorrect in that cephalhematomas can be bilateral and therefore are not limited to the area over *one* bone. *Each* swelling, however, is limited to the area over one bone. Since all other choices are totally incorrect, **(B)** is the *best* choice, even if imperfectly worded.] *(Oski:278)*

56. (C) Most of the serious disorders of organic acid metabolism (eg, maple syrup urine disease, methylmalonic acidemia) present with acidosis, vomiting, and coma, often proceeding to death. Renal failure, intestinal obstruction, and cardiac arrhythmias are not part of the clinical picture of any of these disorders. Although poor growth can be seen in infants with organic acidemia, it is unlikely to be the presenting complaint in the first week of life, especially since infants *normally* lose weight in the first few days of life. [*Note:* Again, attention to every qualifying word or phrase, such as, *in the first week of life*, is very important.] *(Rudolph:304–310)*

57. (C) About 10% of infants born to mothers with myasthenia have transitory weakness lasting several weeks. This results from transplacental passage of maternal IgG antibodies directed against acetylcholine receptors. As the infant's level of maternal antibodies wanes, neuromuscular function recovers. Choice **(B)** is incorrect; although these infants may present with apnea, if they do, they are then unlikely to do well without continued support (artificial ventilation or anticholinesterase drugs) for at least some days to weeks. *(Rudolph:1799–1802; Hathaway: 714)*

58. (C) Term infants usually maintain their blood glucose levels above 30 mg/dL, and 20 mg/dL appears to be the lower level ordinarily encountered for premature and low-birth-weight infants. It is believed, however, that these levels, although frequent, are unphysiologic and may cause symptoms. It has been suggested that 40 mg/dL be considered the lower limit of normal for all newborns. *(Rudolph:184; Hathaway:1101)*

59. (D) Talipes equinovarus deformities have an incidence of about 1 per 1,000 live births and account for about 95% of congenital clubfeet. In this deformity the foot is plantar flexed and inverted. If the diagnosis is established promptly at birth and treatment (casting) is initiated at that time, surgery will be required only rarely. *(Rudolph:1932–1933; Hathaway:633)*

60. (E) The most consistent features of Pierre Robin syndrome are micrognathia, glossoptosis, and cleft palate. The basic embryologic defect is poor growth of the mandible (micrognathia), which forces the developing tongue upward (blocking the medial fusion of the palatine ridges, causing cleft palate) and backward (glossoptosis). The most urgent problem in these infants is upper airway obstruction from glossoptosis. Turning the infant prone often permits the tongue to fall forward, relieving the obstruction. *(Rudolph:171,433,1470; Hathaway:359–360)*

61. (B) So-called pyridoxine dependency is a group of rare, inborn metabolic errors that cause severe neonatal seizures that respond to pharmacologic (as opposed to physiologic) doses of pyridoxine. Although the disorder is extremely rare, it has given rise to the practice of sometimes empirically administering an intravenous dose of pyridoxine to infants with unexplained and otherwise uncontrollable seizures. *(Oski:323)*

62. (A) The cranium of the child grows at right angles to several sutures, primarily the sagittal, coronal, lambdoidal, and temporal. Isolated premature closure (craniosynostosis) of the sagittal suture results in a long and narrow skull (scaphocephaly) with a slightly greater than normal total circumference. With early fusion of a single suture there usually are no signs of increased intracranial pressure, and the problem is chiefly cosmetic. Craniosynostosis of multiple sutures, however, often is associated with increased intracranial pressure. Hydrocephalus and subdural effusions are not related to premature fusion of cranial sutures. *(Oski:462–467; Hathaway:690)*

63. (E) Most infants who experience fetal bradycardia during labor are not severely asphyxiated at birth and ultimately have a good neurologic outcome. Likewise, most infants who fail to breathe initially or are cyanotic at birth and have a low 1-minute Apgar score recover promptly and do well neurologically. Although a low 5-minute Apgar score indicates more prolonged asphyxia and correlates somewhat better with outcome than does the 1-minute score, most of these infants also will be normal. In contrast, up to 80% of newborns with seizures in the first 36 hours of life will show neurologic abnormalities on long-term follow-up. *(Rudolph:1710–1711,1720)*

64. (C) The lesions described are typical for neonatal acne (acne neonatorum), a not uncommon skin eruption occurring during the first few weeks of life, probably secondary to transplacental maternal hormones. Adenoma sebaceum, one of the several cutaneous manifestations of tuberous sclerosis, bears a superficial resemblance to acne, with a similar facial distribution, but can be differentiated by the absence of pustules and comedones. Furthermore, tuberous sclerosis is a rare disease, and in most cases adenoma sebaceum is not present in the neonatal period. The distribution of the rash in this patient and the presence of comedones are not typical of congenital syphilis, impetigo, or pustulosis. *(Rudolph:919,1872; Hathaway:270)*

65. (E) Within a few hours of birth, the skin of the normal infant often assumes an intense red color that may last for several hours. Although some localized petechiae and ecchymoses may reflect birth trauma, generalized edema and hemorrhagic phenomena always are abnormal. Cyanosis is not uncommon in the normal neonate but usually is present at or soon after birth and clears within a few hours rather than first appearing at that time. Also, cyanosis in the *normal* infant usually is limited to the extremities (acrocyanosis) rather than being generalized. *(Rudolph:168; Hathaway:53)*

66. (C) Late-onset neonatal tetany results from hyperphosphatemia rather than from primary hypocalcemia. The elevated serum phosphate level,

in turn, results from the combination of low phosphate clearance by the kidneys (renal immaturity) and the high phosphate load of unmodified cow milk. Both breast milk and current prepared infant formulas simulating breast milk have a lower phosphate load and a more favorable calcium-phosphorus ratio than does cow milk. *(Rudolph:1782; Hathaway:95)*

67. (C) Necrotizing enterocolitis (NEC) occurs especially frequently among low-birth-weight infants who have had repeated episodes of hypoxia or poor perfusion. It is believed that hypoxia and ischemia of the bowel during these episodes set the stage for invasion of the bowel wall by certain bacteria. The usual signs of NEC are abdominal distention, bloody stools, vomiting, hypothermia, and lethargy. Intussusception is rare in the neonatal period. Volvulus and aganglionosis are unrelated to low birth weight or to hypoxia and usually are associated with failure to pass stool. *Shigella* infection is very uncommon in the nursery. *(Rudolph:1020–1021; Hathaway:90–91)*

68. (B) Most capillary or cavernous hemangiomas are small or even invisible at birth. During the first weeks or months of life, they begin to grow and may become very large before finally starting to regress after a few years. Spontaneous regression is usually (but not invariably) complete or nearly so. Recognition of the natural history of this lesion permits reassurance of parents and avoidance of unnecessary therapy. The best cosmetic results are achieved by natural regression. Active intervention (surgery, x ray, or laser therapy) should be advised only when a complication such as platelet trapping or erosion of tissue is a problem. *(Rudolph:170,913,1086; Hathaway: 272)*

69. (B) Scalded skin syndrome (toxic epidermal necrolysis) is caused by a circulating toxin released by certain strains of *Staphylococcus aureus*. The staphylococci frequently are not growing in the involved areas of skin but may have infected or colonized the pharynx or umbilicus. The disease is most frequent in young infants but is not restricted to neonates. Infants with scalded skin syndrome have no discernible immunologic abnormality. The rash of scalded skin syndrome occasionally may be confused with the rash of Leiner's disease, which is characterized by a more chronic, seborrheic dermatitis. Patients with Leiner's disease have a defect in the fifth component of complement. *(Rudolph:170,612; Oski:446,850; Hathaway:277)*

70. (B) Characteristically, the lesions of erythema toxicum (erythematous papules and vesicles) are loaded with eosinophils. The cause of this transient disorder of term newborns is unknown, and the lesions resolve spontaneously within 1 or 2 days. Cultures of the lesions are sterile. It is important not to confuse this totally benign condition with the rash of serious disorders such as staphylococcal pustulosis or disseminated viral infection. *(Rudolph:170,879–881; Hathaway:270–271)*

71. **(B)** Infants born to mothers with hyperparathyroidism often develop transient hypoparathyroidism, resulting in hypocalcemia and tetany. The mechanism, presumably, is suppression of the fetal parathyroid glands by excessive transplacental maternal parathyroid hormone. Occasionally, the mother's condition may be undiagnosed, and otherwise unexplained hypocalcemia in an infant can lead to the diagnosis of hyperparathyroidism in the mother. *(Rudolph:1647; Hathaway:95)*

72. **(A)** Amnion nodosum suggests oligohydramnios, which, in conjunction with the "Potter's facies" described, is characteristic of bilateral renal agenesis. Esophageal atresia often is associated with polyhydramnios, not oligohydramnios. None of the features of this case are suggestive of congenital heart disease or infection. *(Rudolph:424; Oski:413)*

73. **(C)** Ambiguous genitalia in association with congenital adrenal hyperplasia usually means a female pseudohermaphrodite, since most of the defects result in masculinization of the fetus. The patient described, however, is genetically an XY male. The rare defect of 3β-hydroxysteroid dehydrogenase results in the inability to synthesize testicular androgen and, therefore, failure of normal masculinization of the male fetus, as in this patient. Although the 17-hydroxylase defect also can cause feminization, it is not associated with salt loss. [*Note:* To answer the question correctly, the reader first must note that the patient is XY and then reason that the ambiguous genitalia, therefore, must result from feminization rather than masculinization.] *(Rudolph:1597)*

74. **(B)** Infants born to women with active and untreated Graves's disease may be hyperthyroid at birth, presumably as a result of transplacental passage of long-acting thyroid stimulator (LATS) or a similar substance. If the mother is receiving antithyroid medication, this also crosses the placenta, and the infant generally will be euthyroid or even hypothyroid at birth. Yet because the plasma half-lives of these agents are much shorter than that of LATS, thyrotoxicosis may begin a week or so after birth. Iodides administered to the mother during pregnancy can cross the placenta and block the function of the fetal thyroid. Such infants have been born with huge goiters, but they are either euthyroid or hypothyroid rather than hyperthyroid. *(Rudolph:1640)*

75. **(A)** Epiphyseal dysgenesis with irregular or stippled ossification centers is characteristic of hypothyroidism (although it also is seen in some other conditions). The development of ossification centers is retarded in hypothyroidism, but since the ossification center of the hamate does not normally appear until the age of 4 months, x ray examination of the wrist is of no value in the newborn period. Roentgenographic demonstration of absence of the distal femoral epiphyses (normally evident at 34 to 36 weeks of gestation) in a term infant would be suggestive of hypothyroidism. Although cardiomegaly from myxedema of the heart can be seen rarely, there are so many other, much more common causes of cardiomegaly in the newborn that an enlarged heart would not be suggestive of hypothyroidism. *(Rudolph:1631)*

76. **(E)** Infants born to mothers addicted to heroin tend to be small for gestational age, whereas those born to phenobarbital-addicted mothers are usually of normal size. Both groups of infants have tremors and other signs of withdrawal, and both have a low incidence of neonatal jaundice, presumably because these drugs induce hepatic enzymes, including glucuronyltransferase. Phenobarbital withdrawal symptoms tend to develop later than heroin withdrawal, frequently appearing after day 10 of life. (Pediatrics *48:178,1971; Schaffer:238,446)*

77. **(A)** The most common cause of neonatal meningitis in most hospitals today is group B streptococci. *E. coli* generally is the second leading cause. *Listeria* is less frequent but not uncommon. *Hemophilus influenzae* and *Streptococcus pneumoniae* are uncommon causes of meningitis during the first month of life. *(Oski:480; Hathaway:83)*

78. **(E)** More than 95% of *term* infants will have passed their first meconium stool by the age of 24 hours, and 99.8% by 48 hours. In a term infant, failure to pass meconium by 24 to 48 hours should suggest problems such as intestinal obstruction, Hirschsprung's disease, or hypothyroidism. In contrast, as many as 20% of infants less than 1,500 g at birth may fail to pass meconium by 48 hours of life. (Pediatrics *60:457–459,1977; 79:1005–1007,1987; Rudolph:183)*

79. **(E)** The description and location of the lesion ("beneath fading forceps marks") are typical of subcutaneous fat necrosis, which may follow trauma (forceps) or cold exposure. Buccal cellulitis caused by *H. influenzae* frequently has a violaceous color but is exceedingly rare in the newborn period. *(Hathaway: 271; Schaffer:994–995)*

80. **(D)** The initial lesions of incontinentia pigmenti are inflammatory bullae that eventually evolve into pigmented lesions. The majority of affected patients are female. Mental retardation and seizures are common. The disease also involves the heart, eyes, and skeletal system. *(Rudolph:893–894,1876; Hathaway:274)*

81. **(A)** The premature infant is born with a smaller total hemoglobin mass than the term infant. Since

most of the iron stores at birth are contained in the circulating hemoglobin, the premature infant starts life at a serious disadvantage in regard to iron stores. In cases of hemolysis (as with ABO incompatibility), the liberated iron is not lost from the body, so the risk of iron deficiency is not increased. The same is true of physiologic hyperbilirubinemia. *(Rudolph:1100)*

82. **(D)** Fetal hemoglobin binds poorly to 2,3-DPG. Because 2,3-DPG binding decreases the affinity of hemoglobin for oxygen, fetal hemoglobin, unbound to 2,3-DPG, has an increased affinity for oxygen. Prenatally this works to the advantage of the fetus in obtaining oxygen from the maternal blood (across the placenta), but postnatally it is to the infant's disadvantage in releasing oxygen at the tissue level. *(Rudolph:1095)*

83. **(C)** The mass shown is a typical example of an encephalocele. These lesions, which consist of herniation of the meninges, with or without brain tissue, through a defect in the skull, occur most commonly in the occipital region. The mass is far too large to be an abscess. There is no such entity as posterior hydrocephalus. Hydroceles are limited to the scrotum. Diastematomyelia is a defect in the spinal cord that leads to neurologic signs but is unassociated with an external mass. *(Rudolph:1696–1697)*

84. **(C)** The density represents a normal thymus. The sharp lower border and the lateral rim of radiolucency (lung) constitute the appearance of the classic thymic sail sign. Right upper lobe pneumonia would extend to the edge of the thorax. Furthermore, pneumonia would be unusual in an asymptomatic infant. Lobar emphysema would appear as a radiolucency rather than a radiodensity. *(Pediatr Clin North Am 26:679,1979; Rudolph:1472–1473)*

85. **(C)** The roentgenogram reveals absence of the radius and suggests the thrombocytopenia absent radii (TAR) syndrome, in which disorder thrombocytopenia and bleeding occur early. In Fanconi's syndrome (absent radii and pancytopenia), the hematologic abnormalities usually become manifest after the first or second birthday rather than immediately in the newborn period. *(Rudolph:1161; Oski:2007)*

86. **(A)** Most urinary tract infections in the first few weeks of life are caused by *E. coli*. Other organisms include *Klebsiella, Enterobacter, Proteus,* enterococci, *S. aureus, S. epidermidis,* and occasionally group B streptococci. Anatomic obstruction is a very important diagnostic consideration but is present in only a minority (about 5%) of cases. Renal vein thrombosis is a very rare complication. Catheterization or suprapubic bladder tap is generally the preferred method of establishing the diagnosis because of the difficulty in the young infant of obtaining an uncontaminated bag or voided specimen. *(Rudolph:1289; Schaffer:911–914)*

87. **(B)** Neither cataracts nor myocarditis is a recognized manifestation of congenital syphilis, although an interstitial keratitis is seen in the *late* stages of the disorder. There are a variety of highly characteristic skin manifestations, including bullous lesions on the palms and soles and a diffuse copper-colored maculopapular rash, most intense on the face, palms, and soles. Pneumonia and hepatitis may occur but also are seen in many other neonatal infections. *(Rudolph:619–621; Hathaway:891–892)*

88. **(A)** Physiologic jaundice results from unconjugated hyperbilirubinemia. Although there are many factors contributing to physiologic jaundice, the most important is hepatic immaturity, which is more marked in premature than in term infants. Physiologic jaundice does not appear in the first 24 hours of life. It is not associated with hemolysis and, therefore, is not associated with anemia or reticulocytosis. It is a common problem in infants of all races. *(Rudolph:1055; Schaffer:753–754)*

89. **(D)** Since the infant in question had more than 38 weeks of gestation, he is not premature. He is, however, of low birth weight (below 2,500 g). Therefore, he must be significantly small for his gestational age. This can be confirmed by the use of standard intrauterine growth charts. [*Note:* Answer **(C)** is a true statement, but **(E)** is the one *best* answer because it is most complete. Even though an answer seems correct, it is important to examine all choices.] *(Rudolph:167–169; Hathaway:50–51)*

90. **(D)** Subdural hemorrhage over the cerebral cortex is uncommon in premature infants, who, because of their small size, are less likely than term infants to have trauma to, or molding of, the skull during the birth process. Intraventricular hemorrhages occur primarily in premature infants. Hemorrhagic disease of the newborn can occur in either premature or term infants who do not receive vitamin K prophylaxis but is not more common in term infants. Both congenital infection and neonatal sepsis are more common in premature than term infants. *(Schaffer:422; Hathaway:100)*

91. **(B)** A serum potassium value of less than 4 mEq/L is unusual in the first few days of life. The normal range is 4 to 7.5 mEq/L, depending on gestational age, and is higher in premature infants. Serum sodium concentration also tends to be elevated in the first few days of life, as does the blood urea. Blood glucose in the first few days of life normally ranges from 40 to 90 mg/dL. *(Hathaway:1101–1103)*

92. **(D)** Tachypnea, retractions, cyanosis, and grunting are common findings in the neonatal respiratory distress syndrome (RDS). Wheezing is uncommon in the newborn in general and is not a feature of RDS. *(Rudolph:1486–1487)*

93. (B) Electronic fetal heart rate monitoring (EFM) can be helpful in assessing the oxygenation status of the fetus in utero. The fetal heart rate is usually over 100/minute with considerable beat-to-beat variation. A rate less than 100/minute is unusual and worrisome. A fixed heart rate or decreased beat-to-beat variability often indicates fetal hypoxia (fetal distress). Accelerations of the rate are normal and of no concern. Decelerations may be of no consequence or may be ominous depending on their temporal relationship to uterine contractions. Early decelerations are usually benign, whereas late or variable decelerations frequently indicate fetal distress. *(Schaffer:85; Rudolph:159–163)*

94. (D) There is no direct association between intraventricular hemorrhage and renal vein thrombosis. Recognized factors predisposing to renal vein thrombosis include dehydration, anoxia, shock, birth injury, and polycythemia. Renal vein thrombosis also is especially frequent in infants of diabetic mothers. *(Rudolph:1287)*

95. (D) Cholelithiasis and cholecystitis are not features of extrahepatic biliary atresia. Indeed, in most cases the gallbladder is severely atrophic or absent. Interestingly, jaundice is usually not evident until the second or third week of life. Most cases of extrahepatic biliary atresia do not represent congenital malformations. Rather, there is evidence to suggest that an inflammatory condition of the liver or bile ducts is present before or at birth and that this leads to atrophy and fibrosis of the ducts a short time later. If not treated in a timely fashion, these patients eventually develop biliary cirrhosis, hepatosplenomegaly, ascites, and esophageal varices. Even with treatment (hepatoportoenterostomy; Kasai procedure), many do poorly and eventually require liver transplantation. *(Rudolph:1070–1072; Hathaway:579)*

96. (C) Iron deficiency anemia is essentially unheard of in the newborn period. Even if the mother is severely iron deficient, the fetus usually will not be anemic. Abruptio placentae can result in blood loss from the infant as well as from the mother. Fetal-maternal transfusion can cause neonatal anemia, and twin-to-twin transfusion can cause anemia in one twin and polycythemia in the other. Maternal-infant blood group incompatibility disease (isoimmune hemolytic anemia) is an important cause of anemia in the newborn period. *(Oski:432–435; Hathaway:92)*

97. (C) Hypertrophic pyloric stenosis rarely occurs in the immediate newborn period. Vomiting usually begins about a week after birth. The other conditions listed—duodenal atresia, volvulus, annular pancreas, and meconium ileus—all are important causes of intestinal obstruction and vomiting in the first day of life. *(Oski:371–377; Hathaway:540)*

98. (C) The presence of fetal hemoglobin does not cause or exaggerate cyanosis. Because fetal hemoglobin binds oxygen more avidly than does adult hemoglobin, it will tend to minimize cyanosis, even when the arterial oxygen tension is low. Polycythemia, on the other hand, will increase the likelihood of cyanosis because of the increased mass of reduced hemoglobin. Methemoglobinemia causes cyanosis by preventing hemoglobin from picking up oxygen in the lung. Shock, whether hypovolemic, septic, or cardiogenic, often causes central as well as peripheral cyanosis through a variety of mechanisms. *(Rudolph: 1095)*

99. (E) The most important consequence of polycythemia is hyperviscosity and impaired perfusion of vital organs such as brain and kidney. Increased resistance to blood flow through the lungs often leads to pulmonary hypertension with right-to-left shunting through the foramen ovale and the ductus arteriosus. Signs and symptoms usually first appear a few hours or more after birth, when water normally shifts from intravascular to extravascular space, with a resultant increase in hematocrit. Causes of neonatal polycythemia include chronic intrauterine hypoxemia (high-altitude pregnancy, placental insufficiency, postmaturity, carbon monoxide exposure from heavy maternal smoking), twin-to-twin and maternal-to-fetal transfusion, and maternal diabetes. *(Hathaway:92)*

100. (D) Congenital eye defects (cataracts, glaucoma), cardiac defects (patent ductus arteriosus, ventricular septal defect), and deafness are common manifestations of congenital (intrauterine) rubella infection. Thrombocytopenia also occurs occasionally and usually is transient. Renal abnormalities have not been described. *(Rudolph:689–690; Hathaway:85)*

101. (D) A number of factors appear to lower the threshold for kernicterus: prematurity, asphyxia, respiratory distress syndrome, hypoglycemia, acidosis, sepsis, and hypothermia. Some of these factors, such as acidosis, are believed to exert their effect by interfering with albumin binding of bilirubin. For other factors, the exact mechanism is unknown. Postmaturity itself does not appear to increase the risk of kernicterus. *(Rudolph:1056–1057)*

102. (D) Small-for-gestational-age or small-for-dates infants have an increased incidence of hypoglycemia, polycythemia, and convulsions as well as congenital malformations and pulmonary hemorrhage. *Term* infants, however, have little risk of developing the neonatal respiratory distress syndrome, even if small for gestational age. *(Oski:304–306; Rudolph:199–201)*

103. (B) Infants born to diabetic or prediabetic mothers are often polycythemic. They frequently develop hypoglycemia and hypocalcemia. These infants do have a greater than normal incidence of congenital malformations, including microcolon. They also have an increased incidence of cardiomyopathy manifested as asymmetric septal hypertrophy. *(Rudolph:202–205; Hathaway:93)*

104. **(C)** Some degree of tremors with crying and other activity in the first few days of life is within normal limits. Such tremors may be fine or coarse. Unlike the movements of seizures, the movements of tremors can be elicited by stimulation and can be stopped by holding the affected limb. Although tremors with activity are usually normal, they can be the result of hypocalcemia, maternal drug abuse, or other neurologic problems. Tremors at rest usually are abnormal. When there is a specific cause, tremors may progress to convulsions, but this is the exception rather than the rule. (Pediatr Clin North Am 33:91–109, 1986; Rudolph:176)

105. **(A)** Increased portal blood flow is not a factor in neonatal physiologic hyperbilirubinemia. In fact, it has been suggested that the discontinuance of well-oxygenated umbilical venous blood flow to the liver may be a partial explanation of physiologic jaundice. Increased production of bilirubin secondary to the relative polycythemia of the newborn (mean hemoglobin 17 g/dL) and the relatively decreased survival time of neonatal erythrocytes (80 days), increased enterohepatic circulation, and decreased hepatic conjugation of bilirubin have all been shown to contribute to physiologic neonatal jaundice. *(Rudolph: 400–401; Hathaway:78)*

106. **(B)** Trisomy 18 (Edwards's syndrome) is characterized by severe retardation of growth and mental development. Most of the patients die in early infancy. Characteristic abnormalities include low-set and malformed ears, nail hypoplasia, abnormal fisting with index finger overlying third finger, and rocker-bottom feet. The abnormalities of the hands and feet are clinically distinctive features. Congenital heart disease is usual, most commonly a ventricular septal defect or a patent ductus arteriosus. The face is round with a narrow forehead, frontal bossing, hypertelorism, micrognathia, and antimongoloid palpebral fissures. *(Oski:2008; Hathaway:1022–1023)*

107. **(A)** The cardinal features of trisomy 13 (Patau's syndrome) include cleft lip and palate, holoprosencephaly, and severe mental retardation. Holoprosencephaly is an incomplete development of the forebrain, often associated with absence of the corpus callosum, fusion of the frontal lobes, and a single ventricle. Other features of trisomy 13 include ocular abnormalities, congenital heart disease, and cutaneous defects of the scalp, which can be diagnostic. *(Oski:2008; Hathaway:1023)*

108. **(D)** Down's syndrome is a rather common chromosomal abnormality, occurring in about 1 in 770 live births. Fewer than 5% of patients have a translocation rather than an extra (47) chromosome. Hypotonia and hyperextensible joints are characteristic. Mental retardation is present in all patients but is less severe than in other trisomy syndromes (i.e., trisomies 13 and 18). Clinodactyly, especially of the fifth finger, simian creases of the palm, an increased distance between the first and second toes, upward slanting palpebral fissures, epicanthal folds, flat nasal bridge, and flat occiput are some of the physical findings associated with this syndrome. Many of these patients have serious congenital malformations such as congenital heart disease or duodenal atresia. Brushfield spots (tiny white spots that form a ring in the midzone of the iris) are present in the majority of Down's syndrome children but also are present in up to 25% of normal individuals, especially those with blue eyes. *(Oski:1944; Rudolph:295–296)*

109. **(C)** The cri du chat (cry of the cat) syndrome is so named because of the characteristic cry, which is reminiscent of a mewing cat. This characteristic cry is present in infancy but disappears as the child grows and usually is gone by the age of 1 or 2 years. The cry is high pitched and distinctive and results from a small, narrow, hypoplastic larynx. These patients also have microcephaly, severe mental retardation, epicanthal folds, hypertelorism, antimongoloid slant of palpebral fissures, and low-set ears. The syndrome is associated with a deletion of the short arm of chromosome 5. [Note: The student who understands French has an obvious advantage in answering this question.] *(Oski:1993–1994)*

110. **(E)** Features of Turner's syndrome, 45,X or X0, in the older child include short stature, lack of development of sexual characteristics, primary amenorrhea, webbing of the neck, cubitus valgus (wide-carrying angle of the arms), and short fourth metacarpals. Pathologically, there is ovarian dysgenesis. In the newborn period, redundant skin at the nape of the neck, a low posterior hair line, and edema of the dorsum of the feet are characteristic. Cardiac defects (especially coarctation of the aorta) and renal anomalies are common. Intelligence usually is normal, but perceptual difficulties are frequent and can be severe. *(Oski:2009; Hathaway:1023–1024)*

111. **(C)** In general, regardless of the cause of the hyperbilirubinemia, an unconjugated bilirubin concentration of over 15 mg/dL in the first 24 hours of life is a relative indication for exchange transfusion to prevent higher levels and the risk of kernicterus; a level of 20 mg/dL or greater is an absolute indication. Although phototherapy is not a substitute for exchange transfusion in such an infant, its use *following* exchange transfusion might prevent the need

for subsequent exchange transfusions. Such an infant, therefore, is apt to receive both treatments. *(Hathaway:79–80; Oski:402–407)*

112. (D) A serum bilirubin concentration of 5 mg/dL at the age of 3 days is within normal limits and requires neither phototherapy nor exchange transfusion. *(Hathaway:79–80; Oski:402–407)*

113. (C) The serum concentration of unconjugated bilirubin generally should not be permitted to exceed 20 mg/dL. A level of 25 mg/dL generally requires immediate exchange transfusion followed by phototherapy. *(Hathaway:79–80; Oski:402–407)*

114. (B) A serum bilirubin concentration greater than 12.9 mg/dL in the first few days of life is generally an indication for phototherapy except in the initial 24 hours after birth, during which time an exchange transfusion might be required. The earlier the hyperbilirubinemia occurs, the more likely it is to exceed 20 mg/dL eventually. The later jaundice occurs and the more slowly serum levels of bilirubin rise, the more likely that phototherapy alone will suffice. *(Hathaway:79–80; Oski:402–407)*

115. (D) Mild hyperbilirubinemia beyond the first week of life requires investigation to rule out causes such as infection, hepatitis, biliary atresia, and hemolysis. Treatment of mild hyperbilirubinemia itself at this age, however, usually is unnecessary. *(Hathaway:79–80; Oski:402–407)*

116. (D) A bilirubin level of 2 mg/dL at the age of 24 hours is within normal limits. Since phototherapy acts to decompose bilirubin, it would not be useful in the presence of such a minimal serum level of bilirubin. If the serum level of bilirubin were to increase, then phototherapy would be indicated. Some infants with mild ABO incompatibility never become jaundiced despite a positive Coombs's test. [*Note:* The astute reader should have realized that *any* condition warranting an exchange transfusion also will warrant the use of phototherapy *after* the exchange. Choice **(A)**, therefore, was not a viable choice for any of the questions in this series.] *(Hathaway:471; Rudolph:1092–1094)*

117. (D) Although platelet counts in the newborn period may be slightly lower than usual adult levels, a value below 100,000/mm^3 should be considered abnormal. A value of 50,000/mm^3 is not properly matched to the normal infant of any age. *(Hathaway: 471; Rudolph:1092–1094)*

118. (B) For the reason described in the previous answer, the reticulocyte count falls from a high of 3 to 7% at birth to 1% or less by the age of 1 week. *(Hathaway: 471; Rudolph:1092–1094)*

119. (A) The bone marrow, which has been hyperactive in regard to erythropoiesis before birth, shuts off promptly after birth. Nucleated red blood cells normally are present in the peripheral blood smear at birth but disappear by 2 to 4 days of life. *(Hathaway: 471; Rudolph: 1092–1094)*

BIBLIOGRAPHY

Allan WC, Volpe JJ. Periventricular-intraventricular hemorrhage. *Pediatr Clin North Am.* 1989;36:47–63.

Athreya BH, Silverman BK. *Pediatric Physical Diagnosis.* Norwalk, Conn: Appleton-Century-Crofts; 1985.

Brown A. Neonatal jaundice. *Pediatr Clin North Am.* 1962;9:575–603.

Clark DA. Times of first void and first stool in 500 newborns. *Pediatrics.* 1977;60:457–459.

Feigin RD, Cherry JD. *Textbook of Pediatric Infectious Diseases.* 3rd ed. Philadelphia, Pa: Saunders; 1992.

Filler RM, Simpson JS, Ein SH. Mediastinal masses in infants and children. *Pediatr Clin North Am.* 1979;26: 677–701.

Hathaway WE, Groothius JR, Hay WW, et al. *Current Pediatric Diagnosis & Treatment.* 10th ed. Norwalk, Conn: Appleton & Lange; 1991.

Hon EH, Petrie RH. Clinical value of fetal heart rate monitoring. *Clin Obstet Gynecol.* 1975;18:(4):1–23.

Jhaveri M, Kumar SP. Passage of the first stool in very low birth weight infants. *Pediatrics.* 1987;79:1005–1007.

Nicolaides KH, Rodeck CH. Rhesus Disease: the model for fetal therapy. *Br J Hosp Med.* 1985;34:141–148.

Oski FA, DeAngelis CD, Feigin RD, et al. *Principles & Practice of Pediatrics.* Philadelphia, Pa. JB Lippincott; 1990.

Painter MJ, Bergman I, Crumrine P. Neonatal Seizures. *Pediatr Clin North Am.* 1986;33:91–109.

Rudolph AM, Hoffman JIE, Rudolph CD. *Pediatrics.* 19th ed. Norwalk, Conn: Appleton & Lange; 1991.

Rudoy RC, Nelson JD. Breast abscess during the neonatal period: a review. *Am J Dis Child.* 1975;129:1031–1034.

Sahn DJ, Friedman WF: Difficulties in distinguishing cardiac from pulmonary disease in the neonate. *Pediatr Clin North Am.* 1973;20:293–301.

Schaffer R, Avery, ME. *Schaffer and Avery's Diseases of the Newborn.* 6th ed. Philadelphia, Pa: Saunders; 1991.

Smith DH, Peter G. Current and future vaccines for the prevention of bacterial diseases. *Pediatr Clin North Am.* 1972;19:387–412.

Wald ER, Bergman I, Taylor HG, et al. Long-term outcome of Group B streptococcal meningitis. *Pediatrics.* 1986;77: 217–221.

CHAPTER 4

Feeding and Nutrition
Questions

Historically as well as currently, the topic of feeding and nutrition has special importance in pediatrics because of the rapid growth and development of the pediatric patient, especially the infant. This rapid growth and development results in both quantitatively and qualitatively different nutritional needs than exist for the adult. Quantitatively, for example, the newborn and young infant require more calories and more protein relative to body size than do older individuals. In a qualitative sense, for example, certain amino acids are essential for low-birth-weight and preterm infants but not for children or adults or even for normal term infants. Certain fats are essential for brain growth during the first few years of life but not thereafter.

Furthermore, infants are always fully dependent on their caregivers for the provision of food and nutrients. At no other time of life is the *normal* individual so dependent on others to determine exactly what and how much he shall eat. The practice of infant *feeding* has only recently come into line with the science of infant *nutrition*. It is now recognized that the two are inseparable. We have finally acknowledged that what is best for infant cows is not best for human infants.

Malnutrition secondary to medical or socioeconomic problems remains an important problem in infants and children in the United States. Obesity is a very prevalent disorder. Although specific nutritional deficiencies, except for iron, are uncommon in the developed countries, deficiencies of vitamins or protein still do occur and are a major problem in undeveloped countries. It is for that reason that questions about diseases such as scurvy and pellagra continue to appear on examinations.

DIRECTIONS (Questions 1 through 25): Each of the numbered items or incomplete statements in this section is followed by answers or by completions of the statement. Select the ONE lettered answer or completion that is BEST in each case.

1. It generally is recommended that beikost (infant foods other than milk) be introduced into the infant's diet at about

    (A) 3 weeks
    (B) 6 weeks
    (C) 3 months
    (D) 6 months
    (E) 1 year

2. Developmental readiness for the introduction of beikost into the diet is based on all of the following EXCEPT

    (A) the ability to chew solid foods
    (B) the ability to communicate the degree of satiety
    (C) the ability to sit without support
    (D) good neuromuscular control of the head and neck
    (E) loss of the extrusion reflex

3. The recommended daily dietary allowance of vitamin A for an infant is

    (A) 50 μg (160 IU)
    (B) 100 μg (320 IU)
    (C) 200 μg (650 IU)
    (D) 400 μg (1,300 IU)
    (E) 1,000 μg (3,300 IU)

4. Undernutrition during the first year of life

(A) has no permanent effect on physical growth or development of intelligence
(B) can have permanent effects on physical growth but not on development of intelligence
(C) can have permanent effects on development of intelligence but not on physical growth
(D) can have permanent effects on both physical growth and development of intelligence
(E) can have permanent effects on both physical growth and development of intelligence, but only if coupled with psychosocial deprivation

5. The administration of parenteral vitamin K is indicated for

(A) all newborn infants
(B) infants below 2,500 g
(C) infants of less than 36 weeks' gestation
(D) jaundiced infants
(E) infants born outside of hospital

6. A 10-week-old child weighing 5 kg is being fed only commercial infant formula. To satisfy both his fluid and caloric requirements, the daily intake ought to be at least

(A) 12 ounces
(B) 18 ounces
(C) 28 ounces
(D) 36 ounces
(E) 48 ounces

7. Which of the following statements is most accurate?

(A) The vitamin K content of breast milk is about a third that of cow milk
(B) The vitamin K content of cow milk is about a third that of breast milk
(C) The amounts of vitamin K in cow milk and in breast milk are about the same and are adequate for most infants who have received parenteral vitamin K as newborns
(D) Neither cow milk nor breast milk contains adequate amounts of vitamin K even for infants who received parenteral vitamin K as newborns
(E) There is no vitamin K in either breast milk or cow milk

8. The recommended daily dietary allowance of vitamin D for a young infant is

(A) 2.5 µg (100 IU)
(B) 10 µg (400 IU)
(C) 20 µg (800 IU)
(D) 40 µg (1,600 IU)
(E) 100 µg (4,000 IU)

9. Supplementation with which of the following vitamins is most important for an exclusively breast-fed infant?

(A) Vitamin A
(B) Vitamin E
(C) Vitamin C
(D) Vitamin B_1
(E) Vitamin D

10. Which of the following statements is most correct?

(A) Both breast milk and cow milk contain between 1% and 2% fat
(B) Both breast milk and cow milk contain between 3% and 4% fat
(C) Breast milk contains about 1% fat, and cow milk about 3%
(D) Breast milk contains about 3% fat, and cow milk about 1%
(E) Breast milk contains about 3% fat, and cow milk about 6%

11. The recommended daily intake of protein for optimal growth during the first 6 months of life is about

(A) 0.2 g/kg
(B) 1.0 g/kg
(C) 2.0 g/kg
(D) 5.0 g/kg
(E) 10.0 g/kg

12. The recommended daily intake of dietary protein for optimal growth at the age of 10 years is about

(A) 0.2 g/kg
(B) 1.0 g/kg
(C) 2.0 g/kg
(D) 5.0 g/kg
(E) 10.0 g/kg

13. Which of the following organs is most likely to decrease in size during a period of undernutrition?

(A) Brain
(B) Heart
(C) Kidneys
(D) Liver
(E) Thymus

14. The calcium requirement for a school-age child is in the order of

(A) 0.1 g/day
(B) 1.0 g/day
(C) 10.0 g/day
(D) 50.0 g/day
(E) 100 g/day

15. Vitamin B_{12} deficiency is most likely to occur in a child with

(A) resection of the jejunum
(B) resection of the ileum
(C) resection of the colon
(D) a colostomy
(E) a gastrojejunostomy

16. Folic acid deficiency is most likely to occur in a child with

(A) malabsorptive disease of the small intestines
(B) hemangioma of the ileum
(C) a rectal polyp
(D) a gastrostomy
(E) gastroesophageal reflux

17. A strict vegan diet (a diet excluding all animal products, even eggs, milk, and milk products, as well as meats) for a young child is likely to be deficient in

(A) vitamin C
(B) vitamin E
(C) vitamin B_1
(D) vitamin B_{12}
(E) vitamin A

18. Dietary supplementation of vitamin E is advisable for

(A) all infants
(B) premature infants
(C) postmature infants
(D) exclusively breast-fed infants
(E) exclusively formula-fed infants

19. An 18-month-old child whose diet is almost exclusively cow milk is very likely to develop

(A) iron deficiency anemia
(B) systemic hypertension
(C) protein deficiency
(D) rickets
(E) folic acid deficiency

20. Which of the following vitamins are fat soluble?

(A) A, D, and C
(B) D, K, and B_1
(C) A, D, K, and E
(D) C, D, K, and E
(E) B_1, K, and E

21. Soy-protein formulas are commonly used in infant feeding. Which of the following statements regarding soy-protein formulas is correct?

(A) Infants fed exclusively with soy-protein formula display growth comparable to infants fed cow-milk-protein formula
(B) The protein in soy-protein formulas is essentially nonallergenic, and clinically significant soy-protein hypersensitivity is extremely rare
(C) Soy-protein formula is most useful in children with well-documented, severe, gastrointestinal allergic reactions to cow-milk protein
(D) Soy-protein formula should not be used in patients with a family history of celiac disease
(E) Infants fed soy-protein formula should receive supplemental dietary calcium

Please note the use of a negative qualifier such as EXCEPT, LEAST, or NOT in each of the following questions (Questions 22 through 25).

22. Which of the following minerals is NOT required for normal growth and development?

(A) Zinc
(B) Selenium
(C) Copper
(D) Lead
(E) Iodine

23. Which of the following is NOT an essential amino acid?

(A) Alanine
(B) Leucine
(C) Valine
(D) Threonine
(E) Phenylalanine

24. Recent concerns about the prevention of atherosclerotic heart disease have lead to recommendations for reducing the fat content, and particularly the cholesterol content, of the diet early in life. This may include the use of skim milk. It is recommended that skim milk NOT be used for infant feeding

(A) until the age of 6 months
(B) until the age of 2 years
(C) beyond the age of 4 years
(D) in the absence of obesity
(E) before puberty

25. All of the following statements are true EXCEPT

(A) unmodified cow milk contains more than twice the protein of breast milk
(B) cow milk contains sucrose
(C) breast milk contains lactose
(D) the ratio of casein to whey is significantly greater in cow milk than in breast milk
(E) both cow milk and breast milk contain lactoglobin

DIRECTIONS (26 through 30): Each set of matching questions in this section consists of a list of 4 to 26 lettered options followed by several numbered items. For each numbered item select the ONE lettered option with which it is most closely associated. Each lettered option may be selected once, more than once, or not at all.

Questions 26 through 30

(A) Carbohydrate
(B) Protein
(C) Fat
(D) Cholesterol
(E) Starch

26. Accounts for the greatest percentage of calories in the normal diet of the school-age child

27. Accounts for the greatest percentage of calories in breast milk

28. Accounts for the greatest percentage of calories in unmodified cow milk

29. Accounts for the greatest percentage of calories in skim milk

30. Accounts for the greatest percentage of calories in fruit juice

DIRECTIONS (Questions 31 through 34): Each group of items in this section consists of lettered headings followed by a set of numbered words or phrases. For each numbered word or phrase, select

A if the item is associated with (A) only,
B if the item is associated with (B) only,
C if the item is associated with both (A) and (B),
D if the item is associated with neither (A) nor (B).

Questions 31 through 34

(A) Vitamin C deficiency
(B) Niacin deficiency
(C) Both
(D) Neither

31. Rash in sun-exposed areas

32. Dementia

33. Leukopenia

34. Bleeding gums

Answers and Explanations

1. (D) Generally, it is recommended that the introduction of nonmilk foods (beikost) be delayed until the age of 4 to 6 months. One stated reason for this is the low intestinal concentration of pancreatic amylase early in life and the desire to avoid the ingestion of starches. The most compelling reason, however, relates to developmental readiness. Admittedly, it often is difficult to convince parents to refrain from introducing solids at an earlier age. *(Oski:548;* Pediatrics *63:52–59,1979)*

2. (A) By about 6 months, most infants are developmentally ready for the introduction of beikost. They can sit without support, have good control of the head and neck, have command of the swallowing muscles, and can communicate a feeling of satiety. The extrusion reflex, which causes the tongue to push forward and reject solids, has disappeared. Since the first foods introduced are semisolid mush such as cereals, there is no need for the infant to be able to chew solids at this time. [*Note:* This question is not grouped with the other *negative* questions because of its relation to question 1.] *(Oski:548)*

3. (D) The recommended daily allowance of vitamin A for an infant is 400 μg (about 1,300 IU). Excessive amounts can be just as dangerous as insufficient amounts. Signs of hypervitaminosis A include anorexia, hepatosplenomegaly, and increased intracranial pressure. *(Oski:534;* Pediatrics *65:893–896, 1980; Hathaway:113)*

4. (D) There is evidence that serious undernutrition during the first year of life may have deleterious and permanent effects, including developmental deficits, on both mental and physical growth and development. This appears to be an organic effect independent of psychosocial deprivation, although *exogenous* undernutrition often is compounded by such deprivation. The recognition of possible permanent effects, including developmental deficits, of malnutrition during infancy and early childhood has led to increased efforts to avoid such undernutrition both in underprivileged children and in those with chronic gastrointestinal disease. *(N Engl J Med 282: 933–939,1970; Oski:972)*

5. (A) Vitamin K is essential for hepatic synthesis of prothrombin (factor II) as well as factors VII, IX, and X. Plasma prothrombin concentrations are low at birth and fall still lower during the first 3 days of life. The parenteral administration of vitamin K will prevent the postnatal fall in concentration of these factors and thereby prevent hemorrhagic disease of the newborn. It is indicated prophylactically for *all* newborn infants. [*Note*: Of course, vitamin K is indicated for infants below 2,500 g and infants of less than 36 weeks' gestation, and in this sense choices **(B)** and **(C)** are true. However, response **(A)** clearly is the best choice since it encompasses the whole truth rather than a partial truth.] *(Oski:440; Hathaway:115)*

6. (C) A 10-week-old infant requires about 100 to 120 calories per kilogram and 120 to 140 ml of fluid per kilogram per day. For a 5-kg infant this represents 500 to 600 calories and 600 to 700 ml (20 to 23 ounces). However, most milks and prepared infant formulas contain 20 calories per ounce, so it would take 25 to 30 ounces to provide the 500 to 600 calories required. *(Oski:538; Hathaway:105)*

7. (A) Although the vitamin K content of breast milk is only a third that of cow milk, clinical deficiency is rare in normal infants fed either type of milk provided that they received prophylactic vitamin K parenterally at birth. There are reports from China and Japan of vitamin K deficiency with intracranial hemorrhage in exclusively breast-fed infants who did *not* receive prophylactic vitamin K at birth. The vitamin K in breast milk may be better absorbed than that in cow milk. Enteric bacteria are an important additional source of vitamin K. [*Note*: Response **(C)** is only half true. Although the amounts in each milk are adequate, the amounts are not equal. When an examination answer contains two parts, the answer should be considered incorrect if either part is false.] *(Rudolph:1960; Hathaway:115–116; J Pediatr 105: 880,943,1984)*

8. **(B)** The recommended daily allowance of vitamin D for an infant is 10 μg or 400 IU. As for vitamin A, too much vitamin D can be toxic and just as dangerous as too little. The major target organ of vitamin D poisoning is the kidney. [*Note*: Unfortunately, some texts and some examinations use micrograms (μg) and others use international units (IU) when referring to vitamins. Most now use the preferred term "recommended daily allowance" rather than the expression "minimal daily requirement," acknowledging that we really do not know the *minimal* requirement.] *(Rudolph:243–244; Hathaway:114–115)*

9. **(E)** Vitamin D is the only vitamin that needs to be provided as a supplement to normal infants being breast fed. The amount of vitamin D in human milk is marginal and might be inadequate for infants with dark skin or infants with little exposure to sunlight. *(Oski:539; Hathaway:114)*

10. **(B)** Both breast milk and cow milk normally contain about 3.8 g of fat per 100 ml. Most of the cow milk marketed in the United States, however, has had its fat content reduced to the legal minimum of 3.3%. This is for economic rather than nutritional considerations. Fat is the major source of calories in both breast and bovine milk. *(Oski:540; Rudolph:1960; Hathaway:120)*

11. **(C)** The *minimum* dietary requirement of high-quality protein in early infancy has been estimated at about 1.9 g/kg. The *recommended* daily allowance is 2.2 g/kg. Insufficient protein intake leads to poor growth, hypoproteinemic edema, and other changes. Excessive intake can result in metabolic acidosis, lethargy, and poor feeding. *(Oski:534; Hathaway:105–106)*

12. **(B)** As the child gets older, growth slows, and protein requirement falls. By the age of 10 years, the *minimum* daily protein requirement has fallen to 1 g/kg of body weight, with a *recommended* daily allowance of 1.2 g/kg. This amount is provided easily by most ordinary American diets. Even this modest amount, however, may not be available in some strict vegan diets, fad diets, or severe low-calorie diets. *(Oski:534; Hathaway:105–106)*

13. **(E)** The thymus dramatically decreases in size during periods of undernutrition. The other organs listed—brain, heart, liver, and kidneys—lose much less weight. Involution of the thymus during starvation accounts for some of the increased susceptibility to infection in these children. *(Pediatrics 59:490–494, 1977)*

14. **(B)** The multiplicity of factors affecting calcium metabolism, not the least of which is the effect of other dietary factors, makes it difficult to give an exact figure for the daily requirement of calcium. For a

school-age child it is estimated to be about 1 g per day. This is easily provided by most ordinary diets, and calcium supplementation is not necessary, even for the child who drinks little or no milk. Eggs, molasses, nuts, and many fish and vegetables are good sources of calcium. A variety of grains and grain products are fortified with added calcium. *(Oski:534; Hathaway:108,110)*

15. **(B)** Vitamin B_{12} is absorbed primarily in the distal portion of the ileum. Vitamin B_{12} deficiency can occur in children who have had surgical removal of this portion of the bowel or in whom this area has involvement by inflammatory disease. In the former case, deficiency is severe and permanent; in the latter situation, deficiency is mild and often transient. Children who have had surgical removal of the distal ileum should receive prophylactic vitamin B_{12}. *(Rudolph:1105)*

16. **(A)** Folic acid is absorbed primarily in the small intestine. Deficiency is seen commonly in chronic diarrhea and malabsorptive states involving the small bowel. Hypersegmentation of neutrophil nuclei on a peripheral blood smear is usually the first abnormality and is a useful aid to early diagnosis. Folic acid deficiency is not associated with any of the other conditions listed. *(Rudolph:1104)*

17. **(D)** A vegan or strict vegetarian diet provides almost no vitamin B_{12} as well as marginal levels of calcium, vitamin D, and iron. The relatively low caloric density of vegetables also means that a large bulk of food must be ingested to provide adequate calories. The content of vitamins other than B_{12} and D, however, is apt to be adequate. *(Rudolph:238; Pediatrics 70:582–586,1982)*

18. **(B)** Vitamin E is present in milk and distributed so widely in ordinary foods that supplementation is necessary only in very few situations. Since vitamin E appears to cross the placenta poorly, and premature infants do not absorb the vitamin well, supplementation is advised for these infants. Additionally, patients with conditions associated with fat malabsorption, such as biliary atresia and cystic fibrosis, may warrant vitamin E supplementation. *(Oski:347,534,1736)*

19. **(A)** Milk contains very little iron, only about 1.2 mg per liter. The average infant requires 1 to 1.5 mg of iron daily. A diet almost exclusively of milk is a common cause of iron deficiency anemia in the older infant and the toddler. This is especially true when the milk is unmodified cow milk. The iron in cow milk is less well absorbed than that in breast milk. Also, a large intake of unmodified cow milk often is associated with microscopic gastrointestinal blood loss. Cow milk, of course, contains adequate amounts of protein and is fortified with additional vitamin D, so the child described would not be at risk for either

hypoproteinemia or rickets. *(Oski:534,1514; Rudolph: 237,1099–1101)*

20. **(C)** The fat-soluble vitamins are A, D, E, and K. Infants or children with fat malabsorption or infants on severely fat-restricted diets may develop deficiencies of these vitamins. *(Oski:536; Hathaway:113–115)*

21. **(A)** Presently available soy-protein-based commercial infant formulas provide adequate nutrition (including calcium), and infants fed these formulas exhibit normal growth. Soy formulas often are prescribed for infants with personal or family history of allergy in the hope of avoiding the development of milk-protein allergy. Unfortunately, severe gastrointestinal allergic reactions to soy protein in infants is well recognized and not rare. For this reason, soy-protein formula is *not* recommended for infants or children *already demonstrating* significant gastrointestinal hypersensitivity to cow-milk protein. These patients are best prescribed a protein hydrolysate formula. *(Pediatrics 72:359–363, 1983)*

22. **(D)** Trace amounts of zinc, selenium, iodine, and copper are required for optimal growth and health. There is no evidence that even trace amounts of lead are required for health, nor has lead been identified in any human enzyme or coenzyme. Presumably, lead has no role in mammalian metabolism and, in fact, is toxic. *(Oski:537–539; Pediatrics 79:457–465,1987; Hathaway:111–112)*

23. **(A)** There are eight essential amino acids: threonine, valine, leucine, isoleucine, lysine, tryptophan, phenylalanine, and histidine. Alanine is not an essential amino acid. In addition, arginine, cystine, and perhaps taurine are essential for low-birth-weight infants. This knowledge has led to the special formulation of commercial preparations designed for the feeding of low-birth-weight infants as well as to modification of some infant formulas meant for routine feeding. *(Rudolph:213,217)*

24. **(B)** Skim milk is essentially free of all fat. If it is used at a time when the infant receives most or all of his calories from milk, this could lead to essential fatty acid deficiency. Fats, especially saturated fats, are essential for myelinization and brain growth. Additionally, since skim milk contains only 10 calories per ounce, the infant would need to consume a very large volume in order to obtain sufficient calories. This large volume would contain excess amounts of protein and minerals, especially sodium. [*Note:* There is a difference between *skim* milk and *low-fat* milks. The former has zero fat, whereas the latter has ½% to 2% fat. Two-percent-fat milk would be permissible at an earlier age than skim milk. The question specified *skim* milk.] *(Pediatrics 72:253–255,1983; Rudolph:237)*

25. **(B)** The sugar in both cow milk and breast milk is the same, namely, lactose. Neither breast milk nor unmod-

ified cow milk contains sucrose. This is important in prescribing for an infant with lactose intolerance. Breast milk contains about 1% protein, whereas unmodified cow milk contains about 3%. Both milks contain lactoglobulin. The ratio of casein to whey is much greater in cow milk, and this results in a heavier, less easily digested curd. *(Oski:540; Pediatr Clin North Am 24:17,1977; Pediatrics 68:435–441,1981)*

26. **(A)** Carbohydrates are the major source of calories in the normal diet throughout life except in the newborn period, when more than half of ingested calories are derived from fat. Excessive carbohydrate intake usually results in obesity. Inadequate intake results in caloric deprivation and undernutrition rather than any specific deficiency syndrome. *(Rudolph:216; Oski:540; Hathaway:105–108)*

27. **(C)** Fat yields about 9 calories per gram, whereas protein and carbohydrate yield only 4 calories per gram. More than 50% of the calories in human breast milk are in the form of fat. *(Rudolph:216; Oski:540; Hathaway:105–108)*

28. **(C)** Fat also accounts for about half of the calories in *unmodified* cow milk. *(Rudolph:216; Oski:540; Hathaway: 105–108)*

29. **(A)** Skim milk is essentially free of fat. About 60% of the calories are provided as carbohydrate, and the other 40% as protein. *(Rudolph:216; Oski:540; Hathaway:105–108)*

30. **(A)** Fruit juice is almost pure carbohydrate, mostly sugar rather than starch. Less than 5% of the calories is derived from protein and fat. Excessive intake of fruit juices by a young infant can result in inadequate protein intake despite adequate total calories. *(Rudolph:216; Oski:540; Hathaway:105–108)*

31. **(B)** Scurvy results from a diet deficient in vitamin C. Pellagra is the syndrome of niacin deficiency, resulting either from a diet poor in niacin or from pyridoxine deficiency, which blocks conversion of tryptophan to niacin. Pellagra is associated with an erythematous rash in sun-exposed areas, which can progress to exudation and ulceration or roughening and keratosis and a follicular hyperkeratosis. *(Hathaway:117)*

32. **(B)** Dementia occurs regularly in pellagra but is not seen in scurvy. *(Hathaway:117)*

33. **(D)** Leukopenia is not part of the clinical picture of either vitamin C or niacin deficiency. *(Hathaway:117)*

34. **(A)** Although pellagra can produce sore mouth, stomatitis, cheilosis, and a red, swollen, and painful tongue, only in vitamin C deficiency do the swollen and sore gums become hemorrhagic. *(Hathaway:117)*

BIBLIOGRAPHY

AAP Committee on Environmental Hazards. Statement on childhood lead poisoning. *Pediatrics.* 1987;79:457–465.

AAP Committee on Nutrition. Nutrition and lactation. *Pediatrics.* 1981;68:435–441.

AAP Committee on Nutrition. Use of whole cow's milk in infancy. *Pediatrics.* 1983;72:253–255.

AAP Committee on Nutrition. Soy-protein formulas: recommendations for use in infant feeding. *Pediatrics.* 1983;72:359–363.

Chase PH, Martin HP. Undernutrition and child development. *N Eng J Med.* 1970;282:933–939.

Fomon SJ, Filer LJ, Anderson TA, et al. Recommendations for feeding normal infants. *Pediatrics.* 1979;63:52–59.

Hambraeus L. Proprietary milk versus human breast milk in infant feeding. *Pediatr Clin North Am.* 1977;24:17–36.

Hathaway WE, Groothius JR, Hay WW, et al. *Current Pediatric Diagnosis & Treatment.* 10th ed. Norwalk, Conn: Appleton & Lange; 1991.

Katz M, Stiehm ER. Host defenses in malnutrition. *Pediatrics.* 1977;59:490–494.

Mahoney CP, Margolis T, Knauss TA, et al. Chronic vitamin A intoxication in infants fed chicken liver. *Pediatrics.* 1980;65:893–896.

Motohara K, Matsukura M, Matsuda I, et al. Severe vitamin K deficiency in breast-fed infants. *J Pediatr.* 1984;105:943–945.

Oski FA, DeAngelis CD, Feigin RD, et al. *Principles & Practice of Pediatrics.* Philadelphia, Pa: JB Lippincott; 1990.

Rudolph AM, Hoffman JIE, Rudolph CD. *Pediatrics.* 19th ed. Norwalk, Conn: Appleton & Lange; 1991.

Shinwell ED, Gorodischer R. Totally vegetarian diets and infant nutrition. *Pediatrics.* 1982;70:582–586.

CHAPTER 5

Accidents, Poisoning, and Drug Abuse
Questions

Trauma (accidental and nonaccidental) is a leading cause of morbidity and *the* leading cause of mortality in children beyond the first birthday in the United States. Motor vehicles account for more than half of accidental pediatric deaths, and drowning is the second leading cause of accidental pediatric deaths. Poisoning is also an important cause of illness and death in the pediatric age group. Because the word *accident* implies bad luck or a random, chance, unavoidable event, there has been an emphasis on conceptualizing the problem as one of *unintentional injury* rather than *accident*. Usage, however, is difficult to change. The student will be expected to be knowledgeable of the epidemiology of trauma as well as the principles of accident prevention and injury protection.

Drug abuse, with its resultant medical and social consequences, is prevalent among teenagers and preteens. Additionally, maternal drug abuse is directly and indirectly (including lack of prenatal care) responsible for many problems in the *newborn infant*.

DIRECTIONS (Questions 1 through 40): Each of the numbered items or incomplete statements in this section is followed by answers or by completions of the statement. Select the ONE lettered answer or completion that is BEST in each case.

1. Poisoning with methyl alcohol is associated with a

   (A) metabolic acidosis with compensatory respiratory alkalosis
   (B) respiratory acidosis with compensatory metabolic alkalosis
   (C) mixed metabolic and respiratory acidosis
   (D) metabolic alkalosis with compensatory respiratory acidosis
   (E) respiratory alkalosis with compensatory metabolic acidosis

2. The major cause of morbidity and mortality in acute poisoning with acetaminophen is

   (A) hepatic injury
   (B) gastric bleeding
   (C) metabolic acidosis
   (D) methemoglobinemia
   (E) hypoglycemia

3. Following closed head injury, which of the following would be most ominous?

   (A) Irritability
   (B) Vomiting
   (C) Dilated, fixed pupils
   (D) Amnesia for the accident
   (E) Drowsiness

4. Most cases of suicide in children and adolescents are associated with

   (A) chronic physical disease
   (B) mental retardation
   (C) depression
   (D) religious fantasy
   (E) homosexuality

5. Child abuse in the United States is

   (A) an unimportant cause of either morbidity or mortality
   (B) an important cause of morbidity but rarely a cause of death
   (C) an important cause of both morbidity and mortality
   (D) the second leading cause of death in the pediatric age group
   (E) declining in incidence

6. Most cases of serious physical child abuse involve children

   (A) less than 1 month old
   (B) between 1 month and 4 years old
   (C) between 5 and 12 years old
   (D) who are neurologically impaired
   (E) of single parent homes

7. Most pediatric cases of symptomatic lead poisoning in the United States occur in children

   (A) less than 6 months old
   (B) between 6 and 12 months old
   (C) between 1 and 3 years old
   (D) between 3 and 5 years old
   (E) between 10 and 15 years old

8. In regard to screening programs, the concentration of whole-blood lead at which one should undertake medical evaluation of the child and consider therapy is

   (A) 1 μg/dL
   (B) 10 μg/dL
   (C) 25 μg/dL
   (D) 60 μg/dL
   (E) 100 μg/dL

9. Which of the following combinations of signs and symptoms is most suggestive of chronic lead poisoning?

   (A) Ataxia, fever, diarrhea, and polycythemia
   (B) Lethargy, vomiting, hallucinations, and vesicular rash
   (C) Anemia, leukopenia, thrombocytopenia, and hepatomegaly
   (D) Lethargy, abdominal cramps, constipation, anemia
   (E) Hypertension, rash, cough, and leukocytosis

10. A 4-year-old child ingested an unknown number of prochlorperazine (Compazine) tablets. About 12 hours later, the child is noted to hold the head in a tilted position and to have uncontrolled, writhing movements of the hands and arms. The child is brought to the emergency room and found to be afebrile and to have a normal physical examination except for the movements described. At this point you should

    (A) perform a head computerized tomography (CT) scan
    (B) perform a lumbar puncture
    (C) administer syrup of ipecac orally
    (D) administer a slurry of charcoal orally
    (E) administer diphenhydramine intravenously

11. New parents should first be counseled about specific items of child safety and injury protection, such as proper cribs, use of smoke detectors, and proper setting for home water heaters,

    (A) during the first trimester of pregnancy
    (B) during the perinatal period
    (C) when the infant is 3 months old
    (D) when the infant is 6 months old
    (E) when they show an interest by asking questions

12. Shellfish poisoning, which is caused by eating shellfish that have ingested toxic dinoflagellates ("red tide"), is characterized by

    (A) blindness
    (B) vomiting and diarrhea

   (C) seizures and coma
   (D) weakness and paralysis
   (E) rash and fever

13. Which of the following drugs is the most useful chelating agent in acute iron poisoning?

    (A) British anti-lewisite (BAL)
    (B) Ethylene diamine tetraacetic acid (EDTA)
    (C) Desferrioxamine
    (D) Hemoglobin
    (E) Penicillamine

14. A 3-year-old child presents with coma, weaknesses, excessive salivation, bradycardia, and constricted pupils. The most likely drug or toxin to cause these signs is

    (A) diphenhydramine
    (B) phenobarbital
    (C) atropine
    (D) a hydrocarbon
    (E) an organophosphate

15. The most common adverse reaction to marijuana is

    (A) convulsions
    (B) coma
    (C) hypotension
    (D) hypertension
    (E) psychologic disturbances

16. Which of the following is most useful for treating a patient having a "bad trip" from an unidentified hallucinogen?

    (A) Atropine
    (B) Chlorpromazine
    (C) Diazepam
    (D) Methadone
    (E) Phenobarbital

17. Morning glory seeds and jimsonweed have entered the drug scene because of their

    (A) hallucinogenic effect
    (B) antihallucinogenic effect
    (C) stimulant effect
    (D) sedative effect
    (E) potentiating effect on other drugs

18. Ingestion of LSD will most likely result in

    (A) convulsions
    (B) euphoria
    (C) hallucinations
    (D) sedation
    (E) tremors

19. A youngster who sniffs spot remover and then engages in stressful physical activity is at risk for

    (A) convulsions
    (B) hypertension

(C) rhabdomyolysis
(D) severe headache
(E) sudden death

20. An adolescent drug abuser who presents with dilated pupils, coma, hypotension, and hypotonia but is not cyanotic or in shock has most likely overdosed with

(A) amphetamines
(B) aspirin
(C) heroin
(D) glutethimide
(E) phenobarbital

21. After being lifted up by one hand, a young toddler refused to use that arm and holds it flexed at the elbow with the forearm midway between pronation and supination. The child most likely has

(A) a shoulder dislocation
(B) a radial head subluxation
(C) a fracture of a carpal bone
(D) avulsion of the ulnar nerve
(E) a fracture of the radius

22. A 4-year-old child falls on an outstretched arm. The child is likely to sustain a

(A) fracture displacement of the radial epiphysis
(B) Colles's fracture
(C) comminuted radial and ulnar fracture
(D) shoulder dislocation
(E) humeral fracture

23. Which of the following sets of blood gas values is most compatible with acute aspirin poisoning in a 16-month-old child?

(A) pH 7.60; PCO_2 40; HCO_3^- 40
(B) pH 7.50; PCO_2 40; HCO_3^- 30
(C) pH 7.25; PCO_2 20; HCO_3^- 8
(D) pH 7.20; PCO_2 45; HCO_3^- 20
(E) pH 7.00; PCO_2 35; HCO_3^- 8

24. Hyperventilation caused by salicylate poisoning

(A) is usually clinically apparent within minutes of ingestion
(B) is characterized by an increase in rate and depth of ventilation
(C) is characterized by an increase in depth of ventilation only
(D) is characterized by an increase in rate of ventilation only
(E) does not occur in young children

25. Which of the following findings would be most suggestive of the form of child abuse referred to as the shaken infant syndrome?

(A) Ecchymoses over the mastoid area
(B) Retinal hemorrhages

(C) Ecchymoses and petechiae over the upper arms and upper trunk
(D) Circumferential ecchymosis around the arms or legs
(E) Cervical spine dislocation

26. A 9-year-old is injured while sledding. On admission, the child appears in shock and is complaining of pain in the left shoulder. Of immediate concern is the possibility of

(A) rupture of the descending aorta
(B) dislocation of the left shoulder
(C) rupture of the spleen
(D) injury to the left brachial plexus
(E) rupture of the left diaphragm

27. A child's success in avoiding injury will depend primarily on his or her own judgment by about age

(A) 2 years
(B) 5 years
(C) 10 years
(D) 15 years

28. A 1-year-old child is brought to the emergency room because of a swollen left thigh. The parents, who appear very concerned, state that they had left the child with a newly hired housekeeper while they were away for the weekend, and when they returned they noted the swelling. Other than tender swelling of the thigh, physical examination is entirely normal. X-ray examination discloses a displaced fracture of the shaft of the femur; skeletal survey reveals no other fractures or abnormalities. The grandparents, who live with the parents and who had accompanied them on their trip, corroborate the parents' story. The most appropriate action for you to take at this time would be to admit the child for treatment of the fracture and

(A) order a computerized tomography (CT) scan of the head
(B) ask the parents to send in the housekeeper so that you can question her
(C) instruct the parents to discharge the housekeeper
(D) ask the parents if they wish to press charges against the housekeeper
(E) report the incident to a child protection agency

29. You are on duty in the emergency room. A mother calls to say that her 2-year-old child has ingested an unknown number of imipramine tablets. The mother does not have a bottle of ipecac at home. You should advise her to

(A) try to induce emesis by gagging the child with a finger and call back in 15 minutes
(B) administer 3 tablespoons of salt in 8 ounces of water to induce emesis and call back in 15 minutes
(C) administer 3 teaspoons of salt in 8 ounces of water to induce emesis and bring the child to the emergency room
(D) bring the child to the emergency room, where you will induce emesis by administration of syrup of ipecac
(E) bring the child to the emergency room, where you will measure the serum level of iron

30. A 4-year-old child is playing in the basement. The child suddenly comes upstairs, screaming of being bitten by a spider. There is a red wheal-like lesion on the child's face. Over the next few hours the lesion becomes larger, more painful, and darker, until it is violaceous. The most likely complication in this child would be

(A) necrosis at the site of the bite
(B) renal failure
(C) hepatic failure
(D) muscle cramps and seizures
(E) a convulsion

31. Induction of emesis by syrup of ipecac is contraindicated for a child who has ingested

(A) aspirin
(B) ibuprofen
(C) iron
(D) phenobarbital
(E) sodium hydroxide

32. A 2-year-old child is retrieved from a near-drowning episode in a pool. The child is apneic on retrieval but is quickly and successfully resuscitated. On arrival in the emergency room, abnormalities that are likely to be present and require immediate attention would include

(A) hyponatremia and hypokalemia
(B) hyponatremia and hyperkalemia
(C) hyperkalemia and acidosis
(D) acidosis and hypoxemia
(E) hypoxemia and hemolysis

33. Important manifestations of acute iron poisoning include

(A) seizures, coma, and increased intracranial pressure
(B) metabolic alkalosis and hypertension
(C) hemolysis and neutropenia

(D) renal, hepatic, and cardiac failure
(E) metabolic acidosis, shock, and hepatic injury

34. Which of the following statements regarding automobile safety for children is correct?

(A) Children beyond the age of 1 year or 20 lb may ride facing either the front or rear of the car
(B) Children over 25 lb can use adult-type restraints
(C) A 1-year-old child held in the lap of a seat-belted adult is almost as safe as in an infant restraint device
(D) Safety restraints are not needed for infants less than 3 months of age or 10 lb of body weight
(E) Infants under the age of 1 year should ride in restraint devices facing the rear of the car

Please note the use of a negative qualifier such as EXCEPT, LEAST, or NOT in each of the following questions (Questions 35 through 40).

35. Which of the following statements regarding accidents is NOT correct?

(A) Accidents are the leading cause of death in children over 1 year of age
(B) More children drown in backyard swimming pools than at beaches or public pools
(C) Motor vehicle accidents are an uncommon cause of death prior to adolescence
(D) Parents of toddlers should be advised to use guards for windows and gates for stairways
(E) Children under the age of 3 years have little sense of danger or self-preservation

36. A patient with heroin overdose might present with any of the symptoms below EXCEPT

(A) pulmonary edema
(B) coma
(C) hyperventilation
(D) cyanosis
(E) constricted pupils

37. Which of the following statements regarding abuse of inhalants or volatile substances is NOT correct?

(A) Low cost and easy availability of the substances is a factor in their abuse
(B) The onset of action is considerably delayed (more than one hour), favoring overdosage
(C) A state of euphoria or a high is a major effect
(D) These are frequently the first substances to be abused by a child or young adolescent
(E) Use tends to decrease with time (age), often being replaced by other drugs

38. Which of the following statements regarding illicit use of heroin is NOT true?

(A) Mood changes are a prominent effect of the drug
(B) The pupillary changes (miosis, pinpoint pupils) cannot be reversed by atropine

(C) It is associated with criminal behavior and/or delinquency

(D) Medical complications include hepatitis, pneumonia, and bacterial endocarditis

(E) Withdrawal symptoms may begin within 24 hours of abstinence

39. The progressive nature of drug abuse in children and adolescents has been classified into four stages, the last of which is characterized by all of the following EXCEPT

(A) use of the drug to feel normal
(B) loss of control and inability to stop use
(C) use of the drug to achieve social, academic, and personal success
(D) paranoia, self-hate, and aggression
(E) physical deterioration

40. The four major categories of child abuse include all of the following EXCEPT

(A) physical abuse
(B) emotional abuse
(C) sexual abuse
(D) intellectual abuse
(E) neglect

DIRECTIONS (41 through 45): Each set of matching questions in this section consists of a list of 4 to 26 lettered options followed by several numbered items. For each numbered item select the ONE lettered option with which it is most closely associated. Each lettered option may be selected once, more than once, or not at all.

Questions 41 through 45

(A) Amphetamines
(B) Amyl nitrate
(C) Cocaine
(D) Codeine
(E) Glutethimide (Doriden)
(F) Marijuana

41. Hash

42. Cibas

43. Crack

44. Poppers

45. Bennies

DIRECTIONS (Questions 46 through 50): Each group of items in this section consists of lettered headings followed by a set of numbered words or phrases. For each numbered word or phrase, select

A if the item is associated with (A) <u>only</u>,
B if the item is associated with (B) <u>only</u>,
C if the item is associated with <u>both</u> (A) <u>and</u> (B),
D if the item is associated with <u>neither</u> (A) <u>nor</u> (B).

Questions 46 through 50

(A) Ethyl alcohol poisoning
(B) Aspirin poisoning
(C) Both
(D) Neither

46. Hypoglycemia

47. Metabolic acidosis and respiratory alkalosis

48. Acute pancreatitis

49. Hypertension

50. Abnormalities of hemostasis

Answers and Explanations

1. **(A)** Methyl alcohol (methanol) is metabolized to formaldehyde and formic acid, which results in a severe primary metabolic acidosis and a secondary, *compensatory* respiratory alkalosis. This is quite different, for example, from the mixed disturbance seen in children with aspirin poisoning, in which case there is a *primary* respiratory alkalosis as well as a *primary* metabolic acidosis. *(Rudolph:802–803)*

2. **(A)** Acetaminophen poisoning in childhood is common. In most cases, the toddler gets into a supply of the medication; infrequently, the poisoning is the result of improper dosage by a parent or other caregiver. The major problem resulting from acute poisoning with acetaminophen is liver injury and hepatic failure. Hypoglycemia as well as myocardial and renal problems may be seen but are less common and rarely, if ever, lethal. Neither metabolic acidosis nor methemoglobinemia is a complication of acetaminophen poisoning. *(Rudolph:788–789;* Pediatr Clin North Am *33:691–702,1986)*

3. **(C)** Following head trauma, eye changes such as fixed, dilated pupils are very serious and usually indicative of increasing intracranial pressure or focal neurologic damage. A history of unconsciousness, irritability, and lethargy, amnesia for the accident, and vomiting all are seen commonly in the absence of major intracranial injury. *(Rudolph:1760–1761;* Pediatrics *62:819–825,1978)*

4. **(C)** Suicide is the second or third leading cause of death in adolescents. Depression appears to be the most common factor in these patients. Relatively few cases are associated with chronic physical disease, mental retardation, or religious fantasy. There are no data to suggest that problems relating to homosexuality are especially common among these youngsters. *(Rudolph:48; Oski:664–666;* J Pediatr *101:118–123,1982;* Pediatrics *66:144,1980)*

5. **(C)** Child abuse is an important and very common cause of injury, hospitalization, and disability for children in the United States. Although it is not the second leading cause of death in the pediatric age, fatalities do occur all too frequently in this condition. Over the past two decades, there has been a dramatic increase in the reported incidences of child abuse. Whether this represents an actual increase in frequency or only an increase in reporting is unclear. In either case, there is nothing to suggest a decline in frequency, with over a quarter of a million cases reported annually. *(Rudolph:839;* JAMA *254:796–800, 1985;* Pediatr Clin North Am *32:41–60, 1985;* Hathaway: *765)*

6. **(B)** Most cases of physical child abuse and almost all deaths from abuse occur in the age group less than 4 years, especially less than 2 or 3 years, before the child can communicate effectively with others. Although neurologically impaired children are at increased risk for abuse, most victims are neurologically normal. The majority of abusing parents are married and young, in their 20s to early 30s. *(Rudolph:840)*

7. **(C)** Cases of lead poisoning in the United States are seen chiefly in the toddler age group. This is understandable, considering the mechanism of poisoning. The major source of lead poisoning in children living in urban areas is old, flaking lead paint, found in pre-1940 buildings. Some children will chronically ingest the paint flakes. The child needs to be developmentally mature enough to walk about and to peel off the paint or pick up flakes that have fallen to the floor, yet too young to understand the dangers involved. Although it is no longer legal to use lead paints indoors, old buildings still may have layers of paint with high lead content beneath the more recent coats of "lead-free" paint. As these old buildings have been razed and replaced, the incidence of symptomatic pediatric lead poisoning has declined. Although dirt and automobile exhaust also are sources of environmental lead contamination, they have not been documented as causing symptomatic poisoning. *(Rudolph:807; Hathaway:947)*

8. **(C)** As severe, overt lead poisoning has become less common, there has been an increased concern about the long-term neurodevelopmental effects of subclin-

ical lead poisoning. Consequently, there has been a progressive lowering of what is considered the acceptable upper limit for blood lead concentrations. Ideally, blood lead concentration should be close to zero.

Concentrations between 10 and 20 or 25 µg/dL are generally viewed as representing environmental contamination and warranting evaluation of the home and surroundings as well as observation and repeat screening of the child.

Concentrations greater than 25 µg/dL should be considered indicative of an excess body burden of lead and the need for a prompt medical evaluation, even though overt clinical symptoms rarely are present at levels less than 60 µg/dL. *(Rudolph:807;* Pediatr Clin North Am *27:843,1980;* Pediatrics *79:457,1987; Hoekelman:223–224)*

9. **(D)** Common signs of lead poisoning include lethargy, abdominal cramps, constipation, and anemia. Vomiting also is common. Ataxia is seen occasionally. The other items listed—fever, diarrhea, rash, hallucinations, hypertension, thrombocytopenia, and cough—are not associated with lead poisoning. [*Note:* In answering this type of question, it is helpful to examine each answer for a clearly false item. Diarrhea and polycythemia rule out choice **(A)** since the opposites, constipation and anemia, are associated with lead poisoning. Rash is not a feature of plumbism, so choices **(B)** and **(E)** can be excluded. Choice **(C)** contains three incorrect items—leukopenia, thrombocytopenia, and hepatomegaly.] *(Rudolph:807–808; Hathaway:947)*

10. **(E)** The child described has developed extrapyramidal symptoms typical of phenothiazine toxicity. These findings may occur with therapeutic as well as excessive dosage and are common in children. Akinesia, trismus, opisthotonos, torticollis, chorea, dystonia, and oculogyric crises may be seen. These symptoms usually respond dramatically to intravenous diphenhydramine (Benadryl) or benztropine mesylate, although relapses are frequent. The clinical picture is so classic that it can be suspected even in the absence of a history of ingestion. There is no need for either a CT scan or a lumbar puncture in this child. Twelve hours after ingestion is too late for either ipecac or charcoal to be of any value. *(Pediatr Clin North Am 33:299–309,1986; Hathaway:950)*

11. **(B)** The first trimester is too early to begin counseling about child safety. There are too many other issues on the parents' minds, and there is always the uncertainty as to how the pregnancy will progress. However, such counseling should not be delayed beyond the perinatal period. Parents should be advised how to make the home safe *before* the birth of the child, and this should be emphasized again before the baby leaves the hospital. The newborn infant should go home from the hospital **properly restrained** in an approved infant automobile **safety** seat. Safety counseling will need to continue **throughout** childhood. *(Hoekelman:262)*

12. **(D)** Shellfish poisoning is characterized by paresthesia and numbness of the mouth and face, generalized weakness, and paralysis. The incubation period is brief, minutes to hours. In severe cases, mechanical ventilatory assistance may be required. Presumably the flagellates ingested by the shellfish produce a neurotoxin that is, in turn, ingested when the shellfish are eaten, accounting for the symptoms. Larger numbers of dinoflagellates in the water where the shellfish are harvested can impart a red or reddish-brown color to the water, the so-called red tide. (N Engl J Med *295:1117–1120,1976)*

13. **(C)** Desferrioxamine is the chelating agent of choice for iron poisoning. It combines with iron to form ferrioxamine, which is excreted in the urine. Parenteral administration (intravenous) is reserved for children with severe poisoning, as the iron–ferrioxamine complexes are potentially toxic. *(Rudolph:806; Hathaway:946–947)*

14. **(E)** The signs described—coma, weakness, excessive salivation, bradycardia, and constricted pupils—are classic for organic phosphate poisoning. Organophosphates are potent and persistent inhibitors of acetylcholinesterase. Excessive salivation is not seen in phenobarbital, diphenhydramine, or hydrocarbon poisoning. Atropine poisoning causes tachycardia, dry mouth, and dilated pupils, the opposite of the findings in this patient. In fact, atropine is a major antidote in the treatment of organophosphate poisoning. *(Rudolph:814–815; Hathaway:945–946)*

15. **(E)** Few physical or pathophysiologic reactions have been documented with marijuana usage. Emotional, psychologic, and behavioral changes such as depressive reactions, panic, and toxic psychosis have been noted. *(Rudolph:792–793; Hathaway:234;* Pediatr Clin North Am *34:305–312,1987)*

16. **(C)** Diazepam is the safest agent for management of a "bad trip" resulting from an unidentified hallucinogen and is preferable to a barbiturate. Chlorpromazine would be contraindicated in the patient who had taken a hallucinogen with anticholinergic properties. A quiet environment, reassurance, and the company of a trusted adult are helpful. Atropine and methadone have no role in the treatment of these patients. *(Pediatr Clin North Am 34:342–346,1987)*

17. **(A)** Morning glory seeds and jimsonweed are abused because of their profound hallucinogenic effect. Many patients also exhibit confusion, bizarre behavior, and anticholinergic effects. Convulsions are infrequent but can be severe and difficult to control.

Although these drugs are less popular than they were a decade ago, their use remains a problem, especially among adolescents and young adults. (Am J Dis Child *138:737,1984;* Pediatr Clin North Am *34:341–347,1987)*

18. **(C)** Hallucinations, especially visual, are the most common and most striking effect of LSD. Sensations are magnified and distorted. The patient may imagine seeing odors or hearing colors. The emotional response can be either positive and pleasurable or negative and frightening. (Pediatr Clin North Am *34: 341–347,1987)*

19. **(E)** Sudden death is not infrequent in youngsters who sniff organic solvents. The risk appears to be especially great if the inhalation involves a halogenated hydrocarbon (frequently used as solvents or spot removers) and is followed by exercise or other vigorous physical activity. It has been postulated that this may be related to sensitization of the myocardium by the volatile hydrocarbons. A lethal arrhythmia is then precipitated by the catecholamine release occasioned by the exercise. (Pediatr Clin North Am *34:333–339,337,1987)*

20. **(D)** The dilated pupils and coma are suggestive of overdose with glutethimide (Doriden), a sedative drug with atropine-like effects. Patients overdosed with heroin or phenobarbital usually have constricted (miotic) pupils unless severely overdosed and hypoxic. Amphetamines cause hypertension rather than hypotension. Aspirin poisoning does not cause pupillary changes. (Fleisher:561,570–572)

21. **(B)** When a young child is lifted off the ground, dragged, or swung by one arm, the youngster's radius may partly escape from the annular ligament at the elbow. This subluxation of the radial head is a common injury, the so-called nursemaid's injury or nurse-maid's elbow. The child holds the injured arm flexed at the elbow and refuses to move it. The subluxation usually is easily reduced by supination of the arm. (Rudolph:1941; Hathaway:643)

22. **(A)** The growth plate or epiphysis is generally the weakest part of a child's bone, weaker even than surrounding ligaments. Trauma that would result in a tear of the ligament in an adult often results in an epiphyseal fracture in a child. A fall onto an outstretched arm, which might result in a Colles's fracture in an adult, is likely to cause a separation fracture of the distal radial epiphysis in a child. Epiphyseal separations are common childhood injuries. (Rudolph:1938–1939; Hathaway:644)

23. **(C)** Aspirin poisoning results in a mixed disturbance of metabolic acidosis and respiratory alkalosis. In adolescents and adults, the predominant abnormal-

ity usually is the respiratory alkalosis. Before the age of 2 years, however, metabolic acidosis is the predominant process, and the net change in arterial pH is generally a decrease. In response to this mixed disturbance, the PCO_2 is invariably lower than one would anticipate as compensation for the metabolic acidosis (decreased bicarbonate) alone. (Rudolph:818–819; Hathaway:952–953; Pediatrics 70:566,1982)

24. **(B)** Salicylate poisoning results in an increase in both rate and depth of ventilation. The latter usually is especially striking. Generally, neither tachypnea nor deep respirations are clinically apparent until several hours after ingestion. Even young infants show this response. (Rudolph:818–819; Hathaway:952–953; Pediatrics 70:566,1982)

25. **(B)** The shaken infant syndrome is a form of child abuse in which manual shaking of the infant results in retinal and intracranial hemorrhage. Generally, there are no external signs of trauma. The infant brain is easily deformed and subject to shearing injuries. Permanent brain damage is not an uncommon feature. (Hathaway:767; Rudolph:843; Pediatrics 54:396–403,1974)

26. **(C)** The child described probably has sustained an injury to the spleen. Splenic trauma, with or without rupture, is a common sledding injury. Shock may occur rapidly or some time later. Pain in the left shoulder is common and reflects irritation to the left diaphragm. The current approach to management is conservative, with every attempt to salvage, rather than remove, the spleen. (Rudolph:1153)

27. **(B)** In infancy and early toddlerhood, a child's physical safety depends almost entirely on the environment and his caregivers. As the child gets older, injury avoidance is dependent more and more on the youngster's own judgment. Children's activities generally need to be supervised until about 5 years of age. By the age of 6 years, the child's safety will depend on his or her own judgment 90% of the time. (Hoekelman:263)

28. **(E)** All states have laws requiring any person having reason to suspect child abuse or neglect to report the case to the proper child protective authority. Proof of abuse is not a prerequisite for reporting. Who committed the abuse, whether it is a single incident or part of a chronic pattern, and whether or not the parents wish to press charges are irrelevant. It is not the physician's role to play detective. In this particular case, since the neurologic and physical examinations other than of the thigh are normal, there is no indication for a CT scan of the head. (Rudolph:840; Hathaway:765; Am J Dis Child 133:691–696,1979)

29. **(D)** Attempts to induce emesis by gagging the child with a finger or tongue blade or by administration of

salt water are ineffective and essentially useless. In addition, the ingestion of large amounts of salt water has resulted in hypernatremia, an example of the cure being worse than the disease. It is important to induce emesis effectively and as quickly as possible. This is best accomplished by administration of syrup of ipecac, 15 to 20 mL for a young child and 30 mL for an adolescent. The dose should be repeated once if emesis has not occurred in 15 minutes. If the second dose fails, gastric lavage is indicated. Used in this manner, ipecac is safe and effective. *(Rudolph:786; Hathaway:932–933;* Pediatr Clin North Am *26:827–836,1979)*

30. **(A)** The most likely villain in this case is the brown recluse spider (fiddler spider, *Loxoseles reclusa*). Envenomation is characterized by severe local reaction, often leading to local tissue necrosis. Renal and hepatic failure have not been noted, nor have seizures been noted. Painful muscle cramps are characteristic of black widow spider (*Latrodectus mactans*) bite, in which case there is little local reaction, although local pain is common. *(Rudolph:775,822)*

31. **(E)** Induction of emesis is contraindicated in patients who have ingested caustic materials such as strong acids or alkali. Sodium hydroxide is a strong alkali found in home products used to clean drainpipes. Emesis often will result in further esophageal injury. Emesis also is contraindicated in patients who are comatose or have a depressed gag reflex. Lavage or induction of emesis is not contraindicated in patients who have ingested aspirin, ibuprofen, barbiturates, or iron. It is controversial whether or not emesis or lavage is contraindicated in children who have ingested hydrocarbons, which were, therefore, not included as a choice in the question. Since aspiration pneumonia is the most common toxic effect of these agents, theoretically, one would imagine that emesis or lavage might increase the risk of aspiration. Most studies, however, have failed to confirm this theoretical risk. *(Rudolph:786; Hathaway:932;* Pediatrics *29:648–674,1962;* Can Med Assoc J *111:537–538, 1974;* Pediatrics *59:788,1977)*

32. **(D)** The most immediate concern in patients successfully resuscitated from a near-drowning episode is correction of hypoxia and acidosis. The consequences of cerebral hypoxia, with acute brain swelling, are the major causes of morbidity and mortality. Aspiration pneumonia is common. Life-threatening electrolyte disturbances are quite rare in patients who survive to the emergency room. Most victims of near-drowning aspirate relatively late in the immersion episode, after they have become severely hypoxic secondary to apnea. Aspiration of large quantities of fluid, therefore, is rare. [*Note:* A key to answering this question correctly is attention to the phrase "require immediate attention."] *(Rudolph:829;* Pediatr Clin North Am *32:113,1985)*

33. **(E)** The clinical manifestations of iron poisoning have been organized into four stages. The first stage is characterized by gastrointestinal (vomiting, diarrhea, and abdominal pain) and neurologic (coma and seizures) signs. This is followed by a second stage of deceptive quiescence, of up to 48 hours, and then a third stage characterized by shock and metabolic acidosis, with or without evidence of hepatic injury. Leukocytosis is common. Late sequelae (stage 4) include pyloric or antral stenosis and hepatic cirrhosis. *(Rudolph:805–806; Hathaway:946–947;* Am J Dis Child *134:875–879,1980)*

34. **(E)** The head of an infant is relatively larger (compared to total body size or weight) than that of the older child or adult. For this reason, the neck is subjected to proportionally increased force during a crash. Having the infant face backwards diffuses the blow (deceleration) over the entire back. Infants under the age of 1 should ride facing the rear of the car. All older children should ride properly restrained, facing forward. It has been shown that the force generated by a 1-year-old infant in a front-end crash far exceeds the ability of an adult to hold a child in the lap. The child will be propelled forward into the dash or other obstacle. Because of the relatively weak pelvis and vulnerable abdominal organs of the child, it is recommended that a lap belt (as opposed to a toddler seat) *not be used* until the child weighs at least 40 lb and is 4 or 5 years old. *(Rudolph:31;* Pediatr Clin North Am *32:87,1985)*

35. **(C)** Accidents are the leading cause of death in children beyond 1 year of age. The fact that most drowning deaths occur in backyard pools is important in regard to public health measures (fencing laws) and anticipatory guidance (counseling of parents) to prevent such deaths. Motor vehicle accidents are a major cause of morbidity and mortality throughout childhood, hence the importance of proper infant and child car restraints. *(Hathaway:149; Rudolph:30)*

36. **(C)** Hypoventilation, rather than hyperventilation, is to be expected with heroin overdosage. Lethargy, coma, cyanosis, and constricted pupils are common. Pulmonary edema is seen occasionally. *(Rudolph:813)*

37. **(B)** Sniffing of glue and other solvents rapidly produces a sense of euphoria. It is this rapid high, euphoria to the point of exhilaration, that leads to addiction. Their low cost and easy availability are important factors in their use by young children, often as the first consciousness-altering drug. Currently, toluene-containing compounds are popular street drugs for inhalation. As children grow older they tend to abandon the volatile substances, often substituting other illicit substances. *(*Pediatr Clin North Am *34:334–335,1987)*

38. **(B)** Heroin is abused for its mood-altering effects, including euphoria. The drug is illegal, expensive, and

has a relatively short duration of action (3 to 4 hours), which necessitates multiple injections each day to avoid symptoms of withdrawal. This combination of factors forces most users into some type of criminal activity. Medical complications related to intravenous use include viral hepatitis, pneumonia, and bacterial endocarditis. HIV infection is also a risk. The pupillary effects of the drug are reversed by atropine. *(Pediatr Clin North Am 34:354–359,1987)*

39. (C) The final stage of drug abuse is characterized by a need to use the drug just to feel normal; the user finds it progressively more difficult to get high or to achieve euphoria. Compulsion to use the drug is maximal, with loss of control and inability to stop even briefly. Serious behavioral changes are evident—paranoia, self-hate, aggression, and suicidal gestures—and there is profound mental, social, and physical deterioration. Although use of the drug to achieve social success (peer approval, relief of anxiety) may be an early or initial factor, it has been long abandoned by the final stages. *(Oski:747; Hathaway:233)*

40. (D) Child abuse has been classified as physical abuse, emotional abuse, sexual abuse, and neglect. This last group includes lack of nurturance, lack of supervision, and lack of provision of, for example, food, shelter, school, or medical care. Intellectual abuse has not yet been recognized as a category of child abuse. *(Rudolph:839; Hathaway:765–766)*

41. (F) The drug street scene changes so frequently and rapidly that it is difficult for a textbook to remain current regarding popular drugs and their street names. It is important, nevertheless, for the physician to be aware of what is currently being sold and used and what the drugs are popularly called. Knowledge of the drugs and their pharmacology and toxicity will help in identifying and treating cases of overdose and toxic reactions. Knowledge of the street names of the drugs is helpful in taking a history, especially in the emergency room, where, for example, a friend accompanying a comatose drug user may know only the street name of the drug taken. Hash, grass, and hemp are street names for marijuana. *(Pediatr Clin North Am 20:1035–1045, 1973; Fleisher: 561,563–564)*

42. (E) Doriden capsules are referred to as Cibas. *(Pediatr Clin North Am 20:1035–1045,1973; Fleisher:561,563–564)*

43. (C) Crack is cocaine that has been worked into a solid cake, pieces of which are smoked. *(Pediatr Clin North Am 20:1035–1045,1973; Fleisher:561,563–564)*

44. (B) Poppers refers to amyl nitrate. The vial or pearl is crushed, and the vapor inhaled. *(Pediatr Clin North Am 20:1035–1045,1973; Fleisher:561,563–564)*

45. (A) Bennies are the street name for amphetamines. Other names for this drug include peaches, dominoes, and brownies. *(Pediatr Clin North Am 20:1035–1045,1973; Fleisher:561,563–564)*

46. (C) Hypoglycemia is seen in both ethyl alcohol and aspirin poisoning, especially in young children. It is important to monitor blood sugar in these children, as lethargy or coma may be attributed incorrectly to the toxin, and the hypoglycemia may go unrecognized. *(Rudolph:801,819)*

47. (B) A mixed metabolic acidosis and respiratory alkalosis is characteristic of aspirin poisoning. Neither disturbance is seen in ethyl alcohol ingestion. *(Rudolph:801,819)*

48. (D) Pancreatitis is not seen with either *acute* alcohol ingestion or with aspirin poisoning in children. It is sometimes seen with acetaminophen poisoning. *(Rudolph:801,819)*

49. (D) Hypertension is not associated with either alcohol or aspirin poisoning. Hypotention may occur as a late effect of either drug. *(Rudolph:801,819)*

50. (B) Alcohol does not cause any abnormalities of hemostasis. Aspirin, even in small doses, impairs platelet function, and larger doses also interfere with prothrombin production by the liver. *(Rudolph:801,819)*

BIBLIOGRAPHY

AAP Subcommittee on Accidental Poisoning. Co-operative kerosene poisoning study. *Pediatrics.* 1962;29:648–674.

AAP Committee on Adolescence. Teenage suicide. *Pediatrics.* 1980;66:144–146.

Brown RT, Braden NJ. Hallucinogens. *Pediatr Clin North Am.* 1987;34:341–347.

Caffey J. The whiplash shaken infant syndrome. *Pediatrics.* 1974;54:396–403.

Council of Scientific Affairs, AMA. AMA diagnostic and treatment guidelines concerning child abuse and neglect. *JAMA.* 1985;254:796–800.

Eason JM, Lovejoy FH. Efficacy and safety of gastrointestinal decontamination in the treatment of oral poisoning. *Pediatr Clin North Am.* 1979;26:827–836.

Fleisher GR, Ludwig S. *Textbook of Pediatric Emergency Medicine.* 2nd ed. Baltimore, Md: Williams & Wilkins; 1988.

Gaudreault P, Temple AR, Lovejoy FH. The relative severity of acute versus chronic salicylate poisoning in children. *Pediatrics.* 1982;70:566–572.

Hathaway WE, Groothius JR, Hay WW, et al. *Current Pediatric Diagnosis & Treatment.* 10th ed. Norwalk, Conn: Appleton & Lange; 1991.

Hodgman CH, Roberts FN. Adolescent suicide and the pediatrician. *J Pediatr.* 1982;101:118–123.

Hoekelman RA, Friedman SB, Nelson NM, et al. *Primary Pediatric Care.* 2nd ed. St. Louis, Mo: Mosby Year Book; 1992.

Hughes JM, Merson MH. Fish and shellfish poisoning. *N Eng J Med.* 1976;295:1117–1120.

King P, Coleman JH. Stimulants and narcotic drugs. *Pediatr Clin North Am.* 1987;34:349–362.

Knight ME, Roberts RJ. Phenothiazine and butyrophenone intoxication in children. *Pediatr Clin North Am.* 1986;33:299–309.

MacKenzie RG. A practical approach to the drug-using adolescent and young adult. *Pediatric Clin North Am.* 1973;20:1035–1045.

McHugh MJ. The abuse of volatile substances. *Pediatr Clin North Am.* 1987;34:333–339.

Mofenson HC. New correct answer to an old question on kerosene ingestion (letter to the editor). *Pediatrics.* 1977;59:788.

Ng RC, Darwish H, Stewart DA. Emergency treatment of petroleum distillate and turpentine ingestion. *Can Med Assoc J.* 1974;111:537–538.

Oski FA, DeAngelis CD, Feigin RD, et al. *Principles & Practice of Pediatrics.* Philadelphia, Pa: JB Lippincott; 1990.

Piomelli S, Graziano J. Laboratory diagnosis of lead poisoning. *Pediatr Clin North Am.* 1980;27:843–853.

Reece RM, Grodin MA. Recognition of nonaccidental injury. *Pediatr Clin North Am.* 1985:32:41–60.

Robertson LS. Motor vehicles. *Pediatr Clin North Am.* 1985;32:87–94.

Robothman JL, Lietman PS. Acute iron poisoning: a review. *Am J Dis Child.* 1980;134:875–879.

Rudolph AM, Hoffman JIE, Rudolph CD. *Pediatrics.* 19th ed. Norwalk, Conn: Appleton & Lange; 1991.

Rumack BH. Acetaminophen overdose in children and adolescents. *Pediatr Clin North Am.* 1986;33:691–701.

Schmitt BD. Current pediatric roles in child abuse and neglect. *Am J Dis Child.* 1979;133:691–696.

Schwartz RH. Marijuana: an overview. *Pediatr Clin North Am.* 1987;34:305–312.

Singer HS, Freeman JM. Head trauma for the pediatrician. *Pediatrics.* 1978;62:819–825.

Spyker DA. Submersion injury. *Pediatr Clin North Am.* 1985;32:113–125.

CHAPTER 6

Infectious and Communicable Diseases
Questions

Infectious diseases account for such a large proportion of pediatric morbidity and mortality and such a large proportion of the questions on any pediatric exam that a chapter devoted to this topic is clearly warranted. One reason that infectious diseases are so common in the pediatric population is that an individual's first contacts with the more common pathogenic organism (eg, group A and group B beta-hemolytic streptococci, influenza virus, measles virus, CMV) generally occur during infancy and childhood. The newborn and young infant's immunologic system is inexperienced, immature, and sluggish. Another reason is the child's exposure to many individuals in day care and in school. Finally, infectious diseases assume a major importance in children because after early infancy (when prematurity-related problems and congenital abnormalities account for significant disease and death), there are relatively few other major non-traumatic causes of serious illness. Cancer, although the second leading cause of death in children beyond the second birthday (trauma is number one), is still rare. Heart disease, stroke, and hypertension are uncommon in children and, when they do occur, are associated with different etiologies than in adults. Percentagewise, therefore, infectious disease assumes an even greater importance in children than in adults.

In studying infectious diseases, the student should pay attention to different organisms likely to cause specific infections in each pediatric age group. The most common causes of bacteremia, pneumonia, and meningitis are quite different in the neonate than in the older infant or child. For example, *Mycoplasma pneumoniae* is a common cause of pneumonia in the school-age child but is uncommon in the infant or very young child. The examinee also needs to be aware of the effect of the child's age on the manifestation of particular infections. The clinical picture of gonococcal infection in the prepubescent girl is very different from that in the adolescent female.

DIRECTIONS (Questions 1 through 84): Each of the numbered items or incomplete statements in this section is followed by answers or by completions of the statement. Select the ONE lettered answer or completion that is BEST in each case.

1. Frequent features of staphylococcal toxic shock syndrome include

   (A) pneumonia and pleural effusion
   (B) scarlatiniform rash and conjunctivitis
   (C) exudative tonsillitis and cervical adenitis
   (D) arthritis and myositis
   (E) anemia and leukopenia

2. The usual portal of entry of histoplasmosis in the young child is the

   (A) gastrointestinal tract
   (B) urinary tract
   (C) respiratory tract
   (D) skin
   (E) conjunctiva

3. Most of the serum immunoglobulins of a normal infant at birth are

   (A) immunologically inactive
   (B) derived from the mother
   (C) derived from the infant's thymus
   (D) in the IgM fraction
   (E) in the form of isohemagglutinins (anti-A and anti-B)

4. Which of the following parasites gains entry by direct larval penetration of the skin?

(A) *Enterobius vermicularis*
(B) *Trypanosoma gambiense*
(C) *Trichinella spiralis*
(D) *Strongyloides stercoralis*
(E) *Taenia solium*

5. Infants with congenital rubella infection

(A) are virus-free by the time of birth
(B) have virus in their blood but not in their pharyngeal secretions
(C) excrete virus in urine and pharyngeal secretions for a few hours or days after birth
(D) excrete virus but are not infectious
(E) excrete virus and may be infectious for several weeks or months after birth

6. Currently, the U.S. Public Health Service recommends that smallpox vaccination in the United States

(A) be given to all children before 1 year of age
(B) be given to all children at the time of school entry
(C) be accompanied by vaccinia immune globulin
(D) be given only to travelers to Africa and India
(E) not be performed

7. Among nonimmunized and poorly nourished infants and young children in an undeveloped country, which one of the following infections would be most severe and have the highest morbidity and mortality?

(A) Measles
(B) Mumps
(C) Roseola
(D) Rubella
(E) Varicella

8. Ordinarily, the first dose of live attenuated measles vaccine (as MMR) should be administered

(A) at about 3 months of age
(B) at 6 to 9 months of age
(C) at 15 months of age
(D) at about 24 months of age
(E) at the time of school entry

9. The use of combined diphtheria-tetanus-pertussis (DPT) vaccine for primary immunization of young children

(A) should be restricted to underdeveloped countries
(B) is acceptable practice, although clearly inferior to the use of separate vaccines
(C) is the procedure of choice for immunization of normal children
(D) is advisable only for catch-up immunization of children behind the recommended schedule
(E) is no longer acceptable

10. The standard method of immunizing normal infants and children against polio in the United States involves the use of

(A) inactivated vaccine alone
(B) live oral vaccine alone
(C) inactivated vaccine followed by live vaccine
(D) live vaccine followed by inactivated vaccine
(E) inactivated and live vaccines simultaneously

11. In tuberculous meningitis, the exudate tends to be most severe

(A) over the frontal regions of the brain
(B) at the base of the brain
(C) around the cerebellum
(D) in the ventricles
(E) over the temporal lobes

12. Mosquitoes are recognized vectors in the transmission of encephalitis caused by

(A) arbovirus
(B) coxsackievirus
(C) enterovirus
(D) influenza virus
(E) mumps virus

13. A 3-year-old child has a positive tuberculin test. Which of the following would be most suggestive of miliary tuberculosis?

(A) Fever
(B) Hilar lymphadenopathy on roentgenograph
(C) Cough
(D) Elevated erythrocyte sedimentation rate
(E) Hepatosplenomegaly

14. In addition to respiratory symptoms and rash, infection with *Mycoplasma pneumoniae* has been associated most commonly with

(A) hepatic complications
(B) renal complications
(C) neurologic complications
(D) aplastic anemia
(E) immunologic suppression

15. Acute bronchiolitis is

(A) usually associated with high fever and rash
(B) usually associated with bilateral infiltrates on chest roentgenogram
(C) commonly associated with retractions, tachypnea, and wheezing
(D) characterized by the absence of cough despite respiratory distress
(E) most common between 2 and 5 years of age

16. On routine tuberculin skin testing, a well 5-year-old is found to have 8 mm of induration to 5 tuberculin units (TU) of purified protein derivative (PPD).

There is no history suggestive of contact with tuberculosis. This reaction probably indicates

(A) sensitivity to the diluent
(B) subcutaneous rather than intradermal injection of test material
(C) cross-sensitivity to atypical mycobacteria
(D) tuberculous infection without disease
(E) active tuberculosis

17. Infants and children with uncomplicated primary pulmonary tuberculosis

(A) are highly infectious
(B) are moderately infectious
(C) are rarely infectious
(D) are infectious to other children but not to adults

18. Children with enteric fever secondary to *Salmonella* infection frequently have

(A) leukocytosis and tachycardia relative to the degree of fever
(B) leukocytosis and bradycardia relative to the degree of fever
(C) leukopenia and tachycardia relative to the degree of fever
(D) leukopenia and bradycardia relative to the degree of fever

19. Children with chronic granulomatous disease have a defect in

(A) leukocyte migration
(B) synthesis of collagen
(C) capillary permeability
(D) tissue repair following injury
(E) the ability of leukocytes to kill certain phagocytosed bacteria

20. The rash of typhoid fever

(A) is pruritic
(B) is rarely seen in children
(C) characteristically involves the face
(D) usually begins on the first day of fever
(E) consists of small (1- to 6-mm) maculopapules

21. Which of the following is seen most commonly as a complication of gastrointestinal *Shigella* infection?

(A) A generalized erythematous rash
(B) Arthritis
(C) Encephalopathy
(D) Endocarditis
(E) Pneumonia

22. A characteristic of the cutaneous manifestations of congenital syphilis is

(A) that the lesions are sterile
(B) that lesions are most numerous on the trunk
(C) a fleeting salmon-pink macular rash

(D) a papular purpuric eruption on the legs and buttocks
(E) bullous lesions of the palms and soles

23. The most common manifestation of renal involvement in congenital syphilis is

(A) nephritis with nephrotic syndrome
(B) obstructive uropathy
(C) vesicoureteral reflux
(D) acute renal failure
(E) sterile pyuria

24. Congenital syphilis is characterized by

(A) involvement of the long bones
(B) a primary chancre of the umbilicus
(C) a high incidence of cardiovascular involvement
(D) the absence of serum antibodies against the *Treponema pallidum*

25. The most common manifestation of infection with *Neisseria gonorrhoea* in prepubertal girls is

(A) arthritis
(B) conjunctivitis
(C) peritonitis
(D) salpingitis
(E) vaginitis

26. Symptomatic gonococcal urethritis in the male child or adolescent is most often characterized by

(A) hematuria
(B) urinary retention
(C) fever and shaking chills
(D) an incubation period of less than 36 hours
(E) burning on urination and urethral discharge

27. Staphylococcal food poisoning

(A) usually is associated with a high fever
(B) usually begins within minutes of ingestion of the toxin
(C) often is accompanied by staphylococcal bacteremia
(D) is characterized by vomiting, abdominal cramps, and diarrhea
(E) is frequently accompanied by a rash

28. Group A streptococcal infection in children below the age of 1 year is likely to present as

(A) meningitis
(B) scarlet fever
(C) peritonsillar abscess
(D) acute rheumatic fever
(E) fever and nasal discharge

29. In scarlet fever

(A) the fever, rash, and sore throat all begin within the first 24 or 48 hours
(B) sore throat precedes the fever and rash by 2 or 3 days
(C) fever precedes the sore throat and rash by 2 or 3 days
(D) fever and sore throat precede the rash by 3 or 4 days
(E) fever and sore throat precede the rash by 5 or 6 days

30. The most useful diagnostic test for scarlet fever is the

(A) blood culture
(B) antistreptolysin titer
(C) complete blood count
(D) throat culture or rapid strep test
(E) monospot test or Epstein-Barr virus titers

31. Pneumococcal pneumonia

(A) is rare before 2 years of age
(B) is rare after 2 years of age
(C) is generally seen only in infants
(D) is usually preceded by, or associated with, a viral respiratory infection
(E) usually presents with an insidious onset, with fever preceding respiratory signs or symptoms for 2 to 5 days

32. Staphylococcal pneumonia is characterized by pneumatoceles, empyema, and pneumothorax. The ultimate outcome in children who survive usually is

(A) complete resolution
(B) chronic bronchiectasis
(C) chronic lung abscesses and empyema
(D) persistent pneumatoceles
(E) pulmonary fibrosis

33. The first clinical manifestation of tetanus neonatorum usually is

(A) fever
(B) vomiting
(C) convulsions
(D) opisthotonos
(E) difficulty sucking and swallowing

34. The characteristic rash of Rocky Mountain spotted fever is

(A) discrete red papules
(B) fleeting or evanescent
(C) vesicular
(D) purpuric
(E) urticarial

35. The usual course of pertussis in an infant is characterized by

(A) 4 or 5 days of high fever followed by cough and whooping
(B) sudden onset of fever, cough, and whooping

(C) gradual onset of cough, followed by abrupt onset of fever and whooping
(D) rhinitis followed by gradual worsening of cough and finally whooping
(E) rhinitis followed by abrupt onset of fever, cough, and whooping

36. Which of the following white blood cell counts is most suggestive of pertussis?

(A) 3,000/mm³ with 75% lymphocytes
(B) 20,000/mm³ with 65% lymphocytes
(C) 7,000/mm³ with 65% polymorphonuclear leukocytes
(D) 25,000/mm³ with 65% polymorphonuclear leukocytes
(E) 12,000/mm³ with 20% eosinophils

37. A 12-year-old child developed fever about 1 week after visiting relatives in India. The fever has persisted for about 10 days. Diarrhea, present for a few days, has cleared, and the child is now constipated. The child appears moderately acutely ill. The liver and spleen are enlarged. There are palpable, small (2–4 mm) erythematous spots on the trunk only. This child probably has

(A) measles
(B) typhoid fever
(C) *N. meningitidis* bacteremia
(D) rat-bite fever
(E) leptospirosis

38. You are working in a clinic in rural Mexico and examine an 8-year-old boy who has a rectal temperature of 38°C (100°F), bilateral tender parotid swelling, and pain when you flex his neck. He has been complaining of a headache. His immunization history is unknown. Your most likely diagnosis is mumps with

(A) aseptic meningitis
(B) pneumococcal meningitis
(C) viral myositis
(D) upper lobe pneumonia
(E) cervical spine arthritis

39. A previously well 3-year-old child has fever, headache, and photophobia. Your major concern is that the child may have

(A) acute glaucoma
(B) optic neuritis
(C) subarachnoid hemorrhage
(D) meningitis
(E) rabies

40. The combination of fever, hemorrhagic skin lesions, and shock in a 6-year-old child is most suggestive of infection with

(A) *Neisseria meningitidis*
(B) *Hemophilus influenzae*
(C) *Streptococcus pneumoniae*

(D) *Staphylococcus aureus*
(E) beta-hemolytic *Streptococcus*

41. Subdural effusions in association with acute bacterial meningitis are

(A) the result of inadequate treatment
(B) indicative of a bleeding disorder
(C) usually fatal
(D) caused by incidental trauma rather than the infection itself
(E) a common occurrence

42. A 5-year-old child presents with fever for 8 days, lymphadenopathy, splenomegaly, and numerous reactive or atypical lymphocytes on peripheral blood smear. The monospot test is negative. A likely cause of this clinical picture is infection with

(A) adenovirus
(B) cytomegalovirus
(C) herpesvirus
(D) respiratory syncytial virus
(E) rubella virus

43. Which of the following drug regimens is the most appropriate prophylaxis for close contacts of a child with meningococcal meningitis?

(A) Tetracycline for 5 days
(B) Penicillin for 3 days
(C) Rifampin for 2 days
(D) A sulfur drug for 7 days
(E) Penicillin and sulfur for 2 days

44. Early-onset group B streptococcal infection in the neonate

(A) is more common in low-birth-weight and premature than in normal infants
(B) usually presents between the third and fifth days of life
(C) typically is indolent and slowly progressive
(D) usually includes bacteremia and pneumonia but only rarely includes meningitis
(E) usually includes bacteremia and meningitis but only rarely includes pneumonia

45. Meningitis caused by *Listeria monocytogenes* in the pediatric age group is seen primarily in

(A) patients receiving broad-spectrum antibiotics
(B) children with chronic otitis media
(C) newborn infants
(D) the southwestern United States
(E) children with ventriculoperitoneal shunts

46. A 3-year-old nonimmunized child is seen in clinic and diagnosed as having measles. There is a 4-month-old sibling at home. Appropriate management of this sibling would include

(A) immediate immunization with live attenuated measles vaccine
(B) immediate immunization with killed measles vaccine
(C) a modifying dose of gamma-globulin
(D) a preventive dose of gamma-globulin
(E) a modifying dose of gamma-globulin and live attenuated measles vaccine at the same time but in opposite sites

47. A young child with fever, cough, hepatosplenomegaly, and eosinophilia has negative examinations of the stool for ova and parasites. The most likely parasite to cause this combination of findings is

(A) *Ascaris lumbricoides*
(B) *Toxocara canis*
(C) *Dracunculus medinensis*
(D) *Enterobius vermicularis*
(E) *Trichuris trichuria*

48. Of the following parasitic infections, which is most likely to present with intestinal obstruction?

(A) *Enterobius vermicularis*
(B) *Necator americanus*
(C) *Ascaris lumbricoides*
(D) *Strongyloides stercoralis*
(E) *Trichuris trichuria*

49. Invasion of the lung by *Ascaris lumbricoides* occurs most frequently

(A) during the initial stage of infection
(B) as a late complication of chronic infection
(C) during treatment
(D) at the time of a viral respiratory infection

50. The rash of measles

(A) is papulovesicular
(B) is urticarial
(C) is maculopapular
(D) appears on the first day of illness
(E) lasts 24 to 48 hours

51. Of the following extragenital complications of gonorrhea in the adolescent female, which is most common?

(A) Arthritis
(B) Carditis
(C) Meningitis
(D) Pneumonia
(E) Ophthalmolitis

52. The three most common bacterial causes of meningitis in childhood (excluding the neonatal period) are

(A) *Neisseria meningitidis, Hemophilus influenzae,* and *Streptococcus pneumoniae*
(B) *Neisseria meningitidis, Streptococcus pneumoniae,* and *Escherichia coli*
(C) *Neisseria meningitidis,* group A *Streptococcus,* and *Staphylococcus*
(D) *Neisseria meningitidis, Hemophilus influenzae,* and *Listeria monocytogenes*
(E) *Hemophilus influenzae,* group A *Streptococcus,* and *Escherichia coli*

53. Acute herpetic meningoencephalitis

(A) is usually mild and self-limited
(B) is seen only in the neonatal period
(C) has a predilection to involve the temporal lobes
(D) is generally seen in recurrent infection with herpesvirus
(E) is a common manifestation of primary herpesvirus infection

54. Fulminant, life-threatening viral hepatitis in the pediatric-age patient

(A) is more common with hepatitis A than hepatitis B infection
(B) is usually manifested by hepatic failure in the first week of clinical illness
(C) has not been reported with non-A, non-B hepatitis
(D) is most common in patients with an anicteric course
(E) it is seen primarily in children with sickle cell disease

55. The preicteric phase of infectious hepatitis B frequently is associated with

(A) leukocytosis
(B) pyuria
(C) arthralgia or arthritis
(D) a papulovesicular eruption
(E) agitation and anxiety

56. Chronic persistent hepatitis B infection

(A) is characterized by elevated serum levels of bilirubin and normal levels of liver enzymes
(B) gradually, but inexorably, progresses to hepatic destruction and hepatic failure
(C) usually presents as persistent abdominal pain, jaundice, and hepatomegaly following acute hepatitis
(D) is associated with persistence of HBsAg in the serum

57. A 10-month-old child has a temperature of 40° (104°F) for 4 days without other signs. On the fourth day, a rose pink maculopapular rash appears, and the temperature returns to normal. The most likely diagnosis is

(A) echovirus infection
(B) juvenile rheumatoid arthritis

(C) measles
(D) roseola
(E) typhus

58. Gonococcal infection

(A) can be prevented by use of a killed vaccine
(B) can only be prevented by use of the live vaccine
(C) confers immunity to subsequent infection only if the initial infection involves extragenital sites
(D) confers no immunity against repeated infection
(E) can be prevented by serum immune globulin

59. Characteristic oral findings in herpangina include

(A) a confluent exudate on the tonsils and uvula
(B) small vesicles or ulcers on the tonsilar fauces, tonsils, uvula, and pharynx
(C) large ulcers on the tongue and gingiva
(D) inflammation and ulceration of the gingiva and buccal mucosa
(E) all of the above

60. Herpangina is usually caused by infection with

(A) adenovirus
(B) *Corynebacterium hemolyticum*
(C) *Corynebacterium parvum*
(D) coxsackievirus
(E) herpes simplex virus

61. You are taking care of a 26-month-old child with bacterial meningitis. Blood and spinal fluid cultures are positive for *H. influenzae.* The child's household consists of the parents, one grandparent, a 6-month-old sibling, a 5-year-old sibling, and a 14-year-old exchange student who has been living with the family for about 1 month. You advise rifampin prophylaxis for

(A) everyone in the household
(B) everyone except the grandparent
(C) everyone except the grandparent and the visiting student
(D) the siblings only
(E) the 6-month-old sibling only

62. The most common neurologic complication of diphtheria is

(A) neuritis with paralysis
(B) convulsions
(C) coma
(D) transverse myelitis
(E) tetany

63. A previously well 12-year-old youngster presents with fever and splenomegaly and is found to have a positive monospot test, a positive serological test for syphilis, and elevated serum transaminase levels. The organism most likely responsible for these findings is

(A) *Treponema pallidum*
(B) hepatitis B virus

(C) rubella virus
(D) Epstein-Barr virus
(E) toxoplasmosis

64. A 15-year-old presents with pain, photophobia, and blurred vision in one eye. Examination reveals chemosis of the affected eye and small vesicular lesions below the eye and on the nose. Application of fluorescein dye reveals branching, dendritic lesions on the cornea. The most likely cause of this clinical picture is

(A) staphylococcal impetigo and ophthalmolitis
(B) adenoviral infection
(C) retinoblastoma
(D) herpes simplex infection
(E) trauma

65. Which of the following occurs in infants with congenitally acquired immunodeficiency syndrome (HIV infection)?

(A) Thrombocytosis
(B) Decreased serum levels of IgG, IgA, and IgM
(C) Chronic Epstein-Barr (EB) virus infection
(D) An increased ratio of CD4 to CD8 T cells

66. In the normal child, the nadir (lowest point) for serum immunoglobulin G concentration occurs

(A) at birth
(B) during the first year of life
(C) during the second year of life
(D) at puberty
(E) 1 or 2 years after puberty

Please note the use of a negative qualifier such as EXCEPT, LEAST, or NOT in each of the following questions (Questions 67 through 84).

67. Primary pulmonary tuberculosis in childhood and preadolescence commonly is manifested by all of the following EXCEPT

(A) fever
(B) hilar lymphadenopathy
(C) cavitary changes in the upper lobes
(D) over 10 mm induration to 5 TU PPD intradermally
(E) development of hypersensitivity to the tubercle bacillus

68. Which of the following rickettsioses is NOT usually spread by arthropods?

(A) Typhus
(B) Rocky Mountain spotted fever
(C) Scrub typhus
(D) Q fever
(E) Rickettsial pox

69. All of the following are common complications of measles EXCEPT

(A) otitis media
(B) pneumonia
(C) arthritis
(D) laryngotracheitis
(E) encephalitis

70. Which of the following is LEAST characteristic of varicella infection?

(A) An incubation period of 14 to 16 days
(B) A rash progressing from papular to vesicular
(C) A tendency for the rash to be heaviest on the arms and legs
(D) Temperature that is usually less than 38.9°C (102°F)
(E) Itching

71. Maternal infection and viremia with rubella virus during the early weeks of pregnancy may result in any of the following EXCEPT

(A) congenital malformations
(B) stillbirth
(C) abortion
(D) macrosomia and a large-for-gestational age infant
(E) chronic infection of the fetus

72. In addition to exudative tonsillitis, cervical adenitis, and splenomegaly, less common but well-recognized clinical findings in infectious mononucleosis include all of the following EXCEPT

(A) easy fatigability
(B) petechiae on the palate
(C) myringitis bullosa
(D) erythematous rash
(E) airway obstruction secondary to enlarged tonsils

73. Clinical manifestations of scarlet fever include all of the following EXCEPT

(A) exudative tonsillitis
(B) white strawberry tongue
(C) hepatosplenomegaly
(D) erythematous punctiform lesions on the palate
(E) red strawberry tongue

74. The rash of scarlet fever is characterized by all of the following EXCEPT

(A) a rough sandpaper-like texture
(B) a tendency to desquamate
(C) a tendency to become generalized within 24 hours
(D) a tendency to spare areas of skin folds such as the axillae and groin
(E) a red, erythematous appearance

75. Recognized dermatologic manifestations of staphylococcal toxins include all of the following EXCEPT

   (A) generalized exfoliative disease in infants
   (B) toxic epidermal necrolysis in children and adults
   (C) localized bullous impetigo
   (D) a papular, pruritic rash
   (E) a scarlatiniform eruption

76. Which of the following is LEAST likely to be a manifestation of congenital toxoplasmosis?

   (A) Cataracts
   (B) Glaucoma
   (C) Chorioretinitis
   (D) Aniridia
   (E) Blindness

77. Which of the following is LEAST common in acquired toxoplasmosis infection?

   (A) Fever
   (B) Arthritis
   (C) Encephalitis
   (D) Lymphadenitis
   (E) Uveitis

78. All of the following clinical features have been noted in infants and young children with acquired immunodeficiency syndrome (AIDS) EXCEPT

   (A) low birth weight and failure to thrive
   (B) autoimmune hemolytic anemia
   (C) lymphadenopathy
   (D) hepatosplenomegaly
   (E) opportunistic infections

79. Which of the following statements about the roentgenographic findings in primary pulmonary tuberculosis is NOT true?

   (A) Cavitary lesions are the most common finding
   (B) Hilar adenopathy without a visible parenchymal focus is common
   (C) Parenchymal shadows may vary from small areas to an entire lobe
   (D) Calcifications may appear within the parenchymal focus as well as within hilar nodes
   (E) Segmental lesions may be unilateral or bilateral

80. Which of the following would be LEAST common in primary pulmonary tuberculosis in a child?

   (A) Positive tuberculin skin test
   (B) Fever
   (C) Pulmonary rales
   (D) Hilar adenopathy on chest roentgenogram
   (E) Cough

81. Which of the following statements regarding the fluid in tuberculous pleural effusion is NOT true?

   (A) The color is usually yellow or greenish yellow, occasionally blood tinged
   (B) Specific gravity and protein usually are elevated
   (C) Acid-fast stain usually reveals tuberculous organisms
   (D) Glucose may be normal but frequently is low
   (E) Leukocytes may predominate early, and lymphocytes later

82. Which of the following is NOT characteristic of rubella infection in young children?

   (A) Mild leukopenia
   (B) Postauricular and occipital lymphadenopathy
   (C) Four to five days of fever before the rash
   (D) A pink-red maculopapular rash
   (E) Mild thrombocytopenia

83. Which of the following infections is LEAST likely in a child who has never lived or traveled outside of New York State?

   (A) Candidiasis
   (B) Coccidioidomycosis
   (C) Cryptococcoses
   (D) Histoplasmosis
   (E) *Yersinia enterocolita* infection

84. Which of the following females is LEAST likely to develop pelvic inflammatory disease secondary to gonococcal infection of the lower genital tract?

   (A) A 20-year-old with an intrauterine contraceptive device
   (B) A pregnant 17-year-old
   (C) A 16-year-old who has just had her menstrual period
   (D) A 15-year-old who is taking birth control pills
   (E) An 8-year-old who has been sexually abused

DIRECTIONS (85 through 95): Each set of matching questions in this section consists of a list of 4 to 26 lettered options followed by several numbered items. For each numbered item select the ONE lettered option with which it is most closely associated. Each lettered option may be selected once, more than once, or not at all.

Questions 85 through 88

The following questions refer to measles:

   (A) Day 1 of illness through day 5 or 6
   (B) Day 3 of illness through day 4 or 6
   (C) Day 4 of illness through day 8 or 9
   (D) Day 2 of illness through day 10
   (E) Day 1 of illness only

85. Rash

86. Fever

87. Cough

88. Koplik's spots

Questions 89 through 92

(A) *Toxocara canis*
(B) *Ascaris lumbricoides*
(C) *Necator americanus*
(D) *Trichuris trichiuria*
(E) *Enterobius vermicularis*

89. Anemia

90. Hepatomegaly

91. Rectal prolapse

92. Rectal itching

Questions 93 through 95

(A) Dogs
(B) Fish
(C) Rats, mice
(D) Pigeons, parakeets
(E) Cattle, swine

93. *Spirillum minus*

94. *Pasteurella multocida*

95. *Chlamydia psittaci*

DIRECTIONS (Questions 96 through 133): Each group of items in this section consists of lettered headings followed by a set of numbered words or phrases. For each numbered word or phrase, select

A if the item is associated with (A) <u>only</u>,
B if the item is associated with (B) <u>only</u>,
C if the item is associated with <u>both</u> (A) <u>and</u> (B),
D if the item is associated with <u>neither</u> (A) <u>nor</u> (B).

Questions 96 through 98

(A) Pulmonary infection with *Chlamydia trachomatis*
(B) Pulmonary infection with *Bordetella pertussis*
(C) Both
(D) Neither

96. Commonly transmitted to infants by siblings or other children

97. Usually associated with high fever and toxic appearance

98. Eosinophilia common

Questions 99 through 103

(A) IgG
(B) IgM
(C) Both
(D) Neither

99. Can be synthesized by a normal newborn infant

100. Transplacental transmission from mother to fetus

101. Normal serum concentration during the first year of life over 250 mg/dL

102. May be undetectable in cord blood

103. Important in resistance to bacterial infection

Questions 104 through 108

(A) Tetanus
(B) Rabies
(C) Both
(D) Neither

104. Trismus

105. Paralysis

106. Almost always fatal

107. Generalized convulsions

108. Heroin addiction

Questions 109 through 116

(A) Measles (rubeola)
(B) German measles (rubella)
(C) Both
(D) Neither

109. Cough, coryza, and conjunctivitis

110. Exanthem

111. Enanthem (intraoral findings)

112. Temperature elevation to 104°F

113. High incidence of secondary bacterial infection

114. Arthritis

115. Encephalitis, often severe, in about 1 per 1,000 cases

116. Live attenuated vaccine available

Questions 117 through 121

(A) Hepatitis A
(B) Hepatitis B
(C) Both
(D) Neither

117. Anorexia, nausea, and abdominal pain

118. Nonparenteral transmission occurs

119. A small but significant number of patients develop chronic persistent hepatitis

120. Anicteric infection may occur

121. Milder in children than in adults

Questions 122 through 127

(A) Hereditary agammaglobulinemia
(B) Hereditary thymic dysplasia (combined immunodeficiency)
(C) Both
(D) Neither

122. May be transmitted as X-linked disorder

123. Hypocalcemia

124. Enlarged lymph nodes

125. Adenosine deaminase deficiency

126. Skin grafts from unrelated donors not rejected

127. Treatment with immune globulin and antibiotics usually permits survival into adulthood

Questions 128 through 133

Regarding the routine immunization of normal children:
(A) First year of life
(B) Second year of life
(C) Both
(D) Neither

128. Three injections of diphtheria-pertussis-tetanus vaccine

129. Two or three doses of trivalent oral polio vaccine

130. Measles immunization in nonepidemic situation

131. Rubella immunization

132. Killed measles vaccine

133. *Hemophilus influenzae* b conjugate vaccine

Answers and Explanations

1. (B) Manifestations of the staphylococcal toxic shock syndrome, which include fever, mental status changes, conjunctivitis, scarlatiniform rash, and multiple organ failure, are caused by a toxin elaborated by the staphylococci rather than by tissue invasion by the organism. The organism usually can be cultured from skin or mucous membrane and only rarely from the blood. The organism has been recovered from the vagina and has been associated with the use of tampons, especially those designed to be changed infrequently. *(Rudolph:613; Hathaway:853)*

2. **(C)** As in adults, the respiratory tract is the portal of entry for histoplasmosis in essentially all cases in children. Inoculation other than by inhalation is exceedingly rare. *(Rudolph:712–713; Feigin:1953)*

3. (B) At birth, almost all of the infant's immunoglobulin is IgG, acquired from the mother by placental transfer. Serum IgA and IgM levels are very low, as are serum titers of isohemagglutinins. In the presence of intrauterine infection, the newborn infant's serum level of IgM might be increased (eg, 25 to 50 mg/dL) but still would be much lower than the serum concentration of IgG (>600 mg/dL). *(Rudolph:452–453)*

4. (D) Like *Ancylostoma duodenale* ("hookworm"), *Strongyloides stercoralis* enters the human host by penetration of the skin by larvae in the soil. The larvae migrate to the intestines, where they set up residency and mature. *(Feigin:2084)*

5. (E) Infants congenitally infected with rubella excrete the virus in urine and pharyngeal secretions and can be infectious for many weeks or months. Such infants pose a definite hazard to nonimmune family members, caretakers, and medical and nursing personnel. Pregnant females who are not certain of their rubella immune status should not handle these infants or their secretions. *(Rudolph:690)*

6. (E) In 1971, routine vaccination against smallpox in the United States was discontinued because the risk of contracting the disease had become so remote that

the potential benefits of the vaccine were outweighed by the small risk of complications following vaccination. The smallpox virus apparently has no host other than the human body. In 1980, as the result of aggressive medical and public health efforts, the World Health Organization was able to declare the entire globe as certifiably free of smallpox. *(Rudolph:691)*

7. (A) Of the so-called common childhood diseases listed in this question, measles (rubeola) clearly is the most severe, with high fever, inflammation of the respiratory mucosa, and general toxicity. It also has the highest incidence of serious complications—primarily pneumonia, laryngotracheitis and encephalitis. In malnourished children in undeveloped countries, the disease carries a very high mortality, usually secondary to pneumonia or diarrhea or bacterial superinfection. *(Rudolph:677–678; Feigin:1593, 1597–1605)*

8. (C) Ordinarily, the first dose of live attenuated measles vaccine (combined with mumps and rubella as the MMR vaccine) should not be administered before the age of 15 months to maximize the likelihood that transplacentally acquired antibodies have disappeared completely from the child's blood. Otherwise, these antibodies may blunt the infant's immunologic response to the vaccine. On the other hand, administration of the vaccine should not be delayed much beyond 15 months because of the seriousness of measles infection. It is now recommended that a second dose of the vaccine be given either when the child enters elementary school or when he enters junior high school. In areas where, or at times when, measles is epidemic, it is recommended that an initial dose of monovalent measles vaccine be given as early as 6 months of age, followed by the two MMRs as noted. *(Hathaway:137)*

9. (C) The use of a combined diphtheria-tetanus-pertussis (DPT) vaccine is routine and is the method of choice for the primary immunization of infants and young children. It entails fewer injections, and the results are as good as, or better than, those with the use of separate vaccines. *(Rudolph:33–34; Hathaway: 133–135)*

10. **(B)** The standard method of immunization against polio for *normal* infants and children in the United States is with live oral vaccine. The inactivated (killed) vaccine is used only for children with immunodeficiency disorders and their siblings. The killed vaccine, however, is still sometimes used as a booster or for primary immunization in adults because of their greater susceptibility to vaccine-induced paralytic disease. Because the oral vaccine has, on rare occasion, resulted in paralytic disease, there is interest in the routine use of a killed vaccine instead. An effective killed vaccine that could be incorporated into the DPT immunization is under development but is not currently in use. *(Hathaway:136; Rudolph:35–36)*

11. **(B)** In tuberculous meningitis, the greatest degree of meningeal involvement and collection of exudate is around the brainstem and at the base of the brain. This is important because it can lead either to involvement of the cranial nerves or to obstruction of the basal cisterns and hydrocephalus, both of which are seen commonly in this condition. *(Rudolph:627,1360)*

12. **(A)** Mumps virus, enterovirus, coxsackievirus, and influenza virus are spread primarily by direct contact (eg, respiratory droplets, hands) and not through an arthropod vector. A number of viruses, notably the arbovirus, are spread by arthropods. Examples in North America include eastern and western equine encephalitis, St. Louis encephalitis, and Colorado tick fever. The first three are spread by mosquitoes, the last, as the name implies, by a tick. *(Feigin:1390–1403)*

13. **(E)** Fever, cough, hilar lymphadenopathy, and elevated sedimentation rate are seen commonly in uncomplicated primary pulmonary tuberculosis. Hepatosplenomegaly is generally not seen in uncomplicated primary pulmonary tuberculosis but does occur in more than 50% of children with miliary disease. *(Feigin:1328–1332; Rudolph:625–627)*

14. **(C)** *Mycoplasma pneumoniae* has long been known to cause pneumonia, bronchitis, otitis media, myringitis bullosa, and nonspecific upper respiratory infection. More recently, this organism also has been recognized as a cause of various nonrespiratory manifestations such as carditis, encephalitis, and meningitis. Other neurologic manifestations reported with *M. pneumoniae* infection include transverse myelitis, psychosis, poliomyelitis-like syndrome, and Guillain-Barré syndrome. *(Rudolph: 693,1841)*

15. **(C)** In infants with bronchiolitis, fever is usually mild, and a rash is not noted. Cough is characteristic

and frequently severe, as are retraction, tachypnea, and wheezing. The disease is most frequent, as well as most severe, in the first 2 years of life. The chest roentgenogram usually reveals hyperaeration only, although pneumonia is an occasional complication. *(Rudolph:1520; Hathaway:376–377)*

16. **(C)** Reactions of less than 5-mm induration to 5 TU are considered negative. Reactions between 5 and 10 mm are considered doubtful and usually represent infection with atypical mycobacterium. Reactions of 10 mm or more induration generally are considered positive and indicative of infection with *Mycobacterium tuberculosis* but do not necessarily mean clinically evident disease. In some geographic areas of the United States (such as the southeast), where atypical mycobacteria are highly endemic, 12 mm has been suggested as the dividing point in interpreting a *routine* PPD in an asymptomatic child without a history of contact with tuberculosis. The point to remember is that the threshold for interpreting a tuberculin skin test as positive is lower for children with signs or symptoms suggestive of tuberculosis or with a history of contact with tuberculosis. *(Rudolph:630; Feigin:1343–1345)*

17. **(C)** In general, children with *uncomplicated* primary pulmonary tuberculosis are noninfectious and do not require isolation. This is believed to relate to the scanty sputum production, lack of expectoration, and the small number of organisms that can be recovered from sputum or gastric culture. In contrast, children with draining cervical lymph nodes are infectious, as are adolescents with cavitary (adult-type) pulmonary disease. *(Rudolph:632)*

18. **(D)** In enteric *Salmonella* infections fever is characteristic; diarrhea may or may not be present. Some features highly suggestive of *Salmonella* infection include leukopenia and a relative bradycardia; that is, the heart rate is slower than would be anticipated for the degree of fever present. *(Rudolph:603; Feigin: 626–628)*

19. **(E)** The defect in chronic granulomatous disease (CGD) is the inability of polymorphonuclear leukocytes to effect intracellular killing of certain phagocytosed bacteria. The neutrophils can ingest bacteria normally but cannot produce the intracellular hydrogen peroxide needed to kill certain organisms. CGD is inherited primarily as a sex-linked recessive trait, although some females with the disorder have been reported. *(Rudolph:1149–1150)*

20. **(E)** The rash of typhoid fever, which usually appears during the second week of illness, is composed of crops of small, nonpruritic maculopapules ("rose spots") distributed primarily on the lower chest and abdomen. The rash is not uncommon in children with this infection. *(Rudolph:603; Feigin:627)*

21. (C) Encephalopathy, characterized by lethargy or coma and convulsions, is a common complication of enteric infection with *Shigella* and presumably is caused by a neurotoxin elaborated by the organisms. Examination of cerebrospinal fluid is normal. Recovery is the rule. Reactive arthritis is a recognized, but very uncommon, complication of enteric infection with *Shigella*. Reiter's syndrome and hemolytic-uremic syndrome also are well-recognized complications. *(Feigin:639–641)*

22. (E) In general, *T. pallidum* can be demonstrated in *any* mucous membrane or cutaneous lesion of congenital syphilis, especially a moist one. All these lesions are capable of spreading the organism and are highly infectious. The classical cutaneous manifestations of congenital syphilis are a copper-colored maculopapular rash and bullous lesions of the palms and soles. *(Rudolph:619)*

23. (A) Renal involvement in congenital syphilis is a type of glomerulonephritis clinically presenting as nephrotic syndrome. Congenital syphilis is an important cause of nephrotic syndrome in infants less than 6 months of age. *(Rudolph:619–620)*

24. (A) A characteristic feature of congenital syphilis is involvement of the long bones. The most common lesions are osteochondritis, periosteal new bone formation, and osteomyelitic lesions. Since the infection is transplacental, a primary chancre and the associated regional lymphadenopathy are absent. Cardiovascular involvement is rare in the congenital form of infection. IgM and IGG antibodies against the *Treponema* usually are detectable at birth. *(Rudolph:619)*

25. (E) Vaginitis is the most common form of gonococcal infection in the prepubertal female. The unestrogenized, alkaline vaginal mucosa of the prepubertal girl is especially vulnerable to colonization and infection with *N. gonorrhoea*. Although spread by fomites such as contaminated rectal thermometers, bed clothing, and linen is generally believed to occur, most cases beyond infancy result from sexual contact (abuse). Ascending infection (salpingitis, peritonitis) occurs, but only rarely in prepubertal children. Arthritis is uncommon, and conjunctivitis is essentially restricted to the newborn period. [*Note:* The key word in this question is *prepubertal*. Many questions are missed and points lost by failure to pay careful attention to all information in the question.] *(Rudolph:580; Feigin:514–517)*

26. (E) Gonococcal urethritis in the male child or adolescent is clinically similar to the same infection in the adult male. Burning on urination and urethral discharge are the most common symptoms. The incubation period is 2 days to 2 weeks. Fever is uncommon. Hematuria and urinary retention are not part of the picture. *(Rudolph:580)*

27. (D) Staphylococcal food poisoning is caused by a toxin elaborated in the spoiled food before ingestion. Bacteremia does not occur, since this is not an infection. Fever is uncommon. Symptoms—vomiting, abdominal cramps, and diarrhea—usually begin within a few hours (not minutes) of ingestion of the toxin. *(Feigin:572–573; Hathaway:853)*

28. (E) Group A streptococcal infection in children less than 1 year old is commonly manifested by persistent fever and mucoserous nasal discharge. This syndrome has been referred to as "streptococcosis." Localized pharyngeal involvement is uncommon in the first year of life. Meningitis caused by this organism is very uncommon at all ages. The clinical picture of scarlet fever is rarely seen in the first year of life. This may, at least partly reflect a protective effect of transplacentally acquired maternal antibodies to the erythrogenic toxin. It also has been suggested that repeated exposure and hypersensitization to streptococcal exotoxins may be needed for expression of this disease (scarlet fever). Acute rheumatic fever is rare before 4 or 5 years of age. *(Feigin:1296–1300)*

29. (A) Scarlet fever is ushered in by fever and sore throat together or within a short period of each other. The characteristic rash appears within 12 to 48 hours of the onset of fever and sore throat. *(Rudolph:615–616)*

30. (D) Scarlet fever is a syndrome of tonsillitis, fever, and rash caused by an erythrogenic toxin-producing *Streptococcus* in a patient lacking antitoxic immunity. The throat culture for group A hemolytic streptococci is therefore the easiest and most useful diagnostic test for scarlet fever. Although the serum ASO titer will rise in 7 to 14 days, the throat culture or one of the rapid strep tests is more immediate and therefore more useful. [*Note:* The question asked for the most *useful* test, not the most accurate or definitive.] *(Rudolph:615–616)*

31. (D) Pneumococcal pneumonia is the most common acute bacterial pneumonia of infants (excluding the neonate) and children. It usually occurs in association with, or as a complication of, a viral upper respiratory illness. The onset of clinical manifestations is usually rapid and abrupt, and although fever is a prominent feature, respiratory signs and symptoms are common and usually are present early. *(Rudolph:1533)*

32. (A) Most children who recover from staphylococcal pneumonia do so completely. Clinical recovery usually is complete within 3 to 6 weeks. Although the chest roentgenogram ultimately also returns to normal, this process may take as long as 3 to 6 months. (*Rudolph:1534*)

33. **(E)** The first signs of tetanus neonatorum are difficulty sucking and swallowing, followed by body stiffness and spasms. Convulsions and opisthotonos are relatively late signs. Fever and vomiting are not common features of this disorder. (*Rudolph:623*)

34. **(D)** The rash of Rocky Mountain spotted fever begins as irregular pink macules that appear first on the extremities. The rash then spreads to the face and trunk and becomes petechial and purpuric. There are no papules or vesicles, and the rash is not evanescent. (*Rudolph:696; Feigin:1851*)

35. **(D)** Pertussis classically begins with a catarrhal stage indistinguishable from a common cold and lasting up to a week. This is followed by gradual worsening of the cough, finally reaching the paroxysmal stage, characterized by thick, tenacious secretions and fits of forceful coughing that often end in a whoop as the child is finally able to take a full breath. Fever is usually mild or absent. (*Rudolph:595; Hathaway:882*)

36. **(B)** Pertussis usually is associated with a marked absolute lymphocytosis. Peripheral white blood cell counts in the range of 20,000 to 30,000/mm^3 with a majority of lymphocytes are characteristic of this infection. This is a useful and important diagnostic feature. (*Rudolph:596; Hathaway:882*)

37. **(B)** Typhoid fever (infection with *S. typhi*) is characterized by an incubation period of 6 to 21 days, followed by fever, malaise, and, in some cases, rose spots. These are small, palpable erythematous lesions on the trunk. (Petechiae are smaller and not palpable.) Diarrhea, if present, usually clears and often is followed by constipation. (*Rudolph:603*)

38. **(A)** Aseptic meningitis is one of the most common complications of mumps virus infection. As a matter of fact, it occurs so frequently that it might be considered a part of the disease rather than a complication. CSF pleocytosis often occurs in mumps infection, even in the absence of signs of meningeal irritation. Infection with mumps virus is generalized, and other target areas besides the parotid gland and the CSF include the heart, the kidneys, the pancreas, and the testicles in males and breasts in females. (*Rudolph:681*)

39. **(D)** Photophobia is a relatively common finding in meningitis, both bacterial and viral. Although photophobia also occurs in other neurologic conditions, such as brain tumor and subarachnoid hemorrhage, these are less common than meningitis. In this patient, the acute onset in association with fever and

headache also favors the diagnosis of meningitis. (*Feigin:408–409*)

40. **(A)** Although the combination of fever, hemorrhagic eruption, and shock can be seen with bacteremic infection caused by a wide variety of organisms including *H. influenzae, S. pneumoniae, S. aureus,* and beta-hemolytic *Streptococcus,* this combination of findings is most commonly seen with meningococcal (*N. meningitidis*) infection. The hemorrhagic skin lesions (purpura) suggest disseminated intravascular coagulation, an ominous prognostic sign. (*Feigin: 1189–1190; Rudolph:595; Hathaway:856*)

41. **(E)** Subdural effusions are a common complication of acute bacterial meningitis, occurring in 30 to 50% of cases. The exact pathogenesis is unknown, but the effusions are more frequent in young infants, usually sterile, and not related either to inadequate therapy or to a bleeding disorder. They are frequently asymptomatic and rarely fatal. (*Feigin:409,417*)

42. **(B)** The monospot test is a measure of heterophile antibodies that develop in most, but not all, children with Epstein-Barr virus infection. A number of viruses other than the Epstein-Barr virus can cause the clinical picture of mononucleosis, including lymphadenopathy, splenomegaly, and atypical (reactive) lymphocytes on peripheral blood smear. Of the viruses listed in the question, however, only cytomegalovirus (CMV) has clearly and frequently been associated with a mononucleosis-like picture. As a matter of fact, many texts use the term CMV mononucleosis. (*Feigin:1536*)

43. **(C)** Although several drug regimens for prophylaxis of contacts of meningococcal disease are acceptable, the primary regimen recommended at this time is rifampin, 10 mg/kg every 12 hours (q12h) for a total of four doses. The comparatively greater success of this antibiotic in eliminating the nasopharyngeal carriage of meningococcus is believed to be the result of its high concentration in secretions, including saliva, tears, and possibly nasopharyngeal mucus. This same feature accounts for the orange tears and saliva sometimes seen in patients taking rifampin. (*Hathaway:857*)

44. **(A)** The group B streptococcus is the leading bacterial cause of neonatal infection in most medical centers in the United States. Two clinical syndromes, early onset and late onset, have been described, although some features do overlap both groups. The early-onset picture is most frequent in high-risk infants (eg, premature, prolonged rupture of membranes) and usually presents as a severe, rapidly progressive illness in the first day or even hours of life. Pneumonia and bacteremia are the most common manifestations, but meningitis occurs in about one-third of cases. Manifestations of late-onset infec-

tion are often indolent and include bacteremia and meningitis as well as other focal infections such as osteomyelitis, septic arthritis, omphalitis, and breast abscess. *(Feigin:1305–1309; Hathaway:847–848)*

45. (C) *Listeria monocytogenes* meningitis is uncommon in childhood except for the newborn period, where in some series it accounts for up to 10% of cases of bacterial meningitis. A few pediatric cases occur in immunodeficient children, and a rare case in the otherwise normal child. There is no geographic preference and no relation to otitis media, the use of antibiotics, or to the presence of a ventriculoperitoneal shunt. *(Feigin:1180–1185)*

46. (D) Active immunization with live measles vaccine at the time of contact is too late to assure protection. Additionally, children should not receive the vaccine before the age of 6 months to assure an adequate immunologic response. The recommended management of susceptible siblings of a contact case is the use of a preventive dose of gamma-globulin (0.25 mg/kg) and later immunization with the live-virus vaccine. In the past, when most women had had natural measles infection, maternal IgG levels of measles antibody were very high, and transplacental IgG afforded the young infant relatively strong protection. Cases of measles infection in this age group were often milder than in older children. Such is not the case now. Many mothers have low levels of measles antibody (from immunization rather than natural infection), and their infants are susceptible to severe measles infection. *(Feigin:1604–1605)*

47. (B) The dog ascarid, *Toxocara canis*, cannot complete its life cycle in the human, and, therefore, eggs or worms are not discharged in the stool. The clinical picture of toxocariasis (often referred to as visceral larva migrans) is characterized by fever, hepatomegaly, and eosinophilia. Less frequently there may be involvement of the lung, central nervous system, heart, or retina. None of the other parasites listed characteristically causes hepatomegaly. *(Feigin:2085–2086)*

48. (C) *Ascaris* is the largest intestinal roundworm, and occasionally intestinal obstruction may result from heavy infection. The incidence of this complication has been estimated at 2 per 1,000 infected children per year. Intestinal obstruction has not been observed with any of the other parasites listed. *(Rudolph:718)*

49. (A) The initial stage of *Ascaris lumbricoides* infection following ingestion of eggs regularly involves hatching of larvae in the duodenum, penetration to the portal vein, and then to the pulmonary circulation. Invasion of the lung results in alveolar hemorrhage and inflammation which, if severe, may present as pneumonia and eosinophilia, often called Loeffler's pneumonia. In contrast, invasion of the lungs by migrating adult worms is rare. *(Rudolph:718)*

50. (C) Fever and other prodromal symptoms precede the rash of measles by several days. The rash is a maculopapular eruption that appears first on the face and head and then spreads downward to the rest of the body over 2 to 3 days. It then takes another 3 to 4 days for the rash to fade (taking on a brownish-coppery discoloration), giving a total duration of the exanthem of 6 to 7 days. *(Rudolph:677,924)*

51. (A) Salpingitis is the most common complication of gonorrhea in the adolescent female. Arthritis is the second most frequent complication and is, by far, the most common distal or extragenital complication and the most common of the choices listed in the question. The other complications listed are infrequent in adults and rare in children and adolescents. *(J Pediatr 85:595–607,1974; Rudolph:580)*

52. (A) The three most common etiologic agents of bacterial meningitis in children beyond the newborn period are *H. influenzae*, *N. meningitidis*, and *S. pneumoniae*. Before the ages of 3 to 5 years, *H. influenzae* has been the leading cause of meningitis, but after 5 years *S. pneumoniae* and *N. meningitidis* are more common. It is possible that the relatively recently introduced vaccines against *H. influenzae* will push this organism from first place, but it is unlikely it will fall out of the top three. *(Rudolph:559)*

53. (C) Acute herpetic meningoencephalitis is an uncommon to rare complication of primary herpesvirus infection. The infection often is rapidly progressive and frequently fatal. The virus has a definite predilection for involvement of the temporal lobes, which can be demonstrated either by electroencephalograph or by CT scan. *(Feigin:1565–1566)*

54. (B) Fulminant, life-threatening hepatitis in the pediatric patient usually is caused by hepatitis B, rarely hepatitis A. It has been reported with non-A, non-B hepatitis. It is usually manifested by hepatic failure within the first week of the onset of signs or symptoms of hepatitis. It is rare in patients with an anicteric course. Most of the victims had been previously well, without obvious underlying disease. *(Feigin:688–689)*

55. (C) Arthralgia or arthritis is common during the preicteric phase of hepatitis, especially type B. This is usually part of an immune-complex, serum-sickness-like syndrome. A rash frequently is present, but is urticarial rather than papulovesicular. Leukopenia is the rule rather than leukocytosis. *(Feigin:682–683)*

56. (D) Chronic hepatitis follows infection with hepatitis B in a significant percentage of cases (10% in one series). Two patterns of disease have been described—chronic persistent and chronic active. Both are associated with persistence of the hepatitis B surface antigen (HBsAg) in the serum, but the former is usually a nonprogressive problem. Although a small number of patients do convert to the chronic active form, others appear to spontaneously clear their infections. Elevation of liver enzymes with few symptoms other than easy fatigability is the usual clinical picture. (Feigin:689–690)

57. (D) High fever without other signs and clearing of the fever on appearance of a rash are characteristic of roseola. In patients with measles, fever continues for several days after the appearance of the rash. The same is true for the several types of typhus. In infection with echovirus, the rash and fever usually appear together. The rash of juvenile rheumatoid arthritis is evanescent and often appears at the time of temperature elevation. (Rudolph:668–670,925)

58. (D) Immunization against the gonococcus has not been achieved. Currently, there is no effective vaccine (live or killed) against gonorrhea and no effective preparation of serum immune globulin. The organism is not a very potent antigen, and even naturally acquired infection does not confer immunity against subsequent infection. (Feigin:544)

59. (B) Herpangina is a syndrome characterized by small vesicles or punched-out ulcers on the tonsils and fauces, uvula, pharynx, and edge of soft palate. The remainder of the mouth and throat usually appear normal on examination. (Feigin:230–232)

60. (D) Herpangina is a specific syndrome (described above) that can be caused by a variety of viral agents. It was originally described in association with coxsackievirus, but it is now realized that echovirus and herpes simplex virus can cause an identical clinical picture. Despite the name herpangina, coxsackievirus is actually the most common cause. (Feigin:230–232; Hathaway:350,822)

61. (A) Since H. influenzae meningitis is most common in the first year or two of life and infrequent after age 4, prophylaxis of household contacts appears justified only if there are one or more high-risk (less than 4 years old) patients in the household. Under these circumstances, however, it is necessary to treat all household contacts in order to eradicate the organism from asymptomatic carriers. Prophylaxis should be provided regardless of immunization status. Incidentally, the patient also should receive rifampin, since treatment of the meningitis with other antibiotics will not eradicate the organism from the patient's oropharynx. (Feigin:2301)

62. (A) Neuritis is essentially the only neurologic complication seen with diphtheria. It almost always presents with paralysis, usually bilateral, rather than sensory changes. Paralysis of the soft palate is most common, but any muscle group may be involved. Involvement of the phrenic nerve can lead to paralysis of the diaphragm and the need for ventilatory support. Occasionally the symptoms can mimic Guillain-Barré syndrome. (Feigin:1113)

63. (D) The clinical and laboratory findings described are most suggestive of infectious mononucleosis from Epstein-Barr virus. Hepatic involvement evidenced by elevated serum transaminase levels is common, and false-positive serologic tests for syphilis occur occasionally with Epstein-Barr virus mononucleosis. (Rudolph:618,648–649)

64. (D) The clinical picture described is typical of herpes simplex keratoconjunctivitis. The associated vesicular lesions on the skin and the dendritic corneal ulcers are almost pathognomonic of this infection. It is important to diagnose herpes keratitis correctly because infection can be recurrent and lead to loss of vision, and because therapy is available. Topical trifluorothymidine (F_3T) is clearly effective. The value of topical acyclovir is questionable. (Feigin:850–853; Hathaway:306)

65. (C) A number of infants with acquired immunodeficiency syndrome (AIDS) have developed chronic Epstein-Barr (EB) virus infection. Chronic cytomegalovirus (CMV) infection also has been reported in these patients. Thrombocytopenia is seen occasionally; thrombocytosis has not been noted. Serum immunoglobulin levels tend to be increased, not depressed, and the ratio of CD4 to CD8 T cells is reversed rather than increased (Am J Dis Child 137:827,1983; Rudolph:472–473)

66. (B) The lowest concentration of serum immunoglobulin G is reached between 2 and 6 months of age. Essentially all of the serum immunoglobulin present at birth is transplacentally acquired maternal IgG, the half-life of which is about 25 days, so the newborn's serum level of 600 to 1,600 mg/dL falls rapidly during the first few months of life. The total IgG level then begins to rise as the infant's own rate of production comes to exceed the rate of destruction of the maternally transmitted immunoglobulin. (Rudolph:452)

67. (C) Upper lobe cavity disease is characteristic of reinfection or reactivation tuberculosis and is seen primarily in adults, occasionally in adolescents. Although progressive primary disease with cavitation can occur in children, it is rather uncommon and is randomly distributed with no predilection for the upper lobes. Fever, hilar adenopathy, and tuberculin hypersensitivity manifested by a positive tuberculin skin test are common findings in children with primary tuberculosis. (Feigin:1328–1334,1341–1342)

68. (D) Q fever usually is spread by inhalation, the other rickettsial disorders by arthropods. Typhus is spread by lice, scrub typhus and rickettsial pox by mites, and Rocky Mountain spotted fever by ticks. Q fever is also unique among rickettsioses in that it is not associated with a rash. *(Rudolph:697)*

69. (C) Although the list of complications of measles is remarkably long, arthritis is not on the list. Recognized complications include otitis media, pneumonia, laryngotracheitis, encephalitis, thrombocytopenia, hepatitis, and even appendicitis. *(Rudolph:678–679)*

70. (C) The rash of varicella is centripetal, with the heaviest concentration of lesions on the trunk rather than the extremities. Following an incubation period of 12 to 16 days there is the onset of a very pruritic rash, with crops of lesions that begin as papules and progress to vesicles. Fever usually is mild to moderate. *(Feigin:1588)*

71. (D) Congenital malformations, stillborns, and abortions all have been reported with rubella infection during pregnancy. Chronic infection of the fetus also occurs. These infants may continue to excrete rubella virus for years after birth. Infants with congenital rubella tend to be small for gestational age. *(Rudolph:688–690)*

72. (C) Myringitis bullosa has not been noted in the infectious mononucleosis syndrome. Petechiae or erythematous macules on the palate are not infrequent. A rash occurs occasionally. Fatigue is common. Airway obstruction secondary to markedly enlarged tonsils is an infrequent but important complication. *(Feigin:1549–1550)*

73. (C) Hepatosplenomegaly is not a usual feature of scarlet fever. The white strawberry tongue results when reddened, edematous papillae project through the white coating of the tongue in the first few days of infection. When the white coat peels off in the later part of the illness, the tongue takes on the red strawberry appearance. Exudative tonsillitis and erythematous punctate lesions on the palate are common features. *(Rudolph:615–616)*

74. (D) The rash of scarlet fever is red and finely papular, with a characteristic sandpaper-like texture. There is a tendency to desquamate, much as a sunburn does. Rather than sparing areas of skin folds, the rash actually is most intense in the creases of the axillae and groin (Pastia's sign). *(Rudolph:615–616)*

75. (D) Certain strains of staphylococci, especially those belonging to phage group II, elaborate a variety of soluble exotoxins that affect the skin. These toxins can result in a scarlatiniform eruption, a generalized exfoliative disease, toxic epidermal necrolysis (scalded skin syndrome), or a localized bullous impetigo. In the first three disorders, the *Staphylococcus* usually is cultured from a site other than the skin itself, the toxin being distributed through the circulation. In the case of bullous impetigo, the organism usually can be recovered from the lesions, and the toxin acts locally only. A papular pruritic rash has not been described. *(Feigin:1254)*

76. (D) The most common ophthalmologic abnormalities in congenital toxoplasmosis are inflammatory retinal lesions (chorioretinitis), which may be present at birth or show up years later. Cataracts and glaucoma are less common. Blindness may be related to these ophthalmologic abnormalities or have a central basis. There is no known association between toxoplasmosis and the congenital abnormality of aniridia. *(Rudolph:436,768)*

77. (B) The clinical signs and symptoms of acquired toxoplasmosis do not include arthritis. Fever, cervical lymphadenitis, and uveitis are common. Meningitis and encephalitis are less-common but well-recognized complications. Many cases of acquired toxoplasmosis are asymptomatic. *(Rudolph:768–769)*

78. (B) Autoimmune hemolytic anemia has not been reported in children or adults with AIDS. Low birth weight and failure to thrive are common, as are lymphadenopathy and hepatosplenomegaly. These children frequently are infected by opportunistic organisms such as *Pneumocystis carinii, Candida,* and *Mycobacterium avium,* as are adult AIDS victims. *(Rudolph:470–474;* Am J Dis Child *137:827,1983)*

79. (A) In primary pulmonary tuberculosis, cavitary lesions are clearly the exception rather than the rule. In adults, cavitary lesions result from activation of a dormant focus, almost always in an upper lobe. In children, these lesions result from a locally progressive primary infection, fortunately an uncommon event. Enlargement of regional (hilar) lymph nodes is a characteristic and important feature of primary tuberculosis in children. The enlarged nodes are generally directly evident by x-ray examination and, in addition, cause extrabronchial or, less commonly, endobronchial obstruction. Segmental lesions are common and usually result from a combination of obstruction and infection. Such lesions usually are unilateral but can be bilateral. Both the segmental lesions and the involved nodes may calcify during healing. *(Rudolph:626; Feigin:1332–1334)*

80. (C) Abnormal physical signs are found only infrequently on physical examination of the lungs of children with primary pulmonary tuberculosis, even when roentgenographic changes are extensive. Many patients are asymptomatic, and the disease is detected by routine tuberculin skin testing. Others may have fever or cough. As explained in the preceding question, hilar adenopathy on chest roentgeno-graph is common. *(Rudolph:626)*

81. **(C)** Tubercle bacilli usually are present in such small numbers in tuberculous pleural fluid that the smear is more likely to be negative than positive. In contrast, examination of pleural biopsy (needle or open) reveals tubercles and organisms in more than half the cases. The mechanism of formation of a tuberculous pleural effusion is believed to be a hypersensitivity reaction to a small pleural tuberculoma that has ruptured into the pleural space. The hypersensitivity reaction and subsequent effusion dilute the concentration of organisms so that positive smears are much less common than are positive cultures. The fluid usually is yellow, occasionally blood-tinged, and has an elevated specific gravity and protein concentration. The glucose concentration frequently is low but may be normal. Leukocytes often are the predominant cell initially but are soon replaced by lymphocytes. *(Rudolph:627; Feigin:1331–1332)*

82. **(C)** In children, the rash and fever of rubella generally begin together, or the rash may precede the fever by a day or two rather than vice versa. In adolescents and adults, however, the rash may be preceded by a few days of low-grade fever and malaise. Mild leukopenia and thrombocytopenia are common. Postauricular and occipital adenopathy are common and may precede the rash. The rash is characteristically pinkish red and maculopapular. *(Rudolph:687; Hathaway:840–841)*

83. **(B)** Coccidioidomycosis in the United States is essentially limited to the southwestern region. Histoplasmosis is worldwide in distribution, although it is especially endemic in the Ohio and Mississippi River valleys. The organisms of candidiasis and cryptococcosis are ubiquitous. *Yersinia enterocolitica* is widely distributed geographically with a predilection for colder climates. *(Rudolph:709; Feigin:1916–1917)*

84. **(E)** The prepubescent vaginal mucosa is much more susceptible to infection by *N. gonorrhoeae*, than the mature vagina. However, gonococcal infection in the prepubertal girl is usually restricted to the vulva and vagina and rarely spreads to the upper tract, presumably because the endocervical glands are not developed. *(Rudolph:580)*

85. **(C)** The rash of measles begins on the fourth or fifth day of clinical illness and lasts through day 8 or 9. *(Rudolph:677)*

86. **(A)** In patients with measles, fever appears on the first day of illness and lasts 5 or 6 days. *(Rudolph:677)*

87. **(D)** Cough is a prominent feature in measles and is present throughout most of the 10 days of clinical illness in measles. *(Rudolph:677)*

88. **(B)** Koplik's spots are diagnostic for measles. They are white dots or specks on a bright red areola that appear on the second or third day of illness, 1 or 2 days before the appearance of the rash, and last for 1 or 2 days. *(Rudolph:677)*

89. **(C)** Anemia is the major and usually the only clinical manifestation of hookworm infection. The two species of hookworm that inhabit the human intestines are *Necator americanus* and *Ancylostoma duodenale*. *(Rudolph:722–723)*

90. **(A)** Hepatomegaly is one of the common manifestations of human infection with *Toxocara canis*, the dog tapeworm. Ingested embryonated eggs hatch in the small intestine, where larvae penetrate the villi and migrate throughout the body. Since the parasite cannot mature in the human host, the larvae migrate about the body for a prolonged period (visceral larva migrans), and there are no adult intestinal worms. *(Rudolph:719)*

91. **(D)** Children heavily infected with *Trichuris trichiura* develop chronic diarrhea, tenesmus, and rectal prolapse. Rectal prolapse is not characteristically associated with any other parasitic infection. *(Rudolph:725)*

92. **(E)** Pruritus of the rectum or perianal region is the most common manifestation of pinworm infection (*Enterobius vermicularis*). Adult, sexually mature worms migrate from the cecum to the rectum. Females exit the rectum and deposit their eggs in the perianal skin, where they induce a reaction that is usually pruritic, occasionally painful. Rarely, a worm may migrate into the vagina, with resultant discharge and pain. *(Rudolph:721–722)*

93. **(C)** *Spirillum minus* and *Streptobacillus moniliformis* are the two organisms that cause rat bite fever, an acute illness characterized by intermittent fever, rash, and adenitis. In the case of *Spirillum minus*, there generally is an indurated lesion that develops at the site of the bite. Cases have been transmitted by mouse bites. *(Rudolph:599)*

94. **(A)** *Pasteurella multocida* causes a variety of infections in the human host. The organism is frequently found in the oral flora of dogs and cats, and one of the most common forms of human disease is localized infection following a dog or cat bite. There is nothing clinically unique about such infections—local swelling, erythema, and tenderness, with or without fever and local lymphadenitis. *(Feigin:1205–1208)*

95. **(D)** Two species of *Chlamydia*, *C. psittaci* and *C. trachomatis*, are known to cause pneumonia in children. The former, which today is less common, is carried and spread to humans by birds, including pi-

geons and parakeets. Although the infected birds often are clinically ill, they may be asymptomatic. *(Feigin:267)*

96. **(B)** *Bordetella pertussis* is easily spread by respiratory droplets. Infected children (or adults) frequently transmit the disease to nonimmunized infants and younger siblings. *Chlamydia trachomatis*, in contrast, usually is acquired by newborn infants by passage through infected genital tracts. *(Rudolph:595)*

97. **(D)** Neither *B. pertussis* infection nor *C. trachomatis* infection is characteristically associated with fever. In fact, the original descriptions of *C. trachomatis* pneumonia in young infants referred to it as the afebrile pneumonia syndrome. *(Rudolph:572,595–596, 1537–1538)*

98. **(A)** Eosinophilia of more than 400 eosinophils per cubic millimeter is seen very commonly in infants with pneumonia caused by *C. trachomatis*, especially during the later stages of the infection. Lymphocytosis, both relative and absolute, is characteristic of infection with *B. pertussis*. Eosinophilia is not characteristic of pertussis syndrome. [*Note:* Although eosinophilia is uncommon in infants with conjunctivitis with *C. trachomatis*, the question does specify "pulmonary infection."] *(Rudolph:572)*

99. **(C)** The newborn infant, even the premature infant, is entirely capable of synthesizing both IgG and IgM (and IgA, as well), although the rates of production normally are low because in the sterile environment in utero there is no stimulus to produce IgG or IgM. *(Rudolph:451–453)*

100. **(A)** IgG is the only class of immunoglobulin to cross the placenta in significant and measurable amounts. *(Rudolph:451–453)*

101. **(A)** Normal serum concentration of IgG during the first year of life is well over 250 mg/dL, although the concentration may occasionally drop as low as 200 mg/dL at the physiologic nadir, sometime between 2 and 6 months of life. In contrast, IgM concentrations do not normally exceed 150 or 200 mg/dL. *(Rudolph:451–453)*

102. **(B)** IgG is always present in cord blood in large amounts, whereas the level of IgM varies from undetectable to 30 mg/dL. *(Rudolph:451–453)*

103. **(C)** Both immunoglobulin G and immunoglobulin M are important for resistance to bacterial infections. *(Rudolph:451–453)*

104. **(C)** Trismus is seen both with tetanus and with rabies. It is more common with tetanus, in which disease it tends to be persistent, while in rabies it is intermittent. *(Rudolph:621–624,684–686)*

105. **(B)** True paralysis may be seen in patients with rabies. In tetanus, severe muscle spasm may prevent voluntary motion, but true paralysis is not seen. (On rare occasions, however, true paralysis has been reported following antitoxin administration.) *(Rudolph:621–624,684–686)*

106. **(A)** The mortality rate in tetanus is about 50%, and in some centers is considerably lower. Rabies, on the other, is almost always fatal; mortality rates in most series are 100%. *(Rudolph:621–624,684–686)*

107. **(C)** Generalized convulsions are seen in both tetanus and rabies. In patients with tetanus, the convulsions are primarily spinal in origin rather than central. *(Rudolph:621–624,684–686)*

108. **(A)** Tetanus is a well-recognized complication of drug abuse. It is especially common in addicts who engage in the practice of "skin popping." Rabies has not been reported in association with drug abuse, although it has been suggested that human-to-human spread of this infection is possible. *(Rudolph:621–624, 684–686)*

109. **(A)** Cough, coryza, and conjunctivitis are prominent features of measles. Cough is not a feature of rubella. Coryza and conjunctivitis are frequent in rubella but usually are mild. *(Feigin:1597–1599,1800–1806; Rudolph:676–680,686–690)*

110. **(C)** A rash or exanthem occurs in both measles and German measles. The rash of measles consists of erythematous macules that eventually become confluent. The rash begins on the head, spreads to the rest of the body within 3 or 4 days, and takes another 3 or 4 days to fade. The rash of rubella also begins on the head but spreads more rapidly and lasts only a few days. *(Feigin:1597–1599,1800–1806; Rudolph:676–680, 686–690)*

111. **(C)** An enanthem occurs in both diseases. In measles the enanthem consists of small, irregular red spots with white centers. These are the pathognomonic Koplik's spots, which are found on the buccal and labial mucosa. In rubella, one finds reddish spots of various sizes on the soft palate. *(Feigin:1597–1599, 1800–1806; Rudolph:676–680,686–690)*

112. **(A)** Rubella generally is a much milder disease than measles. High fever is the rule in measles, but it is rare in rubella. Children with measles generally appear ill. Children with rubella usually appear well. *(Feigin:1597–1599,1800–1806; Rudolph:676–680,686–690)*

113. **(A)** Secondary bacterial infection occurs frequently in measles but is not seen in rubella. The most com-

mon bacterial infections in children with measles are otitis media and pneumonia. *(Feigin:1597–1599, 1800–1806; Rudolph:676–680,686–690)*

114. **(B)** Arthralgia or arthritis is commonly seen in adolescents and adults with rubella but less frequently in children with this disease. Joint involvement is not seen in measles. *(Feigin:1597–1599,1800–1806; Rudolph:676–680,686–690)*

115. **(A)** Encephalitis occurs in about 0.1% of patients with measles and is severe and often fatal. Rubella encephalopathy, in contrast, occurs in only 1 in 6,000 cases and generally is mild, with complete recovery being the rule. *(Feigin:1597–1599,1800–1806; Rudolph: 676–680,686–690)*

116. **(C)** A live attenuated vaccine is available and is in use for both rubella and measles. Current routine practice involves administration of a combined vaccine [mumps-measles-rubella (MMR)] at 15 months. *(Feigin:1597–1599,1800–1806;Rudolph:676–680,686–690)*

117. **(C)** Both viral hepatitis A and B often are associated with anorexia, nausea, and abdominal pain, which usually precede the jaundice. *(Rudolph:671–675)*

118. **(C)** It is now clear that nonparenteral transmission plays an important role in the spread of hepatitis B virus as well as hepatitis A virus. Hepatitis B is especially common among workers in dialysis units and is endemic in Asia and Africa. *(Rudolph:671–675)*

119. **(B)** Chronic hepatitis may follow infection with either hepatitis B or non-A, non-B but has not been documented following hepatitis A. In one series, about 10% of patients with acute hepatitis B developed chronic hepatitis. Of these, about two-thirds had chronic *persistent* disease, and one-third had chronic *active* disease. *(Rudolph:671–675)*

120. **(C)** Most cases of both hepatitis A and B actually are subclinical (asymptomatic), recognized only by elevated serum transaminases or serologic evidence of infection. In addition, a substantial percentage of cases of hepatitis A and B have findings such as nausea and vomiting, fever, and, often, an enlarged and tender liver, but without any overt jaundice. These cases are referred to as anicteric rather than subclinical. *(Rudolph:671–675)*

121. **(C)** Both hepatitis A and hepatitis B infections tend to be less severe in children than in adults. The percentage of cases that are subclinical or anicteric is higher in children. Fulminant hepatitis is less frequent in children than in adolescents or adults. *(Rudolph:671–675)*

122. **(C)** Both hereditary agammaglobulinemia (also referred to as hereditary hypogammaglobulinemia)

and thymic dysplasia (severe combined immunodeficiency) may be transmitted as X-linked defects. Thymic dysplasia, however, also is transmitted in some families as an autosomal recessive disorder. *(Rudolph:393)*

123. **(D)** Neither agammaglobulinemia nor thymic *dysplasia* is associated with hypocalcemia. Thymic dysplasia should not be confused with congenital *aplasia* or absence of the thymus (DiGeorge's syndrome), which is associated with aplasia of the parathyroid glands and resultant hypocalcemia as well as defects in cellular immunity. *(Rudolph:458–460,463–466)*

124. **(D)** Both hereditary agammaglobulinemia and severe combined immunodeficiency are characterized by a paucity of lymphoid tissue. Enlarged lymph nodes are not part of the clinical picture of either hereditary agammaglobulinemia or combined immunodeficiency. Indeed, palpable lymph nodes are rare in children with either disorder. *(Rudolph:458–460, 463–466)*

125. **(B)** About 25% of children with severe combined immunodeficiency have an associated deficiency of adenosine deaminase (ADA), an important enzyme in lymphocyte function. The ADA deficiency is inherited as an autosomal recessive, permitting both heterozygote detection and prenatal diagnosis by amniocentesis. *(J Pediatr 91:48–51,1977; Rudolph:458–460, 463–466)*

126. **(B)** Because of the defect in cellular immunity in patients with thymic dysplasia, skin grafts are not rejected as they are by normal individuals or by those with simple agammaglobulinemia and intact cellular immunity. *(Rudolph:458–460,463–466)*

127. **(A)** Patients with isolated agammaglobulinemia respond fairly well to treatment with gamma-globulin and antibiotics and generally will survive well into adulthood. On the other hand, patients with combined immunodeficiency usually succumb to infections by *Pneumocystis carinii*, fungi, and viruses in early childhood despite these measures. Marrow transplant from a matched sibling donor has been successful in reconstituting some of these patients, permitting long-term survival. *(Rudolph:458–460,463–466)*

128. **(A)** Standard immunization practice calls for three injections of diphtheria-pertussis-tetanus (DPT) vaccine at 2-month intervals during the first year of life. *(Rudolph:32–37)*

129. **(A)** Trivalent oral polio vaccine (TOP) generally is administered two or three times during the first year of life. The third dose is optional and is not intended as a booster but rather to insure a "take" by all three strains of the attenuated virus. *(Rudolph:32–37)*

130. (B) Measles vaccine is best given at 15 months, usually as a combined live vaccine (MMR). If it is given before the age of 15 months, some patients will fail to seroconvert because of persistence of maternally derived immunoglobulins. However, in epidemics, monovalent measles vaccine is given as early as 6 months. *(Rudolph:32–37)*

131. (B) Administration of rubella vaccine also is recommended after 15 months of life and routinely is given combined with measles and mumps vaccines (MMR). *(Rudolph:32–37)*

132. (D) Killed measles vaccine is no longer routinely used for immunization of healthy children, although it is useful for certain immunologically abnormal children, including children with leukemia. The question specified for normal children. *(Rudolph:32–37)*

133. (C) An effective Hib conjugate vaccine is now available for routine use in the first year of life, with a booster dose at 12 to 15 months depending on the strain of vaccine used. *(Rudolph:32–37; Pediatrics 88: 169–172,1991)*

BIBLIOGRAPHY

AAP Committee on Infectious Diseases. *Haemophilus influenzae* type b conjugate vaccines: recommendations for immunization of infants and children 2 months of age and older: update. *Pediatrics.* 1991;88:169–172.

Feigin RD, Cherry JD. *Textbook of Pediatric Infectious Diseases.* 3rd ed. Philadelphia, Pa: WB Saunders; 1992.

Hathaway WE, Groothius JR, Hay WW, et al. *Current Pediatric Diagnosis & Treatment.* 10th ed. Norwalk, Conn: Appleton & Lange; 1991.

Litt IF, Finberg L. Gonorrhea in children and adolescents. *J Pediatr.* 1974;85:595–607.

Rubenstein A. Acquired immunodeficiency syndrome in infants. *Am J Dis Child* 1983;137:825–827.

Rudolph AM, Hoffman JIE, Rudolph CD. *Pediatrics.* 19th ed. Norwalk, Conn: Appleton & Lange; 1991.

Schmalstieg FC, Nelson A, Mills GC. Increased purine nucleotides in adenosine deaminase-deficient lymphocytes. *J Pediatr.* 1977;91:48–51.

CHAPTER 7

Metabolic Disorders (Including Fluid and Electrolytes)
Questions

Acquired metabolic problems such as fluid and electrolyte disturbances are frequent in infants and children. Diarrhea and vomiting are very common in this age group and often lead to dehydration and/or electrolyte problems. Hypoglycemia and hypocalcemia are relatively common in the newborn but uncommon thereafter. Electrolyte problems may occur secondary to disease (renal failure, cystic fibrosis), therapy (diuretics), or environmental factors (inadvertent substitution of salt for sugar in infant feeding).

Although individual inborn metabolic errors are rare, the sum total of all known such errors is not rare. Additionally, inborn metabolic errors are such classic pediatric diseases that they usually appear on examinations more frequently than would be justified on the basis of their incidence alone. Trying to "learn" all the recognized inborn metabolic errors would be an impossible task for the student and a formidable task for the pediatric resident. It would be better for the reader to focus on a few of the more important defects in each area of metabolism (eg, carbohydrate, amino acids, urea cycle) than to attempt to review all described defects.

DIRECTIONS (Question 1 through 43): Each of the numbered items or incomplete statements in this section is followed by answers or by completions of the statement. Select the ONE lettered answer or completion that is BEST in each case.

1. Maintenance fluid requirement for an infant or child

   (A) is 150 mL per kilogram body weight
   (B) is 100 mL per kilogram body weight
   (C) is 50 mL per kilogram body weight
   (D) is 20 mL per kilogram body weight
   (E) cannot be calculated simply on a weight basis

2. What is the approximate daily basal caloric expenditure of a 5-kg infant?

   (A) 1,000 calories
   (B) 750 calories
   (C) 500 calories
   (D) 250 calories
   (E) 50 calories

3. What is the estimated usual fluid requirement per 100 calories expended?

   (A) 25 mL
   (B) 50 mL
   (C) 100 mL
   (D) 150 mL
   (E) 250 mL

4. What is the basal daily fluid requirement for a 5-kg infant?

   (A) 1,000 mL
   (B) 750 mL
   (C) 500 mL
   (D) 250 mL
   (E) 100 mL

5. What is the approximate fluid requirement of a 25-kg child?

   (A) 2,400 mL
   (B) 2,100 mL
   (C) 1,600 mL
   (D) 1,200 mL
   (E) 900 mL

6. What is the normal daily fluid requirement of a 12-kg child?

(A) 1,400 mL
(B) 1,100 mL
(C) 800 mL
(D) 650 mL
(E) 400 mL

7. What is the approximate daily fluid maintenance requirement of a 50-kg child?

(A) 3,000 mL
(B) 2,600 mL
(C) 2,100 mL
(D) 1,600 mL
(E) 1,200 mL

8. Ordinarily, insensible water loss is in the order of

(A) 10 mL/100 calories expended
(B) 20 mL/100 calories expended
(C) 45 mL/100 calories expended
(D) 70 mL/100 calories expended
(E) 90 mL/100 calories expended

9. A reasonable estimate of the amount of water required for renal excretion of metabolic wastes per 100 calories expended is

(A) less than 10 mL
(B) 10 to 20 mL
(C) 30 to 40 mL
(D) 50 to 70 mL
(E) 80 to 100 mL

10. Normal daily sodium requirement per 100 calories expended is

(A) less than 1 mEq
(B) about 1 mEq
(C) about 3 mEq
(D) about 10 mEq
(E) about 25 mEq

11. An 8-kg infant taking no oral feedings, receiving maintenance intravenous fluids, and having no unusual fluid or electrolyte losses will need how much potassium daily?

(A) None
(B) 2 mEq
(C) 10 mEq
(D) 20 mEq
(E) 35 mEq

12. A 9-kg infant with diarrhea appears moderately dehydrated, with poor skin turgor and decreased urine output. The patient, however, is not in shock. The fluid deficit in this child is probably in the order of

(A) 1,900 to 2,000 mL
(B) 1,400 to 1,500 mL

(C) 900 to 1,000 mL
(D) 400 to 500 mL
(E) 200 to 250 mL

13. You are treating a 7-month-old with dehydration secondary to diarrhea. The serum sodium is reported as 185 mEq/L. At this point you should plan to

(A) correct the hypernatremia slowly
(B) administer a hypertonic glucose solution
(C) use a sodium-free solution
(D) administer mannitol
(E) all of the above

14. A 15-month-old infant with diarrhea and moderately severe dehydration would most likely have which of the following sets of arterial values?

(A) pH 7.40; $PaCO_2$ 40; HCO_3^- 24 mEq/L
(B) pH 7.50; $PaCO_2$ 40; HCO_3^- 31 mEq/L
(C) pH 7.10; $PaCO_2$ 60; HCO_3^- 17 mEq/L
(D) pH 7.20; $PaCO_2$ 50; HCO_3^- 17 mEq/L
(E) pH 7.25; $PaCO_2$ 30; HCO_3^- 14 mEq/L

15. Normal serum osmolality is between

(A) 250 and 260 mOsm/L
(B) 285 and 295 mOsm/L
(C) 300 and 310 mOsm/L
(D) 315 and 325 mOsm/L
(E) 330 and 350 mOsm/L

16. Which of the following conditions is most likely to produce polyuria with isotonic or hypertonic urine?

(A) Central diabetes insipidus
(B) Nephrogenic diabetes insipidus
(C) Potassium deficiency
(D) Diabetes mellitus
(E) Hypercalcemia

17. Which of the following is an important cause of death in children and young adults with homocystinuria?

(A) Sepsis
(B) Renal failure
(C) Bowel obstruction
(D) Hepatic carcinoma
(E) Thromboembolic phenomena

18. Of the following glycogenoses (glycogen storage disorders), which has the best prognosis?

(A) Type Ia (von Gierke's disease)
(B) Type Ib (glucose-6-phosphatase microsomal transport defect)
(C) Type II (Pompe's disease)
(D) Type III (debranching enzyme deficiency)
(E) Type IV (brancher enzyme deficiency)

19. The major clinical manifestation of galactokinase deficiency is

(A) cataracts
(B) early neonatal death
(C) hypoglycemia
(D) jaundice
(E) seizures

20. Infants with galactosemia become symptomatic

(A) only if fed cow milk
(B) only if fed breast milk
(C) if fed either cow milk or breast milk
(D) only if fed glucose
(E) if fed glucose, cow milk, or breast milk

21. A child with diabetic ketoacidosis has the following serum values: glucose 1,000 mg/dL; Na^+ 120 mEq/L; K^+ 4 mEq/L; Cl^- 80 mEq/L; HCO_3^- 15 mEq/L; BUN 16 mg/dL. The patient's serum osmolality probably is about

(A) 210 mOsm/L
(B) 230 mOsm/L
(C) 250 mOsm/L
(D) 290 mOsm/L
(E) 320 mOsm/L

22. The onset of insulin-dependent diabetes mellitus (IDDM) in childhood

(A) is unusual
(B) is usually abrupt
(C) is rarely accompanied by ketoacidosis
(D) should suggest the possibility of Cushing's syndrome
(E) usually is associated with the multiple endocrinopathy syndrome

23. An infant with galactosemia is likely to present with

(A) heart failure
(B) severe anemia
(C) a musty odor to the urine
(D) glycosuria and dehydration
(E) jaundice, vomiting, and hepatomegaly

24. The typical course of untreated classic maple syrup urine disease is

(A) death within hours of birth
(B) death within the first weeks of life
(C) death between 2 and 5 years of age
(D) severe mental retardation, with death by 10 years of age
(E) severe mental retardation, but with a normal life expectancy

25. Routine screening of newborns for phenylketonuria is

(A) impractical
(B) practical, but seldom done
(C) required by law in all states
(D) done by request (parent or physician)
(E) presently done only in large medical centers

26. Phenylketonuria is best treated by

(A) a low-protein diet
(B) a diet low in phenylalanine
(C) a diet high in phenylalanine
(D) a diet low in phenylalanine and tyrosine
(E) a diet high in tyrosine and low in phenylalanine

27. Type IIa glycogenosis, Pompe's disease, is characterized by

(A) mitral valve prolapse
(B) the absence of cardiac involvement
(C) mitral regurgitation and death in adolescence
(D) systolic ejection murmur without heart failure
(E) cardiomegaly, congestive heart failure, and death in infancy

28. An infant with elevated serum cholesterol and without clinical disease should be evaluated for

(A) biliary atresia
(B) cystic fibrosis
(C) intestinal lymphangiectasia
(D) type II familial hypercholesterolemia

29. An infant with fat malabsorption, acanthosis of the red blood cells, and ataxia probably has

(A) abetalipoproteinemia
(B) ataxia-telangiectasia
(C) cystic fibrosis
(D) pancreatic pseudocyst
(E) vitamin B_{12} deficiency

30. Type I Gaucher's disease is characterized by splenomegaly or hepatosplenomegaly without nervous system involvement. The diagnosis should be suspected by the finding of

(A) increased serum lipids
(B) decreased serum lipids
(C) increased serum alkaline phosphatase
(D) increased serum acid phosphatase
(E) hypercalcemia

31. You are evaluating a 10-month-old child for recurrent fractures following relatively minor trauma. You note deep blue sclera and bowing of the lower extremities. X-ray examination reveals generalized osteopenia. The child probably has

(A) achondroplasia
(B) histiocytosis X
(C) osteogenesis imperfecta
(D) osteopetrosis
(E) rickets

32. Pyruvate kinase deficiency is a cause of

(A) hereditary muscle weakness
(B) hereditary nonspherocytic hemolytic anemia
(C) cardiomyopathy
(D) mental retardation
(E) hepatic fibrosis

33. The most common presenting sign of Wilson's disease in children less than 8 years old is

(A) convulsions
(B) cirrhosis of the liver
(C) arthritis
(D) ataxia
(E) psychosis

34. An approximation of normal daily fluid requirement based on body surface area would be about

(A) 500 to 1,000 mL/m^2
(B) 1,000 to 1,500 mL/m^2
(C) 1,500 to 2,000 mL/m^2
(D) 2,000 to 2,500 mL/m^2
(E) 2,500 to 3,000 mL/m^2

35. An infant with diarrhea is 10% dehydrated. Before the onset of illness, the weight was 5 kg, and the surface area 0.3 m^2. The child's serum sodium concentration is normal. Assume that the child will not be fed, that the diarrhea will stop, and that you wish to restore the child to a state of normal hydration in the first 24 hours. The total intravenous fluid requirement for the first 24 hours would be approximately

(A) 750 mL
(B) 1,000 mL
(C) 1,250 mL
(D) 1,500 mL
(E) 1,750 mL

36. Hypokalemic alkalosis is most likely to be seen in which of the following conditions?

(A) Chronic renal failure
(B) Renal tubular acidosis
(C) Hypernatremic dehydration
(D) Hypertrophic pyloric stenosis
(E) Congenital adrenal hyperplasia

37. Hypoglycemia of infancy and childhood is most usefully classified into hyperinsulinemic and normoinsulinemic states. Which of the following is an example of a normoinsulinemic cause of hypoglycemia?

(A) Beta-cell hyperplasia
(B) Neisidioblastosis
(C) Ketotic hypoglycemia
(D) Tolbutamide ingestion

38. A child receiving primaquine for malaria suddenly develops jaundice and anemia. The child probably has

(A) sickle beta-thalassemia
(B) hemoglobin S-C disease
(C) pyruvate kinase deficiency
(D) an autoimmune hemolytic anemia
(E) glucose-6-phosphate dehydrogenase deficiency

39. One of the most striking features in children with Lesch-Nyhan syndrome is

(A) blindness
(B) multiple xanthomas
(C) proptosis
(D) self-destructive biting
(E) variegated hair color

Please note the use of a negative qualifier such as EXCEPT, LEAST, or NOT in each of the following questions (Questions 40 through 43).

40. Hereditary fructose intolerance is **associated with all** of the following EXCEPT

(A) diarrhea
(B) vomiting
(C) hypoglycemia
(D) hepatomegaly
(E) a deficiency of hepatic fructose-1-phosphate aldolase

41. Metabolic abnormalities in diabetes mellitus include all of the following EXCEPT

(A) reduced entry of glucose into the cell
(B) increased glycogenolysis
(C) increased oxidation of fatty acids
(D) decreased gluconeogenesis from amino acids
(E) increased production of ketones

42. In monitoring the home control of children with IDDM, which of the following is LEAST important?

(A) Frequent blood glucose measurements
(B) Frequent urine glucose measurements
(C) Periodic measurements of glycosylated hemoglobin
(D) Avoidance of episodes of ketoacidosis
(E) Avoidance of episodes of hypoglycemia

43. Of the following, which is LEAST likely in an infant with absent hepatic glucose-6-phosphatase activity?

(A) Hepatomegaly
(B) Jaundice
(C) Hypoglycemia
(D) Episodes of metabolic acidosis
(E) Hyperlipidemia

DIRECTIONS (44 through 47): Each set of matching questions in this section consists of a list of 4 to 26 lettered options followed by several numbered items. For each numbered item select the ONE lettered option with which it is most closely associated. Each lettered option may be selected once, more than once, or not at all.

Questions 44 through 47

(A) Phenylalanine hydroxylase deficiency
(B) Tyrosinase deficiency
(C) Cystathionine synthetase deficiency
(D) Branched-chain ketoacid decarboxylase deficiency

44. Ectopia lentis, thromboemboli, and mental retardation

45. Reports of intrauterine damage (mental retardation) of heterozygotic infants born to homozygotic mothers

46. Albinism

47. Urinary odor, coma, flaccidity, opisthotonos, and death

DIRECTIONS (Questions 48 through 51): Each group of items in this section consists of lettered headings followed by a set of numbered words or phrases. For each numbered word or phrase, select

    A if the item is associated with (A) <u>only</u>,
    B if the item is associated with (B) <u>only</u>,
    C if the item is associated with <u>both</u> (A) <u>and</u> (B),
    D if the item is associated with <u>neither</u> (A) <u>nor</u> (B).

Questions 48 through 51

(A) Porphyrias
(B) Urea cycle disorders
(C) Both
(D) Neither

48. Genetic enzyme deficiency or abnormality

49. Hyperammonemia

50. Neurologic manifestations

51. Dermatitis

Answers and Explanations

1. **(E)** Fluid requirements in children cannot be related simply to body weight but must be related to metabolic rate in one way or another. If one were to use a single figure per kilogram of body weight to estimate maintenance fluid requirements, one would either drown the older child or dehydrate the younger one. For example, 100 mL/kg would be appropriate for a 4-kg infant (400 mL) but would be excessive for a 60-kg older child (6,000 mL). Similarly, 35 mL/kg would be appropriate for the 60-kg child (2,900 mL), but insufficient (140 mL) for the 4-kg infant. There are a variety of equally satisfactory methods for calculating maintenance fluid requirements based on surface area, caloric expenditure, or a combination of weight and age. The calculations in the following questions are based, generally, on the caloric method. Some questions based on surface area are included because it is also a popular approach to fluid problems. *(Hathaway:1068–1069; Rudolph:229–231)*

2. **(C)** The smaller the subject, the greater the surface area-to-weight ratio and, consequently, the higher the basal metabolic rate. Infants require more calories per unit of body weight than adults. Infants weighing between 3 and 10 kg require approximately 100 calories per kilogram. A 5-kg infant thus has a basal requirement of about 500 calories. *(Rudolph:230)*

3. **(C)** The usual (average) figure for daily fluid requirement is approximately 100 mL of fluid per 100 calories expended. This value of (100 mL per 100 calories) is employed in *maintenance* fluids for infants and children. It cannot be used for calculating fluid losses or deficits, which must be calculated on the basis of body weight, since *deficit* relates to body mass not to surface area or metabolic rate. *(Rudolph:230; Hathaway:1068)*

4. **(C)** Infants weighing less than 10 kg expend an average of 100 calories per kilogram of body weight. A 5-kg infant thus has a basal caloric requirement of 500 calories. The infant needs about 100 mL of water per 100 calories metabolized and, therefore, has a maintenance requirement of about 100 mL of fluid.

Since it happens that fluid requirement is 1 mL per calorie, the calorie is conveniently omitted from the calculation of fluid requirements, but the concept is important in understanding that fluid needs of an infant or child cannot be calculated as for an adult. *(Hathaway:1068; Rudolph:230)*

5. **(C)** One advantage of the caloric method of calculating maintenance fluids is that it does not require the use of tables or nomograms. The clinician need only remember three figures: 100 calories per kilogram for the first 10 kg of body weight, 50 calories per kilogram for between 10 and 20 kg, and 20 calories per kilogram for more than 20 kg. For the first 10 kg of body weight, the child in question needs 100 calories per kilogram, or 100 mL/kg (10 kg × 100 mL/kg = 1,000 mL). For the second 10 kg of weight, he needs 50 mL/kg, or 500 mL. For the next 5 kg, he needs 20 mL/kg; 20 mL/kg × 5 kg = 100 mL. His total fluid requirement, therefore, is 1,000 mL + 500 mL + 100 mL = 1,600 mL. *(Hathaway:1068–1069; Rudolph:230–231)*

6. **(B)** The fluid requirement could be calculated by figuring 100 mL per 100 calories or per kilogram for the first 10 kg of body weight, plus 50 mL/kg for the remaining 2 kg of body weight. Thus, 100 mL/kg × 10 kg = 1,000 mL plus 50 mL/kg × 2 kg = 100 mL, giving a total of 1,100 mL. Notice that this 12-kg child requires much more than half of the requirement of the 25-kg child in the preceding question. *(Hathaway:1068–1069; Rudolph:230–231)*

7. **(C)** For the first 10 kg, 10 kg × 100 mL/kg = 1,000 mL. For the next 10 kg, 10 kg × 50 mL/kg = 500 mL. For the remainder of body weight, 30 kg × 20 mL/kg = 600 mL. Adding these together, 1,000 mL + 500 mL + 600 mL = 2,100 mL, or approximately 2,000 mL. Notice that this 50-kg child does not require twice as much fluid as the 25-kg child in question 5. *(Hathaway:1068–1069; Rudolph:230–231)*

8. **(C)** Ordinarily, insensible water loss is about 45 mL per 100 calories expended, or just about half of basal fluid turnover. Insensible loss is from the skin and respiratory tract and is increased by fever and tachy-

pnea. Unlike urine output, insensible water loss is obligatory and cannot be significantly decreased, even in the face of dehydration and hypovolemia. *(Kempe:1072; Rudolph:196)*

9. **(D)** An allowance of 50 to 75 mL of water per 100 calories is a reasonable estimate for the amount of fluid required for renal excretion of the products of metabolism. This figure permits the excretion of minerals and metabolic wastes without exceeding the kidneys' ability to concentrate or dilute the urine. *(Rudolph: 230)*

10. **(C)** The normal sodium requirement is about 3 mEq per 100 calories expended. Therefore, the child needs approximately 3 mEq of sodium per 100 mL of maintenance fluid, or 30 mEq per liter. This allows for ordinary excretion of sodium in the urine. Sodium loss in the sweat can vary enormously depending on body temperature, ambient temperature, and level of physical activity. *(Rudolph:230)*

11. **(D)** Normal potassium requirements are slightly less than those for sodium, about 2.5 mEq per 100 calories. For an 8-kg infant, this would amount to 8 mEq × 2.5 mEq = 20 mEq. [*Note:* The question asked for a total amount of potassium, not a concentration or a value per kilogram of body weight. It is not uncommon to lose credit for a question by misreading the terms, for example here, to jump to 2 mEq **(B)** misread as 2 mEq/kg.] *(Rudolph: 230)*

12. **(C)** The infant described probably is about 10% dehydrated. In an infant, mild dehydration is about 5%, moderate dehydration about 10%, and severe dehydration about 15% of body weight. (For an older child or adult, comparable figures would be 3%, 6%, and 9%.) Roughly, 10% × 9 kg = 900 mL. To be more precise, however, the deficit should be calculated on the premorbid weight. Since the child is 10% dehydrated and now weighs 9 kg, weight before dehydration can be calculated: wt pre – (wt pre × % dehydration) = wt current; or wt pre × (1 – % dehydration) = wt current; or wt pre = 9/0.09 = 10 kg. The deficit, therefore, is 10% of 10 kg, or 1,000 mL. The deficit also can be calculated as 10 kg – 9 kg = 1 kg or 1,000 mL. [*Note:* Deficit is not the same as total requirement. Daily total fluid requirement is the sum of deficit plus maintenance plus any ongoing abnormal losses. The examinee must interpret all terms precisely.] *(Rudolph:230–231)*

13. **(A)** The chief problem during the treatment of hypernatremic dehydration is the shift of water into the brain, causing cerebral edema and seizures. The key to successful management is *slow* correction of the serum sodium (over 48 hours or more). This generally entails the use of a low-sodium solution, 25 to 40 mEq/L, administered slowly. The use of a sodium-free solution is dangerous and contraindicated. The

addition of 5% glucose to the solution ensures at least isotonicity with plasma. There is no need for hypertonic glucose or mannitol. *(N Engl J Med 289:196–198,1973; Rudolph:231–232; Oski:62)*

14. **(E)** Several factors combine to produce acidosis in the infant with diarrheal dehydration. Diarrheal stools have a high concentration of bicarbonate, often more than 40 mEq/L. The relative caloric deprivation often present in these situations engenders ketosis. The hypovolemia that is part of the dehydration results in decreased renal perfusion and decreased glomerular filtration. This, in turn, causes retention of metabolic acid wastes. Thus, the infant with diarrhea and dehydration usually has a metabolic acidosis (low serum bicarbonate) and a compensatory respiratory alkalosis (low $PaCO_2$). Choices **(C)** and **(D)** represent combined metabolic and respiratory acidosis and therefore are incorrect. *(Rudolph:228–230)*

15. **(B)** Serum osmolality normally is between 285 and 295 mOsm/L with a maximal range of 275 to 300. Generally, serum osmolality is equal to approximately twice the sodium concentration. Glucose and urea, however, also contribute to serum osmolality. In situations where either of these constituents is appreciably elevated, serum sodium alone is not an accurate estimate of serum osmolality. [*Note:* "Normal" is used here in the literal sense, as usual or average, and not as the chemical term denoting 1 gram equivalent or mole per liter.] *(Rudolph:1228)*

16. **(D)** Polyuria with dilute (hypotonic) urine is seen in a variety of conditions associated with an inability to concentrate the urine (hyposthenuria). These include diabetes insipidus (both central and nephrogenic), chronic potassium deficiency, hypercalcemia, and some cases of renal cystic disease. In contrast, in diabetes mellitus the polyuria results from an osmotic diuresis and is associated with an isotonic or moderately hypertonic urine. *(Rudolph:1240)*

17. **(E)** Thromboembolic phenomena, both arterial and venous, with occlusion of coronary, renal, and cerebral vessels, have been well documented in patients with homocystinuria. Routine tests of clotting function are normal, but platelets from these patients are unusually adhesive. *(Rudolph:310)*

18. **(D)** Patients with type III glycogen storage disease (debranching enzyme deficiency) have a relatively good long-term prognosis. Most improve progressively with age (in regard to liver function), and many become asymptomatic by puberty, although some have shown progressive myopathy in later years. Many patients with types Ia and Ib glycogen storage disease die during the first 2 years of life from ketoacidosis or other complications. Those with type II disease (Pompe's disease) generally die in

early infancy of cardiac failure because of the involvement of cardiac muscles. The juvenile form (type IIb) is milder, but most children still die from muscle failure in the first decade of life. Those with type IV (brancher enzyme deficiency) disease also usually die in the first decade of life from hepatic cirrhosis. *(Rudolph:331–334)*

19. **(A)** Cataracts are usually the only clinical manifestation of galactokinase deficiency. Rarely, benign increased intracranial pressure (pseudotumor cerebri) has been noted. This disease is an important cause of familial cataracts, which can be prevented by avoidance of galactose in the diet. Galactokinase deficiency is a very different disease than galactosemia (next question), although both diseases involve the metabolism of galactose. *(Rudolph:320)*

20. **(C)** Both cow milk and breast milk contain the disaccharide lactose, which is broken down to glucose and galactose. The latter, of course, cannot be properly metabolized by infants with galactosemia (deficiency of galactose-1-phosphate deficiency). Affected children, therefore, must be fed a galactose-free diet. Since lactose is the only natural source of galactose, this is not excessively difficult. (Some vegetables have galactose-containing oligosaccharides, but these are not digestible in human intestines.) Glucose is tolerated without problems. *(Rudolph:260)*

21. **(D)** Total serum osmolality in this patient probably is normal, since the elevated serum glucose increases osmolality while the lowered sodium concentration decreases osmolality. It has been calculated that a concentration of 1,000 mg/dL of glucose provides about 50 mOsm/L (more exactly, 180 mg/dL equals 10 mOsm/L). Normal serum glucose is about 100 mg/dL, so this patient has an excess of about 900 mg/dL. This about equals the decrease in osmolality because of the lower sodium and bicarbonate concentrations. Osmolality may be estimated as twice sodium concentration $(120 \times 2 = 240)$ plus the contribution (not *concentration*) of glucose (45 mOsm/L) and urea (4 mOsm/L), or $240 + 45 + 5 = 290$ mOsm/L. The actual *measured* osmolality might be a little lower than this *calculated* figure because some of the ionic material is protein bound and therefore does not actually contribute to osmolality. [*Note:* It is important to recognize that a patient is not necessarily hyperosmolar despite a blood glucose concentration of 1,000 mg/dL or hypo-osmolar despite a low serum sodium.] *(Rudolph:337–338)*

22. **(B)** Onset of insulin-dependent diabetes mellitus (IDDM) in the first decade of life is common and only rarely associated with Cushing's syndrome or multiple endocrinopathies. The onset is usually abrupt, with only a relatively brief period of polyuria and weight loss preceding the development of ketoacidosis. *(Rudolph:336)*

23. **(E)** Vomiting, hepatomegaly, and jaundice are common presenting features of galactosemia. Prompt diagnosis is imperative, as death or mental retardation may result if treatment is delayed. Peculiar urine odors are characteristic of disorders of amino acid metabolism rather than of carbohydrate metabolism. *(Rudolph:321; Hathaway:1002)*

24. **(B)** Maple syrup urine disease is an inborn metabolic error (autosomal recessive) of metabolism of branched-chain amino acids. The disease derives its name from the characteristic odor imparted to the urine by the excretion of ketoacid analogs of the branched-chain amino acids—leucine, isoleucine, and valine. Symptoms of lethargy, poor feeding, coma, and convulsions begin within a few days of birth, and death within the first month is the rule. Although a rare disease, it is important as a model of an error of amino acid metabolism. A milder form of the disease has been observed. *(Rudolph:305)*

25. **(C)** It is mandatory in all states to screen all newborn infants for phenylketonuria (as well as hypothyroidism and several other conditions) before discharge from the hospital. Despite its relative rarity (about 1 in 10,000), the disease is considered important enough as a cause of preventable mental retardation to warrant the expense of population screening. The method, however, is not without limitation because the blood level of phenylalanine may not have risen to diagnostic levels in infants who are discharged early. For this reason, many pediatricians elect to repeat the screening test routinely at the first office visit at the age of 3 to 4 weeks. *(Rudolph:303)*

26. **(B)** There is considerable evidence that a low-phenylalanine diet can prevent mental retardation and other clinical manifestations of phenylketonuria. Such a diet is feasible, and a special infant formula (Lofenalac) is available. Phenylalanine, however, is an essential amino acid, and it is not easy to maintain a diet with neither too little nor too much phenylalanine. Recent data suggest that it may be important to continue the special diet even beyond the fifth or sixth birthday, although it may be acceptable to ease the rigidity somewhat. *(Rudolph:302–303)*

27. **(E)** In Pompe's disease (type IIa glycogen storage disease), cardiac muscle, as well as striated muscle in general, is affected. The etiology of this disorder is a deficiency of alpha-1,4-glucosidase, a lysosomal enzyme. Children show early signs of congestive heart failure and generally die in infancy. Massive cardiomegaly is common, often with the heart seeming to fill the entire chest on roentgenogram. *(Rudolph:333)*

28. **(D)** An elevated serum cholesterol level in an infant or child may indicate that the child is either homozygous or heterozygous for hypercholesterole-

mia (type II hyperlipoproteinemia). Cystic fibrosis is associated with fat malabsorption and low, rather than elevated, serum lipids. Intestinal lymphangiectasia also is associated with normal or low serum lipids. Children with biliary atresia rarely are without signs of clinical disease. *(Rudolph:366)*

29. **(A)** The hallmark of abetalipoproteinemia is the absence from the plasma of the beta-lipoproteins. The clinical picture of this autosomal recessive disorder is characterized by fat malabsorption, failure to thrive, and a spiny appearance to the red blood cells on peripheral smear (acanthocystosis). Other features include ataxia and retinitis pigmentosa. *(Rudolph:371–372)*

30. **(D)** Type I Gaucher's disease is a lipid storage disease. Although the disease is most frequently encountered in individuals of Ashkenazi Jewish ancestry, it is not limited to this group. The disease is characterized by splenomegaly and, later, hepatomegaly. Osteoporosis is common. Serum acid phosphatase is regularly elevated in this disorder and is a useful diagnostic clue. Elevated alkaline phosphatase is relatively nonspecific, may simply reflect liver disease, and is not diagnostically helpful. The diagnosis is established by demonstration of Gaucher's cells in bone marrow aspirate. *(Rudolph:359)*

31. **(C)** The child described probably has osteogenesis imperfecta, a disorder characterized by osteoporotic bones that fracture easily. Blue sclera, present in infancy, is a common feature. Some patients also have **opalescent** dentin (dentinogenesis imperfecta), and many develop conductive hearing loss in adolescence. At least four types have been described, with differing modes of inheritance (autosomal dominant, autosomal recessive) and varying degrees of severity. *(Rudolph:406)*

32. **(B)** Pyruvate kinase deficiency is an abnormality of the Embden-Myerhof pathway in the red blood cells. The disorder is inherited as an autosomal recessive trait. The primary manifestation is a congenital nonspherocytic hemolytic anemia. None of the other choices listed—muscle weakness, hepatic fibrosis, mental retardation, or cardiomyopathy—is a feature of this defect. There are, however, other enzyme defects in the Embden-Myerhof pathway associated with congenital nonspherocytic hemolytic anemia and myopathy (phosphofructokinase deficiency) or mental retardation (phosphoglycerate kinase deficiency). *(Hathaway:485)*

33. **(B)** Wilson's disease in childhood generally presents as hepatic involvement progressing to cirrhosis. Neurologic manifestations such as ataxia, parkinsonism, seizures, and emotional and behavioral changes are uncommon in early childhood. Occasion-

ally, acute hemolytic anemia and jaundice are the first signs of the disease. *(Oski:1760)*

34. **(C)** Earlier in this chapter, several questions dealt with calculation of fluid requirements on the basis of caloric consumption. It also is possible to calculate daily fluid maintenance requirements on the basis of body surface area, using the range of 1,500 to 2,000 mL per square meter of surface area. A commonly used figure is 1,600 mL/m^2. Tables that convert weight to surface area or nomograms that predict surface area on the basis of height and weight are available in most intern and resident "pocket handbooks," as well as many standard texts. *(Hathaway: 1078)*

35. **(B)** The child's maintenance requirements might be calculated either on a caloric basis (5 kg × 100 calories/kg = 500 calories = 500 mL) or on a surface area basis (0.30 m^2 x 1,600 mL/m^2 = 480 mL). The deficit, however, must be calculated on the basis of weight, not surface area: 5 kg × 0.1 = 0.5 kg = 0.5 L = 500 mL. Adding deficit and maintenance: 500 mL + 480 mL = 980 mL, or 500 mL + 500 mL = 1,000 mL. If one chose to use 2,000 mL/m^2 as the figure for maintenance fluid, the calculation would be (0.3 × 2,000 mL) + 500 mL = 1,100 mL. *(Rudolph:229–231)*

36. **(D)** Infants with pyloric stenosis vomit a great deal of pure gastric fluid, which is rich in hydrochloric acid. Because the obstruction is only partial, the infants often vomit for weeks before diagnosis. The chronic loss of gastric acid results in systemic alkalosis, which in turn leads to urinary loss of potassium ion. Hypokalemic metabolic alkalosis is the typical and classic acid-base disturbance found in these infants. All the other conditions listed are associated with acidosis rather than alkalosis. *(Rudolph:229; Oski:72)*

37. **(C)** Ketotic hypoglycemia is an example of substrate-limited hypoglycemia and is associated with normal or low serum levels of insulin. This disorder appears to result from an impairment of gluconeogenesis, possibly an inability to mobilize alanine from skeletal muscle. Symptoms usually appear between the ages of 1½ and 4 or 5 years and remit spontaneously by the age of 8 or 9 years. The disorder is most common in males. All the other conditions listed are associated with hyperinsulinemia. *(Rudolph:327–328)*

38. **(E)** Glucose-6-phosphate dehydrogenase (G6PD) deficiency is characterized by episodes of hemolysis triggered by viral infections or certain drugs or foods. Common items that can precipitate an attack include primaquine and other antimalarial drugs, nitrofurans, sulfonamides, and fava beans. The hemolysis associated with pyruvate kinase deficiency is more chronic and not related to drugs or foods. *(Hathaway:486)*

39. (D) Lesch-Nyhan syndrome is a congenital (X-linked) disorder of purine metabolism associated with hyperuricemia, severe mental retardation, and choreoathetosis. The most striking feature of the disorder is self-mutilating biting behavior. These patients often destroy their lips and even may amputate distal portions of their fingers. None of the other items listed is associated with this syndrome. *(Rudolph:318)*

40. (A) Hereditary fructose intolerance is associated with a deficiency of the liver enzyme fructose-1-phosphate aldolase, resulting in impaired metabolism of dietary fructose. Ingestion of fructose-containing foods results in vomiting, hepatomegaly, jaundice, hypoglycemia, lethargy, coma, and finally death. Diarrhea is not a feature of this disorder. A fructose-free diet will result in resolution of all symptoms. *(Oski:1757)*

41. (D) A basic pathophysiologic abnormality in diabetes mellitus is decreased entry of glucose into the cell because of insulin deficiency. This results in decreased glucose utilization and increased oxidation of fatty acids, producing acetyl-CoA, which in turn produces ketones. There also is increased glycogenolysis and increased gluconeogenesis from amino acids, which further elevate blood glucose. *(Rudolph:335)*

42. (B) Daily measurement of blood glucose levels is critical to proper diabetic control. Sometimes it is necessary to measure blood glucose before each meal and at bedtime. Determination of urine glucose is too imprecise and delayed to accurately reflect blood glucose and plays little or no role in managing these children. Periodic measurement of glycosylated hemoglobin (HbA$_{1c}$) is an important reflection of long-term control (past 2 to 3 months). Avoidance of both ketoacidosis and hypoglycemia is an important measure of appropriate control. *(Rudolph:341)*

43. (B) Absence of the liver enzyme glucose-6-phosphatase is characteristic of type I glycogen storage disease (von Gierke's disease). Deficiency of this enzyme interferes with hepatic glycogenolysis and gluconeogenesis, resulting in hypoglycemia and episodes of metabolic acidosis. Accumulated hepatic glycogen leads to hepatomegaly but not to jaundice, as other aspects of hepatocellular function are relatively undisturbed. The metabolic disturbance also results in increased production of triglycerides, cholesterol, and uric acid. *(Rudolph:331–332)*

44. (C) Ectopia lentis (subluxated or dislocated lens), thromboembolism, and mental retardation are features of homocystinuria. This is an autosomal recessive disorder of amino acid metabolism in which there is defective activity of cystathionine synthetase, the enzyme that catalyzes the metabolism of homocystine and serine to cystathionine. Mental retardation is common, although not always present, and varies from mild to severe. These patients resemble patients with Marfan's syndrome. *(Oski:89)*

45. (A) It is believed that phenylalanine hydroxylase deficiency (phenylketonuria, PKU) is associated with increased accumulation of toxic products of intermediate metabolism that are damaging to the developing nervous system. In the affected (homozygous) infant, this process begins very soon after birth. Detection of PKU by routine screening of all newborns and treatment of affected individuals by a low-phenylalanine diet has led to a population of adult phenylketonuric women with normal intelligence in the reproductive age. Nonaffected (heterozygote) infants born to homozygous mothers and exposed to these toxic byproducts in utero have demonstrated intrauterine nervous system involvement. *(Oski:84)*

46. (B) Albinism results from a variety of genetic abnormalities including a deficiency of tyrosinase, blocking the production of melanin from tyrosine. In universal albinism (autosomal recessive), in addition to milk-white skin and white or yellow hair, the iris also is affected. Photophobia, horizontal nystagmus, and decreased visual acuity are characteristic. As one would anticipate, there is an increased incidence of skin cancer in patients with albinism. *(Rudolph: 304)*

47. (D) The clinical picture described is that of maple syrup urine disease or branched-chain aminoaciduria. In this autosomal recessive disorder, the enzyme deficiency (branched-chain ketoacid decarboxylase) results in the accumulation of branched-chain amino acids and their ketoacid analogs. Excretion of these substances in the urine gives it a characteristic maple syrup or caramel odor. The clinical features of the disease are severe neurologic abnormalities, including coma and death. [*Note:* Although maple syrup urine disease itself is rare, it is especially important as an example or model of a *group* of inborn metabolic errors whose major clinical manifestation is neurologic dysfunction, including coma.] *(Rudolph:304–305; Oski:91–92)*

48. (C) Both the porphyrias (a group of disorders characterized by impairment in the synthesis of heme) and urea cycle disorders (abnormalities in urea cycle metabolism) are the result of genetic abnormalities of specific enzymes in the respective metabolic pathways. *(Rudolph:311–312,383–385)*

49. (B) Deficiencies of urea cycle enzymes result in hyperammonemia, often to very striking levels. In the porphyrias, in contrast, ammonia metabolism is normal. *(Rudolph:311–312,383–385)*

50. **(C)** Neurologic manifestations can occur in both groups of disorders. The urea cycle disorders are commonly associated with lethargy, hypotonia or hypertonia, and convulsions. Several varieties of porphyria, most notably the acute intermittent variety (Swedish type), are associated with neurologic signs and symptoms—hallucinations, seizures, weakness, and paralysis. *(Rudolph:311–312,383–385)*

51. **(A)** Dermatitis, characteristically of a photosensitive nature, is a prominent feature of most types of porphyria other than the acute intermittent variety. Urea cycle defects do not result in a rash. *(Rudolph: 311–312,383–385)*

BIBLIOGRAPHY

Finberg L. Hypernatremic dehydration in infants. *N Eng J Med.* 1973;289:196–198.

Hathaway WE, Groothius JR, Hay WW, et al. *Current Pediatric Diagnosis & Treatment.* 10th ed. Norwalk, Conn: Appleton & Lange; 1991.

Oski FA, DeAngelis CD, Feigin RD, et al. *Principles & Practice of Pediatrics.* Philadelphia, Pa: JB Lippincott; 1990.

Rudolph AM, Hoffman JIE, Rudolph CD. *Pediatrics.* 19th ed. Norwalk, Conn: Appleton & Lange; 1991.

CHAPTER 8

Therapeutics
Questions

Pediatric therapeutics is a good example of the fact that *children are not simply small adults*. Yes, it is true that pediatric dosages *must be learned on a per-kilogram* basis rather than as "four tablets a day or one gram a day," but that is far from the whole story. Not only drugs but also fluid, calories, and protein requirements must be calculated on the basis of body weight or surface area. "Two liters a day" or "a 1,500-calorie diet" just will not do for children. Many drugs have unique kinetics or side effects in certain age groups and may be contraindicated in those age groups. For example, chloramphenicol is so poorly metabolized by the newborn infant's liver that the drug can rapidly accumulate to lethal blood levels. Tetracyclines deposit in growing bones and developing teeth. In the newborn period, drugs that can displace unconjugated bilirubin from binding to albumin are generally contraindicated. Children are very vulnerable to impairment of linear growth from corticosteroids.

In addition, the drugs and other interventions used most commonly for children differ from those used for adults because of the different diseases that occur in these two groups. A few drugs (eg, human growth hormone, silver nitrate eye drops) are used only in pediatrics; many drugs commonly prescribed for adults are rarely, if ever, given to children.

DIRECTIONS (Question 1 through 71): Each of the numbered items or incomplete statements in this section is followed by answers or by completions of the statement. Select the ONE lettered answer or completion that is BEST in each case.

1. A 5-year-old boy with classic hemophilia A presents to the emergency center with hemarthrosis of the right knee. The most important aspect of care for this child would be

   (A) administration of aspirin
   (B) needle aspiration of the joint
   (C) injection of factor VIII concentrate into the joint
   (D) intravenous administration of factor VIII concentrate
   (E) injection of DDAVP (vasopressin analog) into the joint

2. The truly undescended testicle should be brought surgically into the scrotum

   (A) during the first 2 years of life
   (B) between 2 and 5 years of life
   (C) between 5 and 10 years of life
   (D) just before puberty
   (E) just after puberty

3. A young child has swallowed a penny. X-ray examination reveals the coin to be in the stomach. Consequently,

   (A) the child should be given 20 mL of syrup of ipecac to induce vomiting
   (B) the child should be admitted to the hospital and observed for signs of intestinal obstruction
   (C) the child should immediately be operated on to remove the foreign body
   (D) the child should be sent home and the mother instructed to examine the stools for the foreign object
   (E) an attempt should be made to remove the foreign body by flexible fiberoptic endoscopy

4. Methylphenidate (Ritalin) is most commonly prescribed in the management of children with

   (A) poor appetites
   (B) temper tantrums
   (C) seizure disorders
   (D) breathholding spells
   (E) attention deficit disorders

5. Which of the following statements regarding the use of oral acyclovir in the treatment of varicella is correct?

   (A) It is contraindicated in children less than 2 years of age
   (B) Its use is restricted to immunosuppressed patients
   (C) It is well absorbed and is as effective as intravenous administration
   (D) In normal children it is clinically effective if treatment is begun within the first 5 days of appearance of lesions
   (E) Patients receiving the drug do not need to be monitored with blood counts

6. A 10-year-old child with diabetes sustains a fractured femur and is placed in bed in traction. Assuming that his diet remains unchanged, one would expect his daily insulin requirement to

   (A) fluctuate widely
   (B) increase moderately
   (C) decrease moderately
   (D) decrease to zero
   (E) remain the same

7. Congenital nephrogenic diabetes insipidus is treated with

   (A) antidiuretic hormone
   (B) extra salt in the diet or formula
   (C) fluid restriction
   (D) oral bicarbonate
   (E) thiazide diuretics

8. The drug of choice for continuous prophylactic therapy of febrile seizures is

   (A) carbamazepine
   (B) diazepam
   (C) phenobarbital
   (D) phenytoin
   (E) valproic acid

9. An important side effect of propylthiouracil is

   (A) agranulocytosis
   (B) acute renal failure
   (C) hypoglycemia
   (D) pseudotumor cerebri
   (E) seizures

10. The major advantage of alternate-day prednisone therapy in the treatment of diseases such as asthma or nephrosis is that

    (A) it is more effective
    (B) it is more convenient
    (C) there is less adrenal suppression
    (D) it permits use of a lower total dose
    (E) there is less suppression of the immunologic system

11. Frequent periodic blood transfusions are most important in the routine treatment of

    (A) thalassemia major
    (B) thalassemia minor
    (C) sickle cell anemia
    (D) G6PD deficiency
    (E) hereditary persistence of fetal hemoglobin

12. Which of the following antibiotics would be most appropriate for prophylaxis against bacterial endocarditis in a 10-year-old child with mild congenital aortic stenosis undergoing an invasive dental procedure?

    (A) Amoxicillin
    (B) Clindamycin
    (C) Erythromycin
    (D) Oxacillin
    (E) Vancomycin

13. The drug of choice for the treatment of *Mycoplasma pneumoniae* infection in a 4-year-old child is

    (A) cefuroxime
    (B) chloramphenicol
    (C) erythromycin
    (D) penicillin
    (E) tetracycline

14. The most important aspect of the management of acute epiglottitis, caused by *Hemophilus influenzae* type B, and severe respiratory distress is

    (A) administration of an antibiotic effective against *H. influenzae* type B, including ampicillin-resistant strains
    (B) administration of corticosteroids, both intravenously and by aerosol (IPPB)
    (C) establishment of a secure airway
    (D) inspection of the oropharynx with a bright light and adequate-size tongue blade
    (E) performance of a lumbar puncture to rule out an associated meningitis

15. The syndrome of hereditary prolongation of the QT interval is associated with episodes of ventricular fibrillation, syncope, and sudden death. Which of the following drugs has been most useful in preventing such episodes?

    (A) Atropine
    (B) Digitalis
    (C) Lidocaine
    (D) Phenylephrine
    (E) Propranolol

16. When surgical management of gastroesophageal reflux is indicated (failure of medical management), which of the following procedures is most appropriate?

    (A) Esophageal retropositioning
    (B) Fundoplication

(C) Gastrojejunostomy

(D) Gastrostomy

(E) Vagotomy

17. Palliative surgery for the small infant with severe tetralogy of Fallot, deep cyanosis, and paroxysmal dyspnea would be

(A) pulmonary artery banding

(B) atrial septostomy

(C) aorta-to-pulmonary-artery anastomosis

(D) ductal ligation

(E) implantation of a pacemaker

18. Ethosuximide (Zarontin) is most useful in the treatment of

(A) phenobarbital overdosage

(B) absence (petit mal) seizures

(C) akinetic seizures

(D) grand mal seizures

(E) complex partial seizures

19. Propranolol is a useful drug for the treatment of

(A) asthma

(B) allergic rhinitis

(C) cardiogenic shock

(D) tonic-clonic seizures

(E) paroxysmal supraventricular tachycardia

20. A child who has ingested the rodenticide warfarin should be given

(A) vitamin C

(B) vitamin K

(C) copper sulfate

(D) a phenothiazine

(E) atropine

21. Which of the following is most useful in the treatment of methanol poisoning?

(A) Acetazolamide

(B) Ascorbic acid

(C) Ethanol

(D) Ethylene glycol

(E) Glucose

22. Treatment of acute nitrite poisoning may require administration of

(A) hydralazine

(B) morphine

(C) methylene blue

(D) corticosteroids

(E) antihistamines

23. The approximate dose of diphenhydramine (Benadryl) for a young child is

(A) 0.5 mg/kg per 24 hours

(B) 1.0 mg/kg per 24 hours

(C) 2.5 mg/kg per 24 hours

(D) 5.0 mg/kg per 24 hours

(E) 10.0 mg/kg per 24 hours

24. Twenty-five milligrams of cortisone is approximately equivalent (glucocorticoid effect) to how much dexamethasone?

(A) 0.1 mg

(B) 0.75 mg

(C) 1.5 mg

(D) 2.5 mg

(E) 5.0 mg

25. Diazoxide (Hyperstat)

(A) should not be given to prepubertal children

(B) is contraindicated in hypertension secondary to nephritis

(C) may be given by rapid intravenous injection

(D) should not be used concurrently with a diuretic

(E) frequently causes hypoglycemia

26. Proper management of a 2-year-old child with a positive tuberculin test, normal chest roentgenogram, and no evidence of disease would be to

(A) follow the patient with serial chest x-ray examinations every 2 months

(B) repeat the tuberculin test monthly

(C) treat with isoniazid and rifampin for 6 months

(D) treat with isoniazid alone for 7 to 12 months

(E) treat with isoniazid and rifampin for 3 months, followed by isoniazid alone for an additional 6 months

27. Which of the following statements regarding isoniazid (INH) is true?

(A) Administration in adolescent patients should be supplemented with vitamin B_6

(B) It should be given in divided daily dosage, at least twice a day

(C) It should be taken with milk or an antacid

(D) The most common toxic effect is renal injury with proteinuria

(E) It should not be prescribed in conjunction with rifampin

28. A 10-kg, 2-year-old child has ingested an unknown amount of methadone. In the emergency room the child is comatose. After stabilizing the airway, you should administer

(A) aerosolized albuterol

(B) intravenous naloxone

(C) subcutaneous adrenalin

(D) intramuscular atropine

(E) oral sorbitol

29. Hemorrhagic cystitis is seen with large doses of

(A) cyclophosphamide
(B) methotrexate
(C) actinomycin D
(D) L-asparaginase

30. Which of the following would be indicated for a child with rheumatic chorea?

(A) Aspirin
(B) Bed rest
(C) Diphenylhydantoin
(D) Injections of bicillin every 4 weeks

31. Allopurinol is useful in the management of acute leukemia of childhood

(A) to induce remission
(B) to maintain remission
(C) both to induce and to maintain remission
(D) to prevent vomiting from chemotherapy
(E) to prevent hyperuricemia associated with chemotherapy

32. Which of the following agents is effective against central nervous system (CNS) leukemia when administered systemically?

(A) Methotrexate
(B) Prednisone
(C) Vincristine
(D) Cyclophosphamide
(E) Daunorubicin

33. Following an injection of succinylcholine for intubation and induction of anesthesia, a 5-year-old child is noted to remain apneic and paralyzed for an extended period of time. The child most likely

(A) received an excessive dose of the drug
(B) has been receiving aminoglycosides
(C) has impaired renal function
(D) has pseudocholinesterase deficiency
(E) had an allergic reaction to the succinylcholine

34. The beneficial action of tetracyclines on pustular and cystic acne results from

(A) eradication of staphylococci from the lesions
(B) eradication of staphylococci from the skin surface
(C) reduction of population of *P. acnes* in the skin
(D) reduction of population of streptococci in the skin

35. The major indication for the placement of pressure-equalizing (PE) tubes into the middle ear is

(A) acute otitis media
(B) acute mastoiditis
(C) excessive cerumen
(D) chronic draining otitis media
(E) chronic serous otitis media

36. The primary treatment for hepatoblastoma in childhood is

(A) radiation therapy
(B) chemotherapy
(C) chemotherapy and surgery
(D) vitamin B_{12}
(E) a combination of radiation and chemotherapy

37. One tablespoon contains about

(A) 5 mL
(B) 10 mL
(C) 15 mL
(D) 20 mL
(E) 30 mL

38. An appropriate single antibiotic for the empiric treatment of presumed bacterial meningitis in a 6-month-old child would be

(A) ampicillin
(B) cefadroxil
(C) cefotaxime
(D) cefuroxime
(E) penicillin

39. Use of the gluteal area for intramuscular injections in infants and young children is best avoided because

(A) the area is too vascular
(B) hematomas may dissect into the spine or rectum
(C) such injections may injure the sciatic nerve
(D) it is psychologically undesirable
(E) absorption from this site is poor

40. Primary syphilis is best treated by

(A) ampicillin, 3.5 g orally, plus 1 g of probenecid
(B) procaine penicillin G, 4.8 million units intramuscularly (IM) as a single dose, plus 1 g of probenecid
(C) benzanthine penicillin, 2.4 million units IM as a single dose
(D) spectinomycin, 2 g IM as a single dose
(E) cefuroxime, 4 g as a single dose

41. The appearance of a nonurticarial, maculopapular rash during treatment with oral ampicillin

(A) usually indicates too high a dosage
(B) usually is unrelated to the ampicillin
(C) usually does not indicate IgE-mediated hypersensitivity
(D) may not indicate IgE-mediated hypersensitivity but nevertheless places the patient at considerable risk for a severe immediate hypersensitivity reaction if the drug is given again

42. Which of the following organisms is most likely to be resistant to ampicillin?

(A) *Listeria monocytogenes*
(B) *Bordetella pertussis*

(C) *Klebsiella*

(D) *Salmonella*

(E) Group A beta-hemolytic *Streptococcus*

43. The major advantage of phenoxymethylpenicillin over penicillin G is

(A) lower cost

(B) longer shelf life

(C) lower incidence of allergic reactions

(D) more reliable gastrointestinal absorption

(E) broader spectrum of antimicrobial sensitivity

44. The dose of gentamicin recommended for the treatment of sepsis or meningitis in the first week of life is

(A) 0.25 mg/kg per day

(B) 0.5 mg/kg per day

(C) 1.0 mg/kg per day

(D) 2.5 mg/kg per day

(E) 5.0 mg/kg per day

45. Although antibiotic therapy appears not to alter the clinical course of pertussis once cough has begun, it can be of value in protecting siblings and other contacts against the disease. The antibiotic of choice for this purpose is

(A) cefotaxime

(B) erythromycin

(C) gentamicin

(D) penicillin

(E) trimethoprim-sulfamethoxazole

46. The drug of choice for the treatment of meningococcal meningitis is

(A) cefotaxime

(B) ceftriaxone

(C) cefuroxime

(D) chloramphenicol

(E) penicillin

47. Intravenous gamma-globulin (IVGG) is indicated in the treatment of idiopathic thrombocytopenia purpura

(A) only for patients with central nervous system involvement

(B) only in patients with documented persistent viral infection

(C) only for patients who fail to respond to corticosteroids

(D) only in patients more than 10 years old

(E) as primary therapy

48. The parenteral digitalizing dose of digoxin for a premature infant is in the order of

(A) 0.001 mg/kg

(B) 0.01 mg/kg

(C) 0.03 mg/kg

(D) 0.05 mg/kg

(E) 0.1 mg/kg

49. Appropriate treatment of tonsillopharyngeal diphtheria, diagnosed before the occurrence of cardiac or neurologic manifestations, would be

(A) erythromycin

(B) erythromycin and antitoxin

(C) erythromycin, antitoxin, and corticosteroids

(D) erythromycin, antitoxin, corticosteroids, and digoxin

(E) erythromycin, antitoxin, corticosteroids, digoxin, and phenobarbital

50. Overtreatment, posthypoglycemic hyperglycemia, or poor control should be suspected in a child with diabetes whose daily insulin requirement is greater than

(A) 0.1 unit/kg

(B) 0.5 unit/kg

(C) 1.5 unit/kg

(D) 2.5 unit/kg

(E) 5.0 unit/kg

51. In order to control joint or periarticular bleeding in a child with hemophilia, it is necessary to raise the serum level of factor VIII to about

(A) 1 to 2% of normal

(B) 5 to 10% of normal

(C) 10 to 25% of normal

(D) 25% to 50% of normal

(E) 75 to 100% of normal

52. The use of oral pancreatic enzyme replacement therapy is most helpful in patients with

(A) protein-losing enteropathy

(B) celiac disease

(C) cystic fibrosis

(D) ulcerative colitis

(E) alpha-1-antitrypsin deficiency

53. In the treatment of inflammatory bowel disease, corticosteroids are most useful

(A) in treating acute attacks and exacerbations

(B) in long-term prevention of exacerbations

(C) in patients over 15 years of age

(D) in patients with anorexia

(E) in patients with poor growth but without diarrhea

54. The most useful chelating agent for acute iron poisoning is

(A) dimercaprol (BAL)

(B) deferoxamine (Desferal)

(C) versenate (EDTA)

(D) penicillamine

(E) sodium bicarbonate

55. A child has been poisoned by an anticholinesterase-containing insecticide. The nicotinic effects of the poison (paralysis) would likely be diminished or at least reversed by the prompt administration of

(A) atropine
(B) acetylcysteine
(C) pralidoxime
(D) bicarbonate
(E) physostigmine

56. The most important aspect of the treatment of grades I and II vesicoureteral reflux is

(A) internal urethrotomy
(B) external urethrotomy
(C) a program of frequent voiding
(D) continuous prophylactic antibiotics
(E) avoidance of excess fluid to minimize bladder distention

57. With proper therapy, which of the following childhood malignancies has the highest cure rate?

(A) Wilms's tumor
(B) Neuroblastoma
(C) Retinoblastoma
(D) Rhabdomyosarcoma
(E) Non-Hodgkin's lymphoma

58. In treating diabetic ketoacidosis, the usual dosage of insulin by continuous infusion is

(A) 0.01 to 0.02 units/kg per hour
(B) 0.1 to 0.2 units/kg per hour
(C) 1 to 2 units/kg per hour
(D) 2 to 5 units/kg per hour
(E) 5 to 10 units/kg per hour

59. Which of the following is a useful agent for the treatment of intestinal infection with *Entamoeba histolytica*?

(A) Ampicillin
(B) Aziocillin
(C) Aztreonam
(D) Cefotaxime
(E) Metronidazole

60. Systemic therapy with griseofulvin generally is the treatment of choice for

(A) moniliasis
(B) tinea corporis
(C) tinea pedis
(D) tinea capitis

61. Management of a child with maple syrup urine disease includes

(A) avoidance of maple syrup
(B) avoidance of all monosaccharides
(C) dietary supplementation with glucose

(D) dietary supplementation with pyridoxine
(E) dietary restriction of certain amino acids

62. A side effect of tetracycline that is limited to children is

(A) pseudotumor cerebri
(B) hyperglycemia
(C) tremors and convulsions
(D) permanent discoloration of teeth
(E) hematuria and proteinuria

63. Prompt surgical intervention is the treatment of choice for

(A) Caffey's disease (idiopathic cortical hyperostoses)
(B) congenital dysplasia of the hip (CDH)
(C) idiopathic avascular necrosis of the femoral capital epiphysis (Legg-Calvé-Perthes disease)
(D) slipped capital femoral epiphysis (SCFE)
(E) Osgood-Schlatter disease

64. Fluoride supplementation is recommended for

(A) all infants and young children
(B) infants and young children living in areas where the water supply contains less than 10 parts per million of fluoride
(C) infants and young children living in geographic areas of limited sunlight
(D) infants and young children who consume less than a quart of milk per day
(E) adolescents

65. Which of the following would be the most appropriate therapy for acute gonococcal urethritis in an adolescent male?

(A) Ampicillin, 1 g a day orally for 3 days
(B) Doxycycline, 100 mg twice a day for 7 days
(C) Procaine penicillin G, 1.2 million units IM once
(D) Benzathine penicillin, 2.4 million units IM once
(E) Ceftriaxone, 250 mg IM once

66. Toxic reactions to acetaminophen

(A) involve primarily the liver
(B) involve primarily the central nervous system
(C) are most severe in patients less than 2 years of age
(D) are frequently seen with high therapeutic dosage (15 mg/kg)
(E) are treated with intravenous glucose and sodium bicarbonate

Please note the use of a negative qualifier such as EXCEPT, LEAST, or NOT in each of the following questions (Questions 67 through 71).

67. Naloxone (Narcan) is an effective antagonist against all of the following EXCEPT

(A) codeine
(B) dextropropoxyphene (Darvon)

(C) pentazocine (Talwin)
(D) phenobarbital
(E) methadone

68. Side effects of corticosteroids include all of the following EXCEPT

(A) growth retardation
(B) pseudotumor cerebri
(C) cataracts
(D) hypoglycemia
(E) hypertension

69. Splenectomy may be useful in the management of all of the following EXCEPT

(A) congenital spherocytic anemia
(B) thalassemia major
(C) congenital elliptocytosis
(D) hypersplenism
(E) aplastic anemia

70. Which of the following agents is NOT used in the treatment of acute leukemia of childhood?

(A) Prednisone
(B) Methotrexate
(C) Cyclophosphamide
(D) Chlorambucil
(E) Vincristine

71. All of the following are useful in the management of chronic renal failure EXCEPT

(A) phosphate supplements
(B) 1,25-$(OH)_2 D_3$
(C) calcium supplements
(D) biosynthetic human erythropoietin
(E) $CaCO_3$

DIRECTIONS (72 through 76): Each set of matching questions in this section consists of a list of 4 to 26 lettered options followed by several numbered items. For each numbered item select the ONE lettered option with which it is most closely associated. Each lettered option may be selected once, more than once, or not at all.

Questions 72 through 76

(A) Peak effect 2 to 3 hours
(B) Peak effect 8 to 12 hours
(C) Peak effect 14 to 18 hours
(D) Peak effect 24 hours

72. Lente insulin

73. Ultralente insulin

74. Semilente insulin

75. Regular insulin

76. NPH insulin

DIRECTIONS (Questions 77 through 85): Each group of items in this section consists of lettered headings followed by a set of numbered words or phrases. For each numbered word or phrase, select

> A if the item is associated with (A) <u>only</u>,
> B if the item is associated with (B) <u>only</u>,
> C if the item is associated with <u>both</u> (A) <u>and</u> (B),
> D if the item is associated with <u>neither</u> (A) <u>nor</u> (B).

Questions 77 through 81

(A) Cefoxitin
(B) Ceftazidime
(C) Both
(D) Neither

77. Second-generation cephalosporin

78. Effective against most strains of *Pseudomonas*

79. Effective against anaerobes, including *Bacteroides fragilis*

80. Effective against *Listeria monocytogenes*

81. Effective against *E. coli*

Questions 82 through 85

(A) Furosemide
(B) Spironolactone
(C) Both
(D) Neither

82. Useful in treatment of congestive heart failure

83. Potassium sparing

84. Increases systemic arterial blood pressure

85. Side effects include hearing loss and renal stones

Answers and Explanations

1. (D) The most important aspect of treatment of hemarthrosis (and most other bleeding problems) in children with classic hemophilia A (factor VIII deficiency) is intravenous administration of factor VIII concentrate. The goal is to increase the plasma activity of factor VIII in the patient. Ancillary measures such as aspiration of the joint, application of local cold, temporary immobilization, and analgesics (not aspirin or other NSAIDs, which interfere with platelet function) are helpful but do not obviate the need for factor VIII replacement. DDAVP is helpful only for patients with mild hemophilia A and must be given parenterally, not into the joint. *(Rudolph:1163; Hathaway:508)*

2. (A) Most aspects of the treatment of undescended testes are controversial. Hormonal therapy with human chorionic gonadotropin is advocated by many, yet also decried as useless by others. True undescended (cryptorchid) testes must be distinguished from retractile testes. The latter can be brought into the scrotum manually, whereas the former cannot. For true cryptorchidism, orchiopexy should be performed before the age of 2 years. Delay subjects the undescended testes to risk of repeated trauma and torsion. Although it is believed that undescended testes are intrinsically abnormal, it nevertheless is hoped that early orchidopexy will prevent progressive degeneration of spermatogenic function. *(Rudolph:1303)*

3. (D) Foreign bodies that have passed the esophagus and entered the stomach almost always will pass through the rest of the gastrointestinal tract without difficulty. This includes sharp objects such as straight pins. Children who have ingested nonpointed objects need not be admitted to the hospital. Potentially dangerous objects such as lead washers or large button batteries can be removed by gastroscopy with a flexible fiberoptic gastroscope if necessary. There is absolutely no need for removal of a round, smooth, inert object such as a coin. *(Rudolph:999–1000)*

4. (E) Stimulant drugs such as methylphenidate (Ritalin), amphetamines, and pemoline (Cylert) have been shown to have a beneficial effect in many children with attention deficit disorder and hyperactivity. The seemingly paradoxical calming action of stimulant drugs in these children may be related to increased awareness of, and therefore response to, external stimuli, permitting sustained attention. The drugs have no role in the management of seizure disorders, temper tantrums, or breathholding spells. Appetite *suppression* is an important side effect of these drugs. *(Rudolph:1725–1726)*

5. (E) Although varicella in normal children is generally a mild disease, oral acyclovir has been shown to decrease the number of lesions and lessen the severity and duration of the illness. Oral acyclovir has been approved for use in normal children with varicella, but it appears to be effective only if treatment is begun within the first 24 hours of illness. Routine monitoring with laboratory tests is not necessary. The drug is not well absorbed orally, and immunosuppressed patients may require intravenous administration. *(N Engl J Med 325:1539–1544,1991; J Pediatr 120:627–733,1992)*

6. (B) Exercise expedites the entry of glucose into muscle cells and therefore reduces insulin requirement. Bed rest and inactivity have the reverse effect, increasing insulin requirement in the child with diabetes. *(Rudolph:345; Hathaway:813)*

7. (E) Congenital nephrogenic diabetes insipidus is a genetically determined, probably X-linked, abnormality of renal tubular response to antidiuretic hormone (ADH). Symptoms generally begin shortly after birth and include polyuria, polydipsia, fever, vomiting, constipation, dehydration, hyperelectrolytemia, and failure to thrive. There is no response to even large doses of ADH or its analogs. The seemingly paradoxical response to chronic administration of thiazides is believed to result from total body sodium depletion and enhanced proximal reabsorption of glomerular filtrate. Dietary salt restriction is also helpful, but water intake must be generous. *(Rudolph:1283–1284)*

8. (C) Currently, phenobarbital is the drug of choice for *continuous* prophylaxis against febrile seizures in those selected children for whom such therapy is warranted. Phenytoin has not been shown to be effective. Although valproic acid is effective, the potential toxicities outweigh the benefit and prevent its routine use. Intermittent therapy with phenobarbital is ineffective, but diazepam, orally or rectally (suppositories are not currently available in the United States) at the first sign of a fever or an illness, has been shown to have promise in preventing febrile seizures. [*Note:* Attention to the word "continuous" is critical to answering this question correctly.] *(Rudolph:1793; Hathaway:667–668)*

9. (A) Agranulocytosis is one of the most important toxic side effects of propylthiouracil. Patients should be informed about this possibility and advised to obtain a blood count with every febrile illness. Other side effects include hepatitis, purpura, dermatitis, and lymphadenopathy. *(Rudolph:1639)*

10. (C) The major advantage of administering the total 48-hour dose of prednisone at one time ("alternate-day therapy") is that it results in less adrenal suppression than daily administration. Although this dosage schedule is not effective in all diseases for which corticosteroids are used, it is effective for many cases of asthma or nephrotic syndrome. *(Pediatrics 43:277–282,1969; J Pediatr 5:806–814,1973)*

11. (A) Frequent transfusions are required for patients with thalassemia major (homozygous beta-thalassemia). Without transfusion, hemoglobin levels can fall as low as 2 mg/dL. Thalassemia minor (heterozygous beta-thalassemia), G6PD deficiency, and persistence of fetal hemoglobin do not require routine transfusion therapy. In sickle cell anemia, the hemoglobin falls to levels requiring transfusion only infrequently, usually during an aplastic crisis. Although there are programs involving the use of periodic transfusions in sickle cell patients to prevent sickle crisis, such therapy is not routine, and generally only is used for children with specific indications such as a history of stroke. *(Rudolph:1123–1130)*

12. (A) Although many organisms can cause endocarditis following a dental procedure, *Streptococcus viridans* remains one of the most common. Penicillin is highly effective against this organism, but the longer serum half-life of amoxicillin has led to its recommendation as the drug of choice. Patients with rheumatic heart disease who are receiving continuous prophylaxis with penicillin may harbor strains of *S. viridans* that are relatively resistant to penicillin. Therefore, for patients receiving continuous penicillin, an alternate antibiotic regimen (e.g., erythromycin) may be advisable for prophylaxis against endocarditis. *(Rudolph:1420–1421)*

13. (C) Pencillins and cephalosporins are ineffective against *Mycoplasma* organisms. Erythromycin and tetracycline are effective, but the former is preferred in young children because tetracycline is deposited in growing bone and teeth. Although such deposition has not been shown to have significant pathophysiologic effects, it does cause staining of the teeth, which is cosmetically unacceptable. Chloramphenicol is effective. However, the infrequent but lethal side effect of pancytopenia restricts use of this drug to certain serious infections. *(Rudolph:692)*

14. (C) The greatest danger in acute epiglottitis is rapid progression to total airway obstruction. Prompt establishment of an adequate and secure airway is the single most important aspect of care and is the key to survival. Most authors recommend immediate endotracheal intubation as soon as the diagnosis is made; some would treat conservatively if distress is mild or minimal. Manipulation of the mouth or oropharynx with a tongue blade *is contraindicated* in children suspected of acute epiglottitis. Fatalities have occurred under these circumstances. Whether the mechanism of death is development of total airway obstruction or a severe vagal response is not clear. Optimal management would include direct visualization of the upper airway in the operating room under controlled conditions and endotracheal intubation by a skilled endoscopist. Appropriate antibiotics are important but clearly are a lower priority than maintaining the airway. *(Rudolph:585–586; Hathaway:370)*

15. (E) Hereditary prolongation of the QT interval occurs either with deafness (Jervell-Lange-Nielsen syndrome) or without deafness (Romano-Ward syndrome). Both syndromes have been associated with syncope and sudden death. Although propranolol does not alter the electrocardiographic findings, the drug has been helpful in preventing episodes of ventricular fibrillation and death in patients with either syndrome. *(Rudolph:1354–1355; Am J Dis Child 130:320–322,1978)*

16. (B) When surgical management of gastroesophageal reflux is required, the Nissen fundoplication is the appropriate procedure. In this procedure the fundus of the stomach is wrapped around the lower esophagus so as to mechanically prevent reflux of gastric contents. When the fundal region is contracted by a peristaltic wave, it squeezes the esophagus, preventing vomiting or regurgitation. *(Rudolph:994–995)*

17. (C) Tetralogy of Fallot is characterized by ventricular outflow tract stenosis, ventricular septal defect, dextroposition of the aorta, and right ventricular hypertrophy. The major problem in tetralogy is that too little blood reaches the lungs. Palliation consists of establishing a shunt from the systemic circulation to the pulmonary artery, increasing pulmonary blood flow. In small infants an aorta-to-pulmonary-artery anastomosis is required. In larger infants or children a subclavian-pulmonary anastomosis is preferred. Although total intracardiac surgical correction is feasible for most patients, the very small infant with a hypoplastic right ventricle or pulmonary arteries will require a palliative shunt until definitive surgery can be performed at a later date. *(Rudolph:1400)*

18. **(B)** Ethosuximide is one of the drugs of choice in the treatment of absence (petit mal) seizures. This drug has little role in the management of other types of seizure disorders. *(Rudolph:1775; Hathaway:668–669)*

19. **(E)** Propranolol is a beta blocker that is useful in the management of chronic paroxysmal supraventricular tachycardias, especially when associated with the Wolff-Parkinson-White syndrome. The drug is contraindicated in conditions where beta-adrenergic blockade would be disadvantageous, including asthma and cardiogenic shock. Propranolol is not an anticonvulsant. *(Rudolph:1352)*

20. **(B)** Many rat poisons contain warfarin, a coumarin derivative that inhibits the production of prothrombin by the liver, leading to hemorrhage. This hepatic toxicity can be effectively counteracted by large doses of vitamin K. (Pediatr Clin North Am 27:603–612, 1980; Rudolph:790)

21. **(C)** Methanol is metabolized by the enzyme alcohol dehydrogenase to formaldehyde and formic acid, which are extremely toxic. Ethanol competes for alcohol dehydrogenase and is useful in the treatment of poisoning with either methanol or ethylene glycol. (Pediatr Clin North Am 27:603–612,1980; Rudolph:802–803)

22. **(C)** Nitrite poisoning can result from medication overdose or ingestion (amyl nitrate, nitroglycerin) or environmental sources (nitrate food additives, contaminated well water). Nitrites increase the oxidation of hemoglobin, resulting in methemoglobinemia. Methemoglobin can be converted to hemoglobin by a reducing agent such as methylene blue, which is administered intravenously as a 1% solution. (Pediatr Clin North Am 27:603–612,1980; Rudolph:809,1141)

23. **(D)** The dose of diphenhydramine (Benadryl) is approximately 5 mg/kg per 24 hours, to a maximum adult dose of 50 mg every 4 hours. Drowsiness is a frequent side effect. Overdose can result in irritability, lethargy, or coma. Atropine-like side effects (dry mouth, dilated pupils, and flushing) may be seen. *(Hathaway:1084)*

24. **(B)** Dexamethasone is some 30 times more potent than cortisone. Various steroid preparations have different relative potencies in regard to glucocorticoid (antiinflammatory) and sodium retention

effects. Regarding the former, equivalent doses would be cortisone 25 mg, hydrocortisone 20 mg, prednisone 5 mg, prednisolone 4 mg, dexamethasone 0.75 mg. *(Rudolph: 1973)*

25. **(C)** Diazoxide (Hyperstat) is a very useful drug in the treatment of hypertensive emergencies, including those associated with acute glomerulonephritis. The drug may be used even in young children. It is administered by rapid intravenous injection in a dose of 2 mg/kg body weight. Hyperglycemia (not hypoglycemia) is a common side effect. *(Rudolph:1261, 1442; Hathaway:1084)*

26. **(D)** Infants and young children who are found to have a positive tuberculin skin test should be treated with isoniazid (INH) to prevent the development of active disease. Although INH treatment of the asymptomatic patient with a positive tuberculin skin test is not limited to infants and young children, it is especially important in this age group because of the high risk of miliary disease or tuberculous meningitis. There is no need to repeat the chest roentgenogram unless clinical signs of pulmonary involvement develop. Most authors now recommend a 7- to 9-month course of INH for children with positive tuberculin tests. *(Rudolph:632; Hathaway:886)*

27. **(A)** Peripheral neuritis is rarely seen in young children receiving INH but is a problem in adolescents and adults. This complication can be prevented by administration of 10 mg of vitamin B_6 for each 100 mg of INH. It usually is recommended that INH be given as a single daily dose, which is no less effective and no more toxic than divided doses. The major toxic effects are hepatic, not renal. Although concurrent administration of rifampin does increase the risk of drug-induced hepatitis, it is not contraindicated and is a very commonly used combination. *(Rudolph:631,1981; Hathaway:886)*

28. **(B)** Naloxone (Narcan) is a specific opiate antagonist that will reverse narcotic-induced coma or respiratory depression. The drug has a wide margin of safety and may be repeated as frequently as every 5 to 10 minutes. Overdose does not cause respiratory depression. *(Rudolph:813)*

29. **(A)** Hemorrhagic cystitis is a common toxic effect of large doses of cyclophosphamide. It is not associated with any of the other drugs listed. *(Fernbach JD, Vietti TJ: Clinical Pediatric Oncology, 4th ed. St. Louis, Mosby, 1900:152,565,1991)*

30. **(D)** There is no evidence to suggest that rheumatic chorea responds to the usual antirheumatic agents such as salicylates. Bed rest per se is not necessary. The most important aspects of management are quiet, sympathetic care, avoidance of emotional trauma and stress, and the judicious use of tranquil-

izers or phenobarbital. Drugs such as clonazepam and haloperidol appear to be useful in severe cases. Steroids have been suggested by some authors, but there are no data to document efficacy. It is most important that the patient be started on prophylactic penicillin to prevent recurrent attacks of acute rheumatic fever. *(Rudolph:494–495; Hathaway:702)*

31. **(E)** As chemotherapy of leukemia has intensified, hyperuricemia as a complication of cell death (the "tumor-lysis syndrome") has become more frequent. The major danger of this complication is uric acid nephropathy with acute renal failure. Allopurinol interferes with the conversion of xanthine and hypoxanthine to uric acid and is used to prevent hyperuricemia in children at risk for the tumor-lysis syndrome when receiving chemotherapy. Primarily, this includes children with large tumor masses likely to respond to chemotherapy—lymphomas and leukemia with very high peripheral white blood cell counts. *(Fernbach:152,565,1991)*

32. **(B)** With current induction regimens for acute leukemia of childhood, the central nervous system has become a major site of relapse. Of the antileukemic agents listed, only prednisone achieves a therapeutic level in the cerebrospinal fluid when administered systemically. Methotrexate is effective when given intrathecally. Craniospinal irradiation also is very effective, but it is not without late neurologic and intellectual sequela. *(Rudolph:1188)*

33. **(D)** The genetically determined condition of succinylcholine sensitivity is based on an abnormality (decreased activity) of the serum pseudocholinesterase enzyme. Patients with this condition may experience prolonged apnea and paralysis following administration of succinylcholine. These findings can be reversed, either by transfusion of normal plasma or by administration of a purified preparation of human pseudocholinesterase. A similar phenomenon has been reported with children with organophosphate poisoning given succinylcholine in preparation for intubation. *(Ann Emerg Med 16:215, 1987; Arch Neurol 28:274,1973)*

34. **(C)** The mechanism of action of tetracyclines (and other antibiotics) in pustular and cystic acne is reduction of numbers of *P. acnes* in the skin. It is believed that the action of these organisms on lipids in the sebum, releasing irritating free fatty acids, is a major factor in the development of pustules, nodules, and cysts. *(Rudolph:919)*

35. **(E)** Chronic serous otitis media, if unresponsive to more conservative measures (treatment of underlying allergy and infection if present, etc.), is an indication for myringotomy and insertion of tubes to drain the middle ear and to equalize the pressure in the middle ear (hence, "PE" tubes: pressure-equaliz-

ing tubes). Acute otitis media usually can be treated by antibiotics alone. If this is unsatisfactory, simple myringotomy by blade or needle may be indicated. Acute mastoiditis requires antibiotics and often simple mastoidectomy. Chronic draining otitis media may require long-term antibiotic therapy. Since there already is drainage through a perforation in the tympanic membrane, insertion of a tube would accomplish little. *(Rudolph:940; Hathaway:331)*

36. **(C)** Hepatoblastomas in childhood tend to metastasize later than those in adults. Surgery (partial hepatectomy) and chemotherapy is the treatment regimen of choice and carries a 30 to 50% 5-year cure rate. *(Rudolph:1214–1215)*

37. **(C)** The official tablespoon of the American Standards Association contains 14.79 mL, or approximately 15 mL. Home spoons, of course, vary considerably. A teaspoon holds approximately 5 mL. Differences in the size of home teaspoons and tablespoons make this mode of administration unsatisfactory for situations in which accurate dosage is important. Many prescription drugs are dispensed with syringes or calibrated spoons or droppers. This is essential for drugs such as digoxin or furosemide. *(Dorland's:1658,1665)*

38. **(C)** Both cefotaxime and ceftriaxone are effective single agents for the empiric treatment of bacterial meningitis beyond 2 or 3 months of life, when *Listeria monocytogenes* and gram-negative enteric organisms are no longer a concern. Although cefuroxime does enter the CSF and was once thought to be acceptable treatment for bacterial meningitis, subsequent studies showed consistently poorer results than with other regimens. *(Rudolph:560–562; Hathaway:704)*

39. **(C)** Use of the gluteal muscle as a site for injections in the infant or young child is dangerous. Injury to the sciatic nerve may occur, with resultant neuropathy, weakness, and stunting of leg growth. The anterolateral aspect of the thigh is the preferred site in children less than 2 years old. *(Pediatrics: 70:944–948, 1982)*

40. **(C)** Penicillin remains the drug of choice for the treatment of syphilis. Treatment requires that an effective blood level of the antibiotic be maintained for about 10 days. This is conveniently achieved with an appropriate dose of benzanthine penicillin as a single injection. *(Rudolph:619)*

41. **(C)** Most rashes occurring in children receiving ampicillin do not represent an IgE-mediated immediate-type hypersensitivity reaction. These patients are not at risk of a serious immediate reaction if the medication is taken again. As a matter of fact, such nonurticarial rashes generally do not require that

the drug be stopped and do not contraindicate its use again at a later date. Such rashes are especially frequent (up to 90% in some series) when children with Epstein-Barr virus infections receive ampicillin. (Am J Dis Child 125:187–190,1973; Hoekelman:1305)

42. (C) Most strains of *Klebsiella* are resistant to ampicillin. Most strains of *Listeria monocytogenes, Salmonella,* group A *Streptococcus,* and many strains of *Bordetella pertussis* are sensitive to ampicillin, although it is not necessarily the drug of choice for infection caused by these organisms. (J Pediatr 93:337–377,1978)

43. (D) The gastrointestinal absorption of phenoxymethylpenicillin is more reliable than the cheaper form, penicillin G. Shelf life and incidence of allergic reactions are the same for both drugs. Phenoxymethylpenicillin is slightly more expensive than pencillin G. The antimicrobial spectrum is essentially the same. (J Pediatr 93:337–377,1978)

44. (E) The recommended dose of gentamicin for sepsis or meningitis in the first week of life is 5.0 mg/kg per day in two divided doses. For sepsis or meningitis in the infant more than one week of age, the dose should be increased to 7.5 mg/kg per day and divided into three doses. These doses are based on maturation of renal function. (J Pediatr 93:337–377,1978; Rudolph:562)

45. (B) Erythromycin is the drug of choice to prevent spread of pertussis. Administration to the index case generally will eradicate the organism from the tracheobronchial tree and reduce dissemination. Administration to unimmunized infants and children having contact with the index case is advisable. In both cases, a 5- to 7-day course of erythromycin is recommended. (Feigin:1212)

46. (E) Penicillin remains the drug of choice for meningococcal meningitis. It is highly effective, inexpensive, and, except for allergic reactions, generally free of significant side effects. It has been in clinical use for over four decades, and it is unlikely that previously unrecognized toxic effects will be found. Although several of the third-generation cephalosporins are useful for the treatment of *H. influenzae* meningitis and for the treatment of bacterial meningitis prior to identification of the infecting organism, once the organism has been identified as a meningococcus, penicillin becomes the antibiotic of choice. The drug of choice for *prophylaxis* of close contacts, however, is rifampin not penicillin. (Hathaway:587)

47. (E) Intravenous gamma-globulin (IVGG) has been shown to be very effective in the treatment of idiopathic thrombocytopenic purpura (ITP). The response to IVGG is usually much more rapid than the response to steroids and may last for several weeks.

Many children have no further thrombocytopenia after a single treatment. Although expensive, IVGG is appropriate primary therapy for ITP, and its use is not limited to patients who have failed to respond to other treatment. Mild cases may not require any treatment. (Hathaway:500; Oski:155)

48. (C) The dose of digoxin needs to be individualized for every patient, regardless of age. In neonates, in general, the digitalizing dose is less than in older children; the dose is even less for premature infants. The usual digitalizing dose for a premature infant is in the order of 0.035 mg/kg. (Hathaway:425)

49. (B) Antitoxin is the most critical aspect of the treatment of diphtheria regardless of how early the diagnosis is established. Of course, an appropriate antibiotic (erythromycin or penicillin) also should be administered. Although antibiotics have little effect on the clinical course of the disease, they will at least render the patient noncontagious. (Rudolph:578)

50. (C) The usual insulin requirement for a diabetic child or adolescent is in the range of 0.8 to 1.2 units/kg per day. A requirement greater than 1.2 or 1.5 units/kg per day should suggest overtreatment, posthypoglycemic hyperglycemia, or overeating with poor control. Another possible cause of increased insulin requirement is the development of antiinsulin antibodies. Although antiinsulin antibodies are not rare, they are rarely the cause of clinical resistance to insulin and poor control of blood glucose. (Rudolph:344; Hathaway:812)

51. (D) A serum level of factor VIII of 25 to 50% of normal will control most non-life-threatening episodes of bleeding, including hemarthrosis, in patients with hemophilia. It is important to avoid administering excessive amounts of antihemophilic concentrates unnecessarily. The material is expensive and carries the risk of transmission of viral diseases. (Rudolph:1163)

52. (C) Cystic fibrosis is the most common cause of pancreatic insufficiency in childhood. Most patients with this disease have less steatorrhea and improved weight gain when receiving pancreatic replacement therapy. Treatment with oral pancreatic enzymes is of no value for any of the other conditions listed, none of which are associated with involvement of the pancreas. (Rudolph:251–252,1043)

53. (A) Corticosteroids are very useful and a major aspect of treatment for both ulcerative colitis and regional enteritis. They are, however, mainly beneficial in the treatment of acute attacks and exacerbations and have limited value in long-term management. They are generally discontinued in favor of other medications once symptoms have been brought under control. (Rudolph:1026; Hathaway:572)

54. (B) Deferoxamine (desferrioxamine) is the chelating agent of choice for iron poisoning. It effectively binds the metal and is excreted in the urine. Deferoxamine is indicated for severe intoxication—ingestion of more than 25 mg/kg of elemental iron or a serum iron concentration exceeding 350 mg/dL. Dimercaprol (BAL) actually enhances the toxicity of iron and is contraindicated in cases of iron poisoning. *(Rudolph:806)*

55. (C) Organophosphate insecticides are reversible inhibitors of the enzyme acetylcholinesterase. Atropine reverses the muscarinic action and central nervous system effects of the anticholinesterases. A cholinesterase-reactivating oxime such as pralidoxime (PAM) is effective against both the nicotinic (skeletal muscle paralysis) and the muscarinic as well as the central nervous system effects of the poison. Physostigmine is an acetylcholinesterase inhibitor like the organophosphates and would make the patient worse rather than better. *(Rudolph: 814–815)*

56. (D) Most cases of grade III and less reflux will eventually improve or remit without surgical intervention. Invasive techniques of unproven benefit, such as repetitive cystoscopy, meatotomy, and internal urethrotomy, should be avoided unless specifically indicated. Continuous prophylaxis with appropriate antibiotics is recommended and is the most important aspect of management. Frequent voiding schedules as well as double or triple voiding techniques can be considered only adjunctive measures. *(Rudolph:1299)*

57. (A) With the aggressive and coordinated use of surgery, radiotherapy, and currently available chemotherapeutic agents, the outlook for Wilms's tumor is the best of any of the common childhood malignancies. Overall survival is about 80% and may be as high as 90% in patients with favorable histologic features. *(Rudolph:1201; Hathaway:967)*

58. (B) After an initial intravenous bolus of insulin of 0.1 unit/kg, the dosage recommended for treatment of diabetic ketoacidosis is generally 0.1 unit/kg per hour. A few patients will require 0.2 unit/kg per hour. *(Rudolph:339; Hathaway:811)*

59. (E) Metronidazole, chloroquine, diiodohydroxyquin, emetine, and dehydroemetine are effective amebicidal drugs useful in the treatment of enteric infection. Emetine and dehydroemetine are quite toxic (vomiting, abdominal pain, tachycardia, hypotension, and arrhythmias) and generally are indicated only when other, safer agents have failed. Iodoquinol is used for mild or asymptomatic intestinal infection. Metronidazole is employed for more severe intestinal infection and for hepatic abscesses. *(Rudolph:745)*

60. (D) The majority of cases of tinea corporis and tinea pedis will respond to topical antifungal therapy, and systemic treatment with griseofulvin generally is not indicated. Tinea capitis, on the other hand, responds very poorly to local therapy, and oral griseofulvin is standard therapy. Candidiasis does not respond to griseofulvin. [*Note:* Even though griseofulvin is highly effective against tinea corporis, it is not the treatment of choice. Therefore, **(D)** is the *best* answer.] *(Rudolph:927)*

61. (E) Maple syrup urine disease is a disorder of amino acid metabolism involving the branched-chain amino acids leucine, isoleucine, and valine. Because these amino acids cannot be properly metabolized, dietary restriction is mandatory. In infancy, this requires a synthetic diet with carefully controlled quantities of the branched-chain amino acids. Carbohydrate intake need not be controlled. The disease gets its name from a characteristic maple syrup or caramel odor of the urine. *(Rudolph:305)*

62. (D) Increased intracranial pressure (pseudotumor cerebri) is an infrequent but dramatic toxic side effect of tetracyclines that can occur at any age. Tetracyclines deposit in *developing* teeth and bone, and permanent discoloration is common if large cumulative doses are taken prior to 7 or 8 years of age. *(Rudolph:533)*

63. (D) Surgical intervention with pinning currently is the treatment of choice for slipped femoral epiphysis, a condition of unknown origin occurring primarily in pubescent males. The slippage is generally gradual, unrelated to trauma, and not uncommonly bilateral. Initial treatment of both congenital dysplasia of the hip and Legg-Calvé-Perthes disease is conservative, and surgery is indicated only in cases diagnosed late or those for whom medical management has failed. There is no surgical treatment for Caffey's disease, which is a self-limited inflammatory condition of bone of undetermined origin. Osgood-Schlatter disease is an inflammation at the insertion of the patellar tendon on the tibial tubercle and is treated primarily by rest and decreased physical activity. *(Rudolph:1942–44)*

64. (B) Fluoride supplementation is useful from birth to about 8 years of age, when calcification of most of the permanent teeth is complete. Supplementation is recommended for infants and children in areas where the water supply contains less than 1 ppm of fluoride, for infants who are exclusively breast fed, and for infants who are receiving only ready-to-feed formulas. Fluoride requirement is not related to exposure to sunlight. *(Rudolph:28,981; Hathaway:112–113)*

65. (E) Treatment of gonococcal urethritis depends on achieving a high antimicrobial level in the serum for a short time; prolonged treatment is not required. Benzanthine penicillin should never be used, as it will not achieve sufficiently high blood levels. Ampicillin, 3.0 g orally once, with 1 g of probenecid or procaine penicillin, 4.8 million units IM with 1 g of probenecid, is effective against penicillin-sensitive strains. However, penicillin resistance is so common that a single dose of ceftriaxone, 250 mg IM, is generally the treatment of choice. *(Hathaway:860)*

66. **(A)** Liver injury is the major toxic effect of acetaminophen poisoning and generally is seen only with very large overdoses or poisonings. The hepatic damage is not caused by the acetaminophen itself but rather by a toxic metabolic product. The metabolic pathway producing the hepatotoxic metabolite is less well developed in infants and young children, and therefore, the risks of liver injury are actually somewhat less in young children. Treatment involves oral administration of N-acetylcysteine, which minimizes metabolism of the acetaminophen to the toxic metabolite. To be effective, treatment must be started within 24 hours of ingestion. *(Rudolph:788–789)*

67. **(D)** Naloxone is an effective antagonist to, and will reverse the effects of, morphine and its derivatives, including methadone, codeine, pentazocine, and dextropropoxyphene. However, it is not effective against barbiturates. *(Rudolph:813)*

68. **(D)** The numerous side effects of corticosteroids include *hyper*glycemia, growth retardation, hypertension, osteoporosis, central obesity, moon facies, acne, hirsutism, myopathy, pseudotumor cerebri, cataracts, and glaucoma. (Am J Dis Child *132:806–810, 1978*)

69. **(E)** Splenectomy is required frequently in patients with beta-thalassemia major or hereditary spherocytosis and occasionally in patients with hereditary elliptocytosis. In these conditions, removal of the spleen results in less rapid destruction of affected erythrocytes and, therefore, lessening of the anemia. In the case of thalassemia, splenectomy results in the need for less frequent blood transfusions. Hypersplenism is cured by splenectomy, although the underlying disease that led to the splenomegaly and hypersplenism may remain. Splenectomy has no role in the management of aplastic anemia. *(Rudolph:1130,1133–1134)*

70. **(D)** Chlorambucil is used in the treatment of Hodgkin's disease in children but not in the therapy of acute leukemia of childhood. Prednisone, methotrexate, cyclophosphamide, and vincristine are important and commonly used agents. *(Rudolph:1188)*

71. **(A)** The major mechanism in renal osteodystrophy and hypocalcemia is believed to be phosphate retention from a decrease in renal excretion of phosphate. Management includes restricting dietary phosphate and administering phosphate binders such as $CaCO_3$ (calcium carbonate), which decrease intestinal absorption of phosphate. The $CaCO_3$ also is a source of calcium. Most patients also require vitamin D analogs such as $1,25-(OH)_2 D_3$. Recombinant erythropoietin is helpful in treating the anemia of chronic renal failure. *(Rudolph:1249–1250)*

72. **(B)** Three types of insulin preparations are available—short, intermediate, and long-acting. The long-acting forms are used only infrequently for children. Lente is an intermediate insulin preparation, with peak effect at about 8 to 12 hours and duration of action of 18 to 24 hours. *(Rudolph:1981)*

73. **(C)** Ultralente is a long-acting insulin preparation, peaking at about 14 to 18 hours and lasting over 24 hours. *(Rudolph:1981)*

74. **(A)** Semilente insulin is short-acting and peaks at about 2 to 3 hours. The duration of action of semilente insulin is in the order of 6 hours. *(Rudolph:1981)*

75. **(A)** Regular insulin is similar to semilente in action. It peaks in 2 to 3 hours and lasts for about 6 hours. *(Rudolph:1981)*

76. **(B)** NPH insulin is similar to lente. It peaks at 8 to 12 hours and lasts for 18 to 24 hours. Combinations of short- and intermediate-acting insulins (eg, regular plus NPH) in the same injection are used frequently. Once or twice a day injections of such combinations will provide adequate control of blood sugar for most children with diabetes. *(Rudolph:1981)*

77. **(A)** Cefoxitin is a second-generation cephalosporin. Ceftazidime is a third-generation cephalosporin. *(J Pediatr 107:161–168,1985; Rudolph:530–531; Hathaway: 1091)*

78. **(B)** First- and second-generation cephalosporins (including cefoxitin) are not effective against *Pseudomonas* species. Third-generation cephalosporins are effective against *Pseudomonas*, and ceftazidime is the most effective of all. (J Pediatr *107:161–168,1985; Rudolph:530–531; Hathaway:1091*)

79. **(A)** Cephalosporins generally are not clinically effective against anaerobic bacteria. Cefoxitin is the only exception to this rule and is quite effective against most anaerobes including *Bacteroides fragilis*. (J Pediatr *107:161–168,1985; Rudolph:530–531; Hathaway:1091*)

80. **(D)** *Listeria monocytogenes* is uniformly resistant to all currently available cephalosporins. (J Pediatr *107:161–168,1985; Rudolph:530–531; Hathaway:1091*)

81. **(C)** Although third-generation cephalosporins are more effective against *E. coli* than are members of the first and second generations, all cephalosporins

are rated as effective against this organism. *(J Pediatr 107:161–168,1985; Rudolph:530–531; Hathaway:1091)*

82. **(C)** Furosemide (Lasix) and spironolactone (Aldactone) are clinically useful diuretics. The former is much more potent and is available for intravenous and intramuscular as well as oral administration. The latter produces only a mild to moderate diuresis and is available only as an oral preparation. Furosemide is very useful and in general is the diuretic of choice for the acute management of severe congestive heart failure. *(J Pediatr 86:657–669,825–832,1975; Rudolph:1431)*

83. **(B)** Spironolactone usually is employed as an ancillary diuretic (in combination with furosemide or chlorothiazide) and is especially useful because of its potassium-retaining effect, which helps offset the potassium-wasting effect of furosemide or chlorothiazide. *(J Pediatr 86:657–669,825–832,1975; Rudolph: 1431)*

84. **(D)** Neither of these agents increases systemic blood pressure; as a matter of fact, they usually reduce systemic blood pressure. *(J Pediatr 86:657–669,825–832,1975; Rudolph:1431)*

85. **(A)** Side effects of furosemide not shared by spironolactone include ototoxicity and renal stones secondary to hypercalciuria. *(J Pediatr 86:657–669,825–832, 1975; Rudolph:1431)*

BIBLIOGRAPHY

Balfour HH Jr, Rotbart HA, Feldman S, et al. Acyclovir treatment of varicella in otherwise healthy adolescents. The Collaborative Acyclovir Study Group. *J Pediatr.* 1992;120:627–733.

Bergeson PS, Singer SA, Kaplan AM. Intramuscular injections in children. *Pediatrics.* 1982;70:944–948.

Cherington M, Lasater G. Prolonged paralysis in pseudocholinesterase deficiency. *Arch Neurol.* 1973;28:274–275.

Dorland's Illustrated Medical Dictionary. 27 ed., Philadelphia, Pa: WB Saunders; 1988.

Dunkle LM, Arvin AM, Whitley RJ, et al. A controlled trial of acyclovir for chickenpox in normal children. *N Eng J Med.* 1991;325:1539–1544.

Eichenwald HF. Medical progress: antimicrobial therapy in infants and children: update. *J Pediatr.* 1985;107: 161–168.

Eichenwald HF, McCracken GH Jr. Antimicrobial therapy in infants and children. Part I. Review of antimicrobial agents. *J Pediatr.* 1978;93:337–377.

Fernbach JD, Vietti TJ. *Clinical Pediatric Oncology.* 4th ed. St. Louis, Mo: Mosby; 1991.

Frank JP, Friedberg DZ. Syncope with prolonged QT interval. *Am J Dis Child.* 1978;130:320–322.

Hathaway WE, Groothius JR, Hay WW, et al. *Current Pediatric Diagnosis & Treatment.* 10th ed. Norwalk, Conn: Appleton & Lange; 1991.

Hoekelman RA, Friedman SB, Nelson NM, et al. *Primary Pediatric Care.* 2nd ed. St. Louis, Mo: Mosby Year Book; 1992.

Kerns D, Shira JE, Go S, et al. Ampicillin rash in children. Relationship to penicillin allergy and infectious mononucleosis. *Am J Dis Child.* 1973;125:187–190.

Kilham HA. Hospital management of severe poisoning. *Pediatr Clin North Am.* 1980;27:603–612.

Loggie JM, Kleinman LI, Van-Maanen EF. Renal function and diuretic therapy in infants and children. Part II. *J Pediatr.* 1975;86:657–659.

McEnery PT, Gonzales LL, Martin LW, et al. Growth and development of children with renal transplants. Use of alternate-day steroid therapy. *J Pediatr.* 1973;5:806–814.

Oski FA, DeAngelis CD, Feigin RD, et al. *Principles & Practice of Pediatrics.* Philadelphia, Pa: JB Lippincott; 1990.

Rimsza ME. Complications of corticosteroid therapy. *Am J Dis Child.* 1978;132:806–810.

Rudolph AM, Hoffman JIE, Rudolph CD. *Pediatrics.* 19th ed. Norwalk, Conn: Appleton & Lange; 1991.

Sadeghi-Najad A, Senior B. Adrenal function, growth, and insulin in patients treated with corticoids on alternate days. *Pediatrics.* 1969;43:277–282.

Selden BS, Curry SC. Prolonged succinylcholine-induced paralysis in organophosphate insecticide poisoning. *Ann Emerg Med.* 1987;16:215–217.

CHAPTER 9

General Pediatrics
Questions

This chapter deals with those aspects of pediatrics not covered in the preceding chapters. When analyzing pediatric diseases by system or by etiology, the student should recognize that not all systems or etiologic categories are created equal. Infectious diseases, respiratory and gastrointestinal problems, and trauma are the most common disorders of childhood beyond the newborn period. The spectrum of general pediatrics is very different from the spectrum of internal medicine. In contrast to adulthood, for example, cardiac problems are uncommon in childhood, and those that do occur are usually congenital and present early in life. Beyond the newborn period, the most common cause for referral of a child to a cardiologist is a *functional* or *innocent* murmur. There will be proportionately fewer cardiology questions on a pediatric examination than on an internal medicine examination.

DIRECTIONS (Questions 1 through 84): Each of the numbered items or incomplete statements in this section is followed by answers or by completions of the statement. Select the ONE lettered answer or completion that is BEST in each case.

1. The highest death rate in the pediatric age group occurs

   (A) in the first month of life
   (B) between 2 and 12 months of life
   (C) between 2 and 4 years of life
   (D) just before puberty
   (E) during adolescence

2. The use of a blood pressure cuff that covers one-half of the length of the upper arm

   (A) may cause pain and discomfort
   (B) may give an erroneously low reading
   (C) may give an erroneously high reading
   (D) can cause a pulsus paradoxus
   (E) is appropriate in children less than 5 years of age or less than 25 kg of body weight

3. The most common cause of chronic subdural hematoma in infants is

   (A) acute leukemia
   (B) child abuse
   (C) congenital defects of the brain
   (D) hemophilia
   (E) scurvy

4. A 10-year-old boy presents with signs of increased intracranial pressure. Suprasellar calcifications are evident on skull roentgenogram. The most likely cause of these findings is

   (A) toxoplasmosis
   (B) metastatic neuroblastoma
   (C) optic glioma
   (D) pseudotumor cerebri
   (E) craniopharyngioma

5. A 3-year-old child with poor growth and serum IgA antigliadin antibodies probably has

   (A) celiac disease
   (B) chronic renal disease
   (C) cystic fibrosis
   (D) hyperimmunoglobulinemia A
   (E) milk protein hypersensitivity

6. A severely retarded infant is noted to have hepatosplenomegaly and a cherry-red spot in the macula. Of the following, which is most likely the cause of these findings?

   (A) Tay-Sachs disease
   (B) Niemann-Pick disease (type A, infantile)
   (C) Gaucher's disease (infantile)
   (D) Metachromatic leukodystrophy
   (E) Globoid-cell leukodystrophy

7. A 12-year-old girl develops progressive tremors and emotional lability. Ophthalmologic examination reveals a golden-brown discoloration of the limbic region of the cornea. The most likely diagnosis is

(A) Down's syndrome
(B) congenital rubella
(C) glycogen storage disease
(D) Wilson's disease
(E) lead poisoning

8. The diagnosis of Werdnig-Hoffman disease is most likely in an infant with progressive muscular weakness and

(A) normal deep tendon reflexes
(B) seizures
(C) fasciculations of the tongue
(D) recurrent fevers
(E) atrophy of the optic nerve

9. Early diagnosis of cerebral palsy is important because it permits

(A) genetic counseling to prevent subsequent cases
(B) treatment of the underlying lesion and prevention of progression
(C) guidance that may minimize or prevent secondary physical and emotional problems
(D) prophylactic anticonvulsant treatment to be instituted prior to the onset of seizures

10. The most common type of cerebral palsy is

(A) ataxic
(B) athetoid
(C) hypotonic
(D) mixed
(E) spastic

11. A 3-year-old child presents with the relatively sudden onset of truncal ataxia. Other than ataxia and a mild lateral nystagmus, physical and neurological examination are normal. A CT scan of the head is unremarkable. Lumbar puncture reveals a clear fluid with normal pressure. Examination of the cerebrospinal fluid discloses 25 mononuclear cells per cubic millimeter, normal concentrations of protein and glucose, and a negative Gram's stain. It would be most reasonable to advise the parents to expect

(A) fairly rapid improvement
(B) progression of ataxia
(C) progression of ataxia and development of seizures
(D) progression of ataxia and development of dementia
(E) permanent persistence of ataxia

12. Which of the following statements about neuroblastoma is correct?

(A) Adrenal insufficiency is the most common presenting complaint
(B) Survival is best in children in whom the tumor presents beyond age 2 years

(C) Hematuria is a common finding
(D) It usually presents between 4 and 8 years of age
(E) Spontaneous regression has occurred in some children

13. A 2-year-old child with aniridia and an abdominal mass probably has

(A) a hemangioma of the liver
(B) an intestinal duplication
(C) a neuroblastoma
(D) a teratoma
(E) Wilms's tumor

14. The diencephalic syndrome, which may be seen in infants with tumors in or near the hypothalamus, is characterized by

(A) papilledema and an enlarging head
(B) hyperalertness, euphoria, and emaciation
(C) lethargy, increased appetite, and obesity
(D) seizures, mental retardation, and hypertension
(E) aggressive behavior, obesity, and blindness

15. Congenital malformations, other than those of the head and face, most commonly seen in association with craniosynostosis involve the

(A) trachea and esophagus
(B) heart
(C) umbilicus
(D) extremities
(E) spine

16. Rheumatic chorea is associated with

(A) convulsions
(B) a fine tremor at rest
(C) increased intracranial pressure
(D) irregular, jerky, and spasmodic movements

17. The most characteristic EEG finding in complex partial (psychomotor) seizures is

(A) spikes over the temporal lobes
(B) diffuse slowing
(C) generalized spike-and-wave pattern
(D) multifocal spikes
(E) slowing in the occipital regions

18. The arthritis of acute rheumatic fever usually

(A) is monarticular
(B) heals without deformity
(C) appears after the fever subsides
(D) is seen only in patients with concurrent carditis
(E) involves large (ie, ankle, knee, wrist) and small (hands and feet) joints equally

19. Malignant hyperthermia is associated with

(A) cardiovascular collapse during exercise
(B) hyperthermia precipitated by a variety of muscle relaxants and anesthetic agents

(C) high fever during chemotherapy of leukemia or lymphoma

(D) severe metabolic alkalosis

(E) elevated body temperature secondary to a brain tumor

20. A previously well 6-month-old infant is brought to the emergency room because of signs of an upper respiratory infection and because "his heart is beating fast." Examination reveals an uncomfortable appearing infant with tachycardia. Temperature is 38.3°C. An ECG shows a very regular heart rate of 280 beats per minute. It is not clear whether or not P waves are present; the QRS complexes are normal. The infant most likely has

(A) sinus tachycardia secondary to a URI and fever

(B) sinus tachycardia secondary to congenital structural heart disease

(C) supraventricular tachycardia without underlying structural heart disease

(D) supraventricular tachycardia secondary to congenital structural heart disease

(E) supraventricular tachycardia secondary to Wolff-Parkinson-White syndrome

21. The most common organisms to cause bacterial endocarditis in children are

(A) streptococci and staphylococci

(B) streptococci and *Hemophilus* species

(C) *Hemophilus* species and pneumococci

(D) staphylococci and *Salmonella* species

(E) staphylococci and *Hemophilus* species

22. A 2-month-old infant is hospitalized because of severe dyspnea and cyanosis. Chest roentgenogram reveals minimal cardiomegaly and a diffuse reticular pattern of the lung fields. Which of the following best explains these findings?

(A) Acute viral myocarditis

(B) Hypoplastic left heart

(C) Pulmonary artery atresia

(D) Total anomalous pulmonary drainage with venous obstruction

(E) Transposition of the great arteries

23. Balloon atrial septostomy is most useful in infants with

(A) large ventricular septal defects

(B) anomalous pulmonary venous drainage

(C) truncus arteriosus

(D) transposition of the great arteries

(E) endocardial fibroelastosis

24. Which of the following statements regarding brain tumors in childhood is true?

(A) Most are located in the midline and/or below the tentorium cerebri

(B) Brain tumors are a rare type of cancer in childhood

(C) Signs of increased intracranial pressure are rare

(D) Seizures are the presenting complaint in most cases

(E) Most cases occur in the first year of life

25. An 8-month-old child is hospitalized because of vomiting and screaming episodes for 12 hours. During the episodes, the infant draws up his legs as if having abdominal pain. Physical examination reveals a sausage-shaped mass in the right upper quadrant. Temperature is 38°C. White blood cell count is 18,000/mm^3. Which of the following would be most useful?

(A) Passage of nasogastric tube

(B) Examination of a stool specimen for ova and parasites

(C) Blood culture

(D) Renal ultrasound

(E) Barium enema

26. Most cases of pancreatic insufficiency in childhood are caused by

(A) autoimmune disease

(B) biliary atresia

(C) carcinoma

(D) congenital absence of the pancreas

(E) cystic fibrosis

27. A 10-year-old child with muscle weakness, an erythematous, scaly rash on the face, arms, and hands, and heliotrope patches on the eyelids most likely has

(A) dermatomyositis

(B) eczema

(C) Henoch-Schönlein purpura

(D) juvenile rheumatoid arthritis

(E) trichinosis

28. Which of the following conditions is associated with an increased risk of brain abscess?

(A) Chronic renal failure

(B) Idiopathic or familial epilepsy

(C) Congenital cyanotic heart disease

(D) Chronic or recurrent tonsillitis

(E) Tay-Sachs disease

29. A positive serum rheumatoid factor is uncommon in children with rheumatoid disease other than systemic lupus erythematosus. When it does occur, it is most likely in a girl with

(A) the acute systemic form of juvenile rheumatoid arthritis

(B) the pauciarticular form of juvenile rheumatoid arthritis

(C) the polyarticular form of juvenile rheumatoid arthritis

(D) psoriatic arthritis

(E) ankylosing spondylitis

30. The most reliable method of prevention of recurrent episodes of acute rheumatic fever is

(A) prophylactic penicillin for all dental and surgical procedures as well as for trauma and febrile illnesses
(B) prompt treatment with oral or intramuscular penicillin for 10 days for any signs or symptoms of pharyngitis
(C) prompt treatment with oral or intramuscular penicillin for 10 days for any febrile illness
(D) an intramuscular injection of benzathine penicillin every 4 weeks
(E) prompt administration of penicillin and corticosteroids for 14 days for any documented infection with group A beta-hemolytic streptococci

31. A 2-year-old black child presents with anemia and painful swelling of the hands and feet. The most likely diagnosis is

(A) child abuse
(B) congenital syphilis
(C) leukemia
(D) sickle cell disease
(E) vitamin D deficiency

32. Which of the following is most likely to occur as an isolated manifestation of acute rheumatic fever?

(A) Arthritis
(B) Carditis
(C) Chorea
(D) Erythema marginatum
(E) Fever

33. Which of the following is most frequently an important factor in the etiology of iron deficiency anemia in a 2-year-old child?

(A) Use of artificial sweeteners
(B) Lack of fresh fruit in the diet
(C) Intake of large amounts of fruit juice
(D) Intake of excessive amounts of vitamin C
(E) Intake of large amounts of unmodified cow milk

34. The benign lymphangioma known as the cystic hygroma occurs most frequently in

(A) the head and neck
(B) the groin
(C) the mediastinum
(D) the abdomen
(E) the extremities

35. Ultrasound examination of a 2-year-old child with an abdominal mass reveals displacement of the kidney without intrinsic distortion of the calyces or pelvis. The most likely cause of the mass is a(an)

(A) adrenal carcinoma
(B) adrenal hemorrhage
(C) metastatic osteogenic sarcoma
(D) neuroblastoma
(E) Wilms's tumor

36. Bone marrow aspiration is most likely to confirm the diagnosis in a patient with which one of the following malignancies?

(A) Hepatoblastoma
(B) Neuroblastoma
(C) Retinoblastoma
(D) Rhabdomyosarcoma
(E) Wilms's tumor

37. A 6-year-old child is seen because of ear pain. The child is afebrile. The skin of the left ear canal is markedly edematous and moderately inflamed. There is a drop of thick, yellow discharge visible at the external meatus; it is not possible to insert an otoscope into the edematous canal. There is exquisite pain when you move the tragus. The remainder of the examination is unremarkable. The child denies putting anything in his ear but does acknowledge that he has been spending a lot of time in the swimming pool. The most likely diagnosis is

(A) a cholesteotoma
(B) a foreign body
(C) draining otitis media
(D) mastoiditis
(E) otitis externa

38. Intestinal lactase deficiency in infancy

(A) may be either genetic or acquired
(B) often is associated with pancreatitis
(C) causes a strongly alkaline pH of the stool
(D) is a recognized cause of intestinal obstruction
(E) usually leads to malabsorption without clinically evident diarrhea

39. Careful observation and periodic examination are most important for siblings of a child with

(A) Ewing's sarcoma
(B) leukemia
(C) neuroblastoma
(D) osteogenic sarcoma
(E) retinoblastoma

40. Patients with anaphylactoid purpura (Henoch-Schönlein purpura) generally have

(A) a decreased platelet count
(B) a prolonged prothrombin time
(C) a prolonged partial thromboplastin time
(D) a prolonged bleeding time
(E) normal clotting parameters

41. Features of the McCune-Albright syndrome include polyosteotic fibrous dysplasia of bone, abnormal skin pigmentation, and

(A) anemia
(B) deafness
(C) precocious puberty

(D) multiple neurofibromas

(E) chronic glomerulonephritis

42. Which of the following is a feature of congenital hypoplastic anemia (Diamond-Blackfan syndrome)?

(A) Associated malformations, especially of the thumbs, heart, and skeleton

(B) Intrauterine placental transfusion between twins of dissimilar blood types

(C) Microcytosis

(D) Intrauterine infection

(E) Hepatosplenomegaly

43. A patent ductus arteriosus in an otherwise normal 6-month-old infant is likely to be associated with

(A) a right-to-left shunt

(B) a continuous murmur at the second left intercostal space

(C) a narrow pulse

(D) bacterial endocarditis

(E) right ventricular hypertrophy

44. A 3-year-old child with cyanosis and clubbing, a systolic murmur, and a history of squatting during exertion and of episodes of increased cyanosis and loss of consciousness probably has

(A) breathholding spells

(B) cystic fibrosis

(C) cardiomyopathy

(D) pulmonary fibrosis

(E) tetralogy of Fallot

45. Which of the following is most likely to present as congestive heart failure in infancy?

(A) Marfan's syndrome

(B) Endocardial fibroelastosis

(C) Friedreich's ataxia

(D) Ostium secundum atrial septal defect

(E) Sickle cell disease

46. The most common presentation of congenital aganglionic megacolon (Hirschsprung's disease) in the newborn is

(A) an abdominal mass

(B) diarrhea

(C) intestinal obstruction

(D) peritonitis

(E) sepsis

47. Transient erythroblastopenia of childhood

(A) is most common in the first 2 months of life

(B) may be associated with severe anemia requiring transfusion

(C) is associated with macrocytic cells with an increased percentage of fetal hemoglobin

(D) tends to recur repeatedly until adolescence

(E) is most frequently seen in association with anicteric hepatitis B infection

48. Complex partial (psychomotor) seizures are characterized by

(A) lack of alterations in mental state, consciousness, or responsiveness

(B) a brief tonic-clonic phase

(C) automatisms

(D) three-per-second spike-and-wave pattern on EEG

(E) lack of postictal phenomenon

49. Infantile spasms usually are characterized by

(A) persistent, chronic jerking of individual extremities

(B) persistent, chronic twitching of individual muscles

(C) episodes of localized muscle spasm lasting minutes to hours

(D) episodes of sudden and brief spasms of trunk, neck, and extremities

(E) spasms of the small muscles of the face, hands, and feet

50. The most common presenting sign in children with Hodgkin's disease is

(A) hepatosplenomegaly

(B) rash and/or pruritus

(C) localized superficial lymphadenopathy

(D) anemia

(E) failure to thrive

51. Infantile spasms are associated with

(A) a hypsarrhythmic pattern on EEG

(B) a favorable outlook in regard to neurologic and intellectual development

(C) a response to treatment with phenobarbital

(D) hypocalcemia

(E) an abnormality of metabolism of skeletal muscle

52. A systolic heart murmur is heard on routine examination of an asymptomatic 12-year-old child. The electrocardiogram shown in Figure 9–1 is obtained. Which of the following diagnoses is most likely?

(A) Atrial septal defect

(B) Coarctation of the aorta

(C) Endocardial fibroelastosis

(D) Hyperthyroidism

(E) Ventricular septal defect

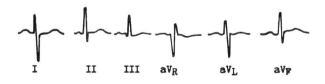

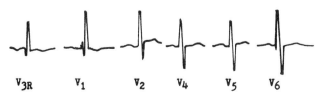

Figure 9–1

53. A 3-month-old infant is admitted because of lethargy and irritability. The roentgenograms shown in Figure 9–2 are obtained on admission. The most likely diagnosis is

(A) child abuse
(B) metastatic neuroblastoma
(C) multifocal osteomyelitis
(D) osteogenesis imperfecta
(E) rickets

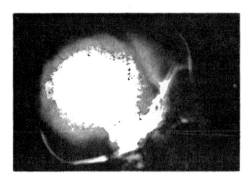

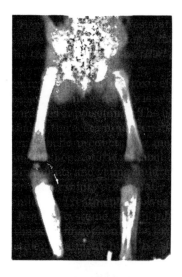

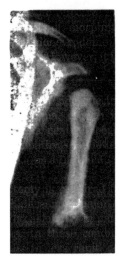

Figure 9–2

54. Megaloblastic anemia may be seen occasionally in infants

(A) with Hirschsprung's disease
(B) being fed goat milk
(C) being fed unmodified cow milk
(D) on a low-fat diet
(E) with cystic fibrosis

55. Familial dysautonomia (Riley-Day syndrome) is seen predominantly in

(A) African blacks
(B) individuals of European Jewish ancestry
(C) individuals of Arab ancestry
(D) individuals of Mediterranean ancestry
(E) Asians

56. Increased intracranial pressure may be seen with

(A) achondroplasia
(B) glycogen storage disease
(C) hypervitaminosis C
(D) galactosemia
(E) juvenile rheumatoid arthritis

57. Werdnig-Hoffman disease (infantile spinal muscular atrophy) is characterized by

(A) weakness, hypertonia, and increased deep tendon reflexes
(B) hypertonia, weakness, and muscle fasciculations
(C) weakness with normal muscle tone and deep tendon reflexes
(D) hypotonia, decreased deep tendon reflexes, and muscle fasciculations
(E) hypotonia, normal strength, and normal deep tendon reflexes

58. The most common ophthalmologic complication in children with juvenile rheumatoid arthritis is

(A) cataracts
(B) ptosis
(C) glaucoma
(D) corneal ulcerations
(E) iridocyclitis

Please note the use of a negative qualifier such as EXCEPT, LEAST, or NOT in each of the following questions (Questions 59 through 84).

59. Which of the following would NOT be expected in a child with pseudotumor cerebri

(A) increased intracranial pressure
(B) papilledema
(C) sixth nerve palsy
(D) coma
(E) headache

60. Spasmus nutans is characterized by all of the following EXCEPT

(A) nystagmus
(B) trismus
(C) head nodding
(D) deviation or tilt of the head
(E) eventual resolution

61. Which of the following statements about non-Hodgkin's lymphoma in children is NOT true?

(A) It is more common than Hodgkin's disease
(B) Abdominal involvement may present with intussusception
(C) Involvement of the central nervous system occurs frequently
(D) Diffuse involvement of bone marrow occurs frequently
(E) Radiation therapy, with or without chemotherapy, is the treatment of choice

62. Which of the following statements regarding leukemia in childhood is NOT correct?

(A) It is the most common form of cancer in childhood
(B) The peak incidence in childhood is in the 12- to 16-year age group
(C) The most common form is acute lymphoblastic leukemia (ALL)
(D) It is more common in white than nonwhite children
(E) There is an increased incidence in children with Down's syndrome

63. Which of the following statements regarding central nervous system involvement by leukemia in children is NOT correct?

(A) CNS involvement may occur while the patient is in bone marrow remission
(B) Signs and symptoms include headache, vomiting, and papilledema
(C) Involvement can be detected in the asymptomatic patient by routine lumbar puncture
(D) Most cases respond to vigorous systemic chemotherapy
(E) Intrathecal methotrexate can be used for both prevention and treatment

64. Which of the following would NOT be expected between acute episodes in a 7-year-old boy with uncomplicated sickle cell disease?

(A) Hemoglobin 5.0 g/dL
(B) Reticulocyte count of 12%
(C) Total white blood cell count of 19,000/mm^3
(D) Macrocytosis of red blood cells
(E) Sickle cells noted on peripheral blood smear

65. Glucose-6-phosphate dehydrogenase deficiency in blacks has been associated with all of the following EXCEPT

(A) acute hemolytic episodes following the ingestion of certain drugs with oxidant properties
(B) neonatal hyperbilirubinemia in the premature infant
(C) hemolysis of young as well as old red cells
(D) reticulocytosis
(E) X-linked recessive pattern of inheritance

66. Which of the following statements comparing periorbital and orbital cellulitis is NOT correct?

(A) Periorbital cellulitis is more likely to occur in an infant or younger child
(B) Periorbital cellulitis is more likely to be associated with an underlying ethmoid sinusitis
(C) Orbital cellulitis is more likely to be associated with proptosis
(D) Orbital cellulitis is more likely to be associated with chemosis (edema of the bulbar conjunctivitis)
(E) Orbital cellulitis is likely to be associated with decreased movement of extraocular muscles

67. Clinical findings in Wilson's disease include all of the following EXCEPT

(A) jaundice and hepatomegaly
(B) hemolytic anemia
(C) congestive heart failure
(D) hypertonia and rigidity
(E) hematuria and glycosuria

68. Congenital intracranial arteriovenous malformations may present as any of the following EXCEPT

(A) congestive heart failure
(B) increased intracranial pressure
(C) meningitis
(D) seizures
(E) subarachnoid hemorrhage

69. Which of the following statements about hepatoblastoma is NOT true?

(A) It usually presents as an abdominal mass
(B) There is an increased incidence of associated abnormalities including hemihypertrophy and the Beckwith-Wiederman syndrome
(C) The peak age of diagnosis is between 5 and 10 years of age
(D) Most patients have elevated serum levels of alpha-fetoprotein
(E) Serum levels of alkaline phosphatase are often elevated

70. According to the revised Jones criteria for the diagnosis of rheumatic fever, which of the following is NOT considered a major manifestation?

(A) Carditis
(B) Erythema marginatum
(C) Subcutaneous nodules
(D) Arthralgia
(E) Chorea

71. Common clinical characteristics of Letterer-Siwe disease include all of the following EXCEPT

(A) a rapidly progressive course, with death usually occurring before 2 years of age
(B) pulmonary involvement
(C) lymphadenopathy, splenomegaly, and hepatomegaly
(D) urticarial-like rash
(E) lytic lesions of the skull and long bones

72. Which of the following statements about sudden infant death syndrome (SIDS) is NOT true?

(A) It is a leading cause of death between 1 and 12 months of age
(B) It is more common among lower socioeconomic and among nonwhite families
(C) Most deaths occur after the noon feeding or during an afternoon nap
(D) There is an increased frequency among infants that were of low birth weight
(E) There is an increased risk among siblings of SIDS victims

73. The prognosis in children with systemic lupus erythematosus is LEAST favorable in those with

(A) fever and leukocytosis
(B) anti-DNA antibodies
(C) polyserositis
(D) nephritis
(E) seizures

74. The natural course of events in ventricular septal defects not corrected surgically may include any of the following EXCEPT

(A) a normal life without symptoms
(B) bacterial endocarditis
(C) development of pulmonary valvular obstruction
(D) spontaneous closure of the defect
(E) increasing pulmonary vascular resistance

75. Findings in the Prader-Willi syndrome include all of the following EXCEPT

(A) obesity
(B) mental retardation
(C) hypogonadism and undescended testes
(D) seizures
(E) hypotonia

76. Which of the following is NOT a clinical feature or recognized complication of tetralogy of Fallot?

(A) Anoxic spells
(B) Brain abscess
(C) Congestive heart failure
(D) Cyanosis
(E) Poor growth

77. Which of the following statements regarding localized coarctation of the aorta is NOT true?

(A) The localized narrowing is in the region of the insertion of the ductus arteriosus
(B) There is an increased incidence in infants with Turner syndrome
(C) Symptoms may appear in infancy or may be deferred until adulthood
(D) Spontaneous closure of the ductus arteriosus in infancy may be associated with temporary improvement in symptoms
(E) Hypertension may develop in untreated cases

78. Which of the following is NOT one of the four cardinal structural or pathophysiologic features of tetralogy of Fallot?

(A) Atrial septal defect
(B) Dextroposition of the aorta
(C) Right ventricular hypertrophy
(D) Right ventricular outflow tract obstruction
(E) Ventricular septal defect

79. Mucocutaneous lymph node syndrome (Kawasaki syndrome) is characterized by all of the following EXCEPT

(A) fever and inflammation of the tongue and/or lips
(B) involvement of coronary arteries
(C) desquamation of skin, especially of hands and feet
(D) a violaceous and purpuric rash, appearing first on the face and trunk
(E) enlarged cervical lymph nodes

80. Which of the following malignancies is LEAST likely to occur in the below-5-year age group?

(A) Retinoblastoma
(B) Neuroblastoma
(C) Hodgkin's disease
(D) Leukemia
(E) Wilms's tumor

81. Congenital absence of the spleen may be associated with all of the following EXCEPT

(A) abnormalities of situs
(B) overwhelming sepsis
(C) congenital malformations, especially of the heart
(D) anemia
(E) Howell-Jolly bodies on peripheral blood smear

82. Thrombocytopenia is seen in association with all of the following EXCEPT

(A) lead poisoning
(B) hemolytic uremic syndrome
(C) giant hemangioma
(D) congenital bilateral absence of the radius
(E) hypersplenism

83. There is an increased risk of malignant neoplasms in all of the following conditions EXCEPT

(A) cystic fibrosis
(B) Down's syndrome
(C) hemihypertrophy
(D) neurofibromatosis
(E) Wiskott-Aldrich syndrome

84. All of the following statements about medulloblastoma are true EXCEPT

(A) the peak incidence is in the first decade of life
(B) spread to the meninges is not uncommon
(C) papilledema is a late and uncommon finding
(D) the prognosis for cure is poor
(E) the tumor is radiosensitive

Directions (85 through 93): Each set of matching questions in this section consists of a list of 4 to 26 lettered options followed by several numbered items. For each numbered item select the ONE lettered option with which it is most closely associated. Each lettered option may be selected once, more than once, or not at all.

Questions 85 through 90

(A) Hb 12 g/dL; WBC 11,500/mm^3; platelets 160,000/mm^3; reticulocytes 1%
(B) Hb 12 g/dL; WBC 11,500/mm^3; platelets 25,000/mm^3; reticulocytes 1%
(C) Hb 5.5 g/dL; WBC 3,000/mm^3; platelets 35,000/mm^3; reticulocytes 0.5%
(D) Hb 5.5 g/dL; WBC 8,000/mm^3; platelets 400,000/mm^3; reticulocytes 0.5%
(E) Hb 8 g/dL; WBC 19,500/mm^3; platelets 170,000/mm^3; reticulocytes 14%

85. Idiopathic thrombocytopenic purpura

86. Normal 2-year-old child

87. Sickle cell disease, not in crisis

88. Iron deficiency anemia

89. Acute lymphoblastic leukemia

90. Acquired aplastic pancytopenia

Questions 91 through 93

(A) Congenital aganglionic megacolon
(B) Duodenal atresia
(C) Jejunoileal atresia
(D) Intestinal malrotation
(E) Meconium ileus

91. Cystic fibrosis

92. Midgut volvulus

93. Enterocolitis

DIRECTIONS (Questions 94 through 136): Each group of items in this section consists of lettered headings followed by a set of numbered words or phrases. For each numbered word or phrase, select

A if the item is associated with (A) only,
B if the item is associated with (B) only,
C if the item is associated with both (A) and (B),
D if the item is associated with neither (A) nor (B).

Questions 94 through 98

(A) Friedreich's ataxia
(B) Huntington's chorea
(C) Both
(D) Neither

94. Genetic disorder

95. Cardiac involvement

96. Progressive course

97. Kyphoscoliosis

98. Immunodeficiency

Questions 99 through 105

(A) Grand mal seizures
(B) Absence (petit mal) seizures
(C) Both
(D) Neither

99. Rare before 3 years of age

100. Complications of acute anoxia

101. Three-per-second spike-and-wave pattern on EEG

102. Patient frequently falls to the ground

103. Preceding aura

104. Significant mortality

105. More common in girls

Questions 106 through 109

(A) Normal electrocardiographic findings for a 2-month-old infant
(B) Normal electrocardiographic findings for a 12-year-old child
(C) Both
(D) Neither

106. Rs pattern over right precordium

107. Inverted T wave in V_{3r} and V_1

108. Inverted T wave in V_5 and V_6

109. Inverted P wave in lead I

Questions 110 through 114

(A) Congestive heart failure
(B) Persistent cyanosis
(C) Both
(D) Neither

110. Large ventricular septal defect in a 6-month-old infant

111. Tetralogy of Fallot in a 3-year-old child

112. Transposition of the great arteries with ventricular septal defect

113. Ostium secundum defect in a 3-month-old infant

114. Double aortic arch in a 6-week-old infant

Questions 115 through 120

(A) Bacterial endocarditis
(B) Acute rheumatic fever
(C) Both
(D) Neither

115. Congestive heart failure

116. Appearance of new heart murmurs

117. Subcutaneous nodules

118. Petechiae

119. Erythema marginatum

120. Macrocytic, hypochromic anemia

Questions 121 through 125

(A) Congenital hypertrophic pyloric stenosis
(B) Duodenal atresia
(C) Both
(D) Neither

121. Vomiting in the first 24 hours of life

122. Bile-stained vomitus

123. Metabolic alkalosis

124. Association with Down's syndrome

125. Surgical treatment indicated

Questions 126 through 132

(A) Factor VIII deficiency
(B) Idiopathic thrombocytopenia purpura
(C) Both
(D) Neither

126. Autosomal recessive

127. Petechial rash common

128. Joint hemorrhage common

129. Increased incidence of gram-negative sepsis

130. Response to splenectomy

131. Response to aspirin

132. Relationship to viral infection

Questions 133 through 136

(A) Autosomal recessive polycystic kidney disease
(B) Autosomal dominant polycystic kidney disease
(C) Both
(D) Neither

133. May affect infants and children

134. Associated with congenital hepatic fibrosis

135. Associated with pulmonary emphysema and lung cysts

136. May progress to renal failure

Answers and Explanations

1. (A) The highest pediatric death rate is in the first month of life. Mortality then decreases steadily with increasing age until adolescence, when the death rate rises, primarily from an increase in accidents, homicide, and suicide. More than half of the deaths in the first year of life occur during the first 28 days. Neonatal and infant mortality rates are considerably higher for nonwhites than for whites. *(Rudolph:4–5)*

2. (C) Blood pressure cuffs must be appropriately matched in size to the upper arm of the patient. This is especially true for infants and young children, in whom variations in cuff size can result in greater differences in blood pressure measurements than in adolescents and adults. Too small a cuff will give a falsely high reading. To a much lesser extent, too large a cuff can result in an erroneously low reading. The bladder of the cuff should cover at least two-thirds of the length of the arm and should wrap around at least three-quarters of the circumference. A cuff covering only one-half of the length of the upper arm is likely to give too high a reading. *(Hathaway:625; J Pediatr 91:963–966,1977; 92:934–938,1978)*

3. (B) Deliberate trauma is presently the most common discernable cause of chronic subdural hematomas in infants. This parallels the marked increase in frequency of, or recognition of, child abuse as a cause of infant morbidity and mortality in general. External signs of head trauma may be absent if the injury is caused by forceful shaking rather than a blow. Retinal hemorrhages are a frequently associated finding, reflecting the shaking injury. Irritability, lethargy, vomiting, and failure to thrive are common nonspecific signs. Coma, convulsions, and focal neurologic signs also occur. *(Rudolph:842,1760)*

4. (E) Increased intracranial pressure and radiographically evident calcifications in the region of the sella turcica are common findings in children with craniopharyngiomas. The latter are present in about three-fourths of the patients. Visual defects (involvement of optic nerve or chiasm) and endocrine dysfunction, especially growth failure (involvement of pituitary gland), are other frequent features. The tumor generally presents between 7 and 12 years of age. Optic gliomas usually do not cause increased intracranial pressure and usually do not calcify. *(Rudolph:1743)*

5. (A) Celiac disease is a disorder in which malabsorption and steatorrhea result from an intolerance to certain proteins or peptides (usually gliadin) of the wheat protein moiety, gluten. Atrophy of the intestinal villi is the characteristic pathological finding. Although steatorrhea is usually present, failure to thrive or short stature may occur in the absence of steatorrhea or diarrhea. Circulating IgA antibodies to gliadin have a high correlation with celiac disease and are diagnostically significant. *(Rudolph:1017–1018)*

6. (B) The sphingolipidoses are a group of rare inborn errors of lipid metabolism characterized by the accumulation of lipids in the central nervous system and/or the liver and spleen. The infantile form of Niemann-Pick disease (Type A) results from a defect in the enzyme sphingomyelinase and is characterized by the accumulation of sphingomyelin in the brain, liver, spleen, lungs, and adrenal glands. There is progressive loss of neurologic function and severe psychomotor retardation. A cherry-red spot in the macula is noted in about 30% of patients. Tay-Sachs disease (defective hexosaminidase A) is associated with psychomotor retardation and a cherry-red spot, but there is no hepatosplenomegaly. Macular degeneration and a cherry-red spot are not part of the clinical picture of Gaucher's disease, metachromatic leukodystrophy, or globoid-cell leukodystrophy. *(Rudolph:355)*

7. (D) The Kayser-Fleischer ring is a classical finding in Wilson's disease and is almost pathognomonic for this disease. The ring consists of a greenish or golden brown discoloration of the limbic region of the cornea, resulting from deposition of colored granules in Descemet's membrane. Although best seen by slit-lamp examination, the ring sometimes can be visualized by simple examination with an ophthalmoscope. Wilson's disease is a disorder of copper metabolism characterized by the deposition of copper in the brain, liver, and other organs. Neurologic findings include tremors, spasticity, dysarthria, and emotional lability. Most affected children also have evidence of hepatic involvement and eventually develop cirrhosis. *(Rudolph:387,1079)*

8. **(C)** Werdnig-Hoffman disease is an autosomal recessive disorder affecting the anterior horn cells and the motor nuclei of the brainstem. Loss of motor function begins in infancy and progresses fairly rapidly, leading to ventilatory failure within the first 2 years of life. Clinical features include hypotonia, weakness or paralysis, hyporeflexia, and muscle fasciculations, which are most readily noted in the tongue. Seizures, optic atrophy, and fever are not features of this disorder. There also is a rare, late-onset, more slowly progressive degenerative disorder of the anterior horn cells referred to as Kugelberg-Welander disease. *(Rudolph:1443,1794–1795)*

9. **(C)** The term cerebral palsy refers to a static, nonprogressive abnormality of the central nervous system affecting motor function and resulting from a perinatal (before or during birth or in early infancy) insult. By definition, this is a nonprogressive disorder, and, therefore, treatment can be aimed only at preventing secondary problems rather than preventing progression of the disorder itself. The underlying lesion is the end result of a perinatal injury and as such is not treatable. Since the causes of cerebral palsy are so varied, and since so few cases are related to recognizable genetic disorders, effective genetic counseling to prevent subsequent cases is difficult. Although the risk of developing epilepsy is significantly greater for these children than for the general population, only 25 to 35% will eventually do so, and administration of anticonvulsant drugs prior to the onset of seizures is not indicated. Thus, the importance of early diagnosis is to help the parents understand the infant or child and his or her problem and to minimize or prevent *secondary* physical (primarily contractures) or emotional (e.g., guilt, unrealistic expectations) problems. *(Rudolph:1720–1724)*

10. **(E)** Almost three-quarters of all cases of cerebral palsy are of the spastic type. Involvement rarely may be limited to a single extremity (monoplegia). More frequently, one (hemiplegia) or both (quadriplegia) sides of the body are affected. Findings are those of an upper motor neuron lesion and include increased muscle tone, increased deep tendon reflexes, clonus, and extensor plantar responses. Other, less frequent types of cerebral palsy are dyskinetic (usually athetoid), atactic (ataxic), and mixed. The atonic variety is classified as a subtype of spastic cerebral palsy and is characterized by hypotonia with normal or increased deep tendon reflexes. The most frequent mixed variety is a combination of spasticity and athetosis. *(Rudolph:1720)*

11. **(A)** Although a variety of disorders can present as the relatively sudden onset of ataxia, with or without nystagmus, the child described most likely has acute cerebellar ataxia or acute cerebellitis. This is an acute, short-lived inflammation of the cerebellum, usually presumed to be viral or postinfectious in origin. The prognosis is excellent; improvement may be evident in less than a week after onset, and recovery is almost always complete. A mild cerebrospinal fluid pleocytosis with mononuclear cells is present in a little less than half of the cases. In the patient described, other causes of ataxia are less likely: the normal CT scan rules out a posterior fossa tumor; the CSF pleocytosis eliminates drugs such as alcohol, phenobarbital, or phenothiazines as well as metabolic disorders such as Hartnup disease; and the normal physical exam makes a neuroblastoma unlikely. *(Rudolph:1820–1821; Hathaway:696–700)*

12. **(E)** Most neuroblastomas arise from the adrenal gland or from sympathetic neural tissue in the chest or abdomen. The median age at diagnosis is 2 years, with most cases presenting before 5 years. Survival is best in infants and young children. In one series there was a 74% survival rate for infants diagnosed before a year of age and only 12% survival for those diagnosed after the second birthday. Spontaneous regression and remission have been noted with this tumor, especially in infants under 6 months of age and infants with metastases limited to liver, skin, or bone marrow. Differentiation of the tumor to a benign ganglioneuroma also has been observed. Abdominal mass is the usual presenting complaint. Adrenal insufficiency is not a regular feature of this disorder. *(Pediatr Clin North Am 32(3):764–768,1985; Rudolph:1201–1202)*

13. **(E)** Aniridia is a congenital absence or hypoplasia of the iris; cases occur on an autosomal dominant, autosomal recessive, and sporadic basis. Sporadic cases are at risk for the development of a Wilms's tumor, which occurs in up to 20% of such children. This association has been referred to as the Miller or aniridia-Wilms' tumor syndrome and has been linked to a deletion of the p13 band of the short arm of chromosome 11. Children with aniridia should be followed closely with repeated physical examination and ultrasound examination of the abdomen and kidneys for the first few years of life unless a positive family history clearly indicates that the patient's aniridia is not of the sporadic variety. *(Rudolph:1199,1905)*

14. **(B)** The cardinal features of the diencephalic syndrome are hyperalertness, euphoria, and severe failure to thrive or weight loss. The syndrome is secondary to a lesion, usually a glioma, in the hypothalamic region. Other findings include vomiting, optic atro-

phy, nystagmus, and occasionally polyuria. The reason for the emaciation is not clear. Vomiting and hyperactivity may be contributing factors but by themselves seem not to be an adequate explanation. The syndrome appears restricted to infants; older children and adults with lesions in the hypothalamus usually develop obesity rather than emaciation. *(Rudolph:1738–1739)*

15. **(D)** Craniosynostosis is the condition of premature fusion of one or more of the cranial sutures and occurs both as an isolated abnormality and in association with a wide variety of congenital malformations, syndromes, and chromosomal abnormalities. Excluding abnormalities of the head and face, the extremities are the organs most frequently involved with associated defects. The most common and best known such syndrome is the autosomal dominant Aperts syndrome—craniosynostosis plus extensive syndactyly of the fingers and toes. *(Rudolph:963,1921)*

16. **(D)** Rheumatic chorea is a neurologic dysfunction that occurs as a relatively late sequela of a group A beta-hemolytic streptococcal infection. Although the most striking and most characteristic feature is chorea, there also may be muscle weakness and emotional lability. The weakness usually is mild but occasionally may be marked. The child appears clumsy, and handwriting deteriorates. Facial grimacing is common. The choreiform movements consist of gross writhing, jerking, and irregular movements. Fine tremor is not noted, and convulsions are not associated with this disorder. *(Rudolph:494)*

17. **(A)** Partial complex seizures (psychomotor seizures or temporal lobe seizures) are characterized clinically by automatisms—repetitive complex but purposeless and inappropriate motor activities. There may or may not be changes in consciousness and responsiveness. There may be bizarre behavior, strange feelings, confusion, and fear. The most common electroencephalographic finding is spike waves over the temporal lobes. *(Rudolph:1772)*

18. **(B)** The arthritis of acute rheumatic fever is a painful acute migratory polyarthritis. Although any joint can be involved, it is primarily the large joints of the **extremities** that are affected in most cases. Pain and swelling in one joint subsides as another joint becomes symptomatic. Eventually, all joints heal without deformity or other permanent sequelae. Fever and arthritis usually occur concomitantly but may occur in the presence or absence of carditis. *(Rudolph:493)*

19. **(B)** Malignant hyperthermia is a genetically determined disorder of muscle metabolism, most frequently transmitted by an autosomal dominant pattern. The striking features of the disease are episodes of severe muscle spasm or rigidity, hyperthermia, cardiac arrhythmias (especially ventricular tachycardia), and metabolic acidosis. Attacks most often are triggered by anesthetic agents (especially halothane) or succinylcholine and are life threatening. Serum creatine phosphokinase (CPK) levels are regularly markedly elevated following such episodes but may be either elevated or normal between episodes. Although some patients have muscle weakness and a well-recognized myopathic disorder such as Duchenne muscular dystrophy, most are asymptomatic and are undiagnosed prior to the occurrence of an untoward reaction to anesthesia. *(Rudolph:395,1807)*

20. **(C)** The infant described most likely has supraventricular tachycardia (SVT). Heart rates over 200 beats per minute rarely result from sinus tachycardia. Although SVT may occur any time during childhood, there is a peak incidence of first episodes in early infancy, often in association with a respiratory infection. Preexcitation syndromes, such as Wolff-Parkinson-White syndrome, are found in only a minority of infants with SVT. Most infants presenting with SVT do not have associated structural heart disease, and a specific cause cannot be found in the majority of cases. *(Rudolph:1350–1351)*

21. **(A)** The most common pathogens in bacterial endocarditis in children are streptococci (*S. viridans*, group D streptococci, enterococci) and staphylococci (*S. aureus*, *S. epidermidis*). Almost any organism, however, can cause endocarditis. *S. pneumoniae* occasionally causes endocarditis; *Hemophilus* species rarely do. Although infection of a normal heart can occur, especially with *S. aureus*, most cases occur in previously abnormal hearts, usually secondary to congenital heart disease. *(Rudolph:1418)*

22. **(D)** The clinical findings described are classic for the entity of total anomalous pulmonary venous return with obstruction of the veins. In this condition, the pulmonary veins drain to the right rather than the left atrium. After mixing with systemic venous return in the right atrium, some of the oxygenated pulmonary venous blood shunts across the foramen ovale (which is kept open by the increased right atrial pressure), providing a right-to-left shunt of partially oxygenated blood into the systemic circulation. In many cases, the pulmonary venous return is not directly into the right atrium but rather takes a devious route, often coursing below the diaphragm before reaching the right atrium. In such instances, venous obstruction is the rule, and cyanosis results both from the right-to-left shunt and from wet, congested lungs. A diffuse reticular pattern to the lung fields is characteristically seen on roentgenogram. Although the heart may be considerably enlarged in patients without venous obstruction, it is characteristically normal or only minimally enlarged in those with obstruction. *(Rudolph:1409)*

23. (D) In transposition of the great arteries, the aorta arises from the right ventricle, and the pulmonary artery arises from the left ventricle. This results in two separate circulations, which would be immediately incompatible with life were it not for some mixing or shunting of blood across an atrial or ventricular septal defect or a patent ductus arteriosus. A small amount of blood also shunts through the bronchial circulation. Survival depends on the magnitude of these communications. Shunting at the atrial level can be increased by passing a balloon catheter through the foramen ovale, inflating the balloon and quickly withdrawing it, rupturing the tissues around the foramen and enlarging the communication between the right and left atrium. This procedure, balloon atrial septostomy, can be life saving and can allow delay of surgical correction until the child has grown larger. Balloon septostomy also can be useful in conditions with inadequate pulmonary blood flow (pulmonary and tricuspid atresia) but not in any of the other conditions listed in the question. *(Rudolph:1407)*

24. (A) Brain tumors, although rare in the first year of life, are the second most common type of cancer in childhood, exceeded only by leukemia. More than half of the tumors in children are located below the tentorium, and about three-quarters are in the midline. For this reason, increased intracranial pressure from obstruction of the third or fourth ventricle is a common finding. Seizures can be the presenting complaint but are not in the *majority* of cases. *(Rudolph:1731–1733)*

25. (E) The infant described most likely has an intussusception of the intestine. This condition is most frequent in the second half of the first year of life and involves the telescoping of one segment of bowel into another, most frequently the ileum into the colon (ileocolic intussusception). Intermittent abdominal pain and vomiting are common features. Mild fever and leukocytosis are frequent. Very often the intussusceptum can be palpated as a sausage-shaped mass. Circulation to the intussuscepted bowel can be impaired, resulting in discharge of a bloody, mucous stool—the so-called "currant jelly" stool. Barium enema is the procedure of choice and can be therapeutic as well as diagnostic. Under fluoroscopic visualization, the radiologist usually is able to employ the hydrostatic pressure of the enema to reduce the intussuscepted bowel. *(Rudolph:1034; Hathaway:551)*

26. (E) Cystic fibrosis is the most common cause of pancreatic insufficiency in childhood, accounting for almost all cases. Biliary atresia is not associated with pancreatic insufficiency, and carcinoma of the pancreas is not seen in childhood. Congenital hypoplasia or absence of the pancreas is recognized but rare. Schwachman syndrome is a rare condition of unknown cause characterized by pancreatic insuffi-

ciency and neutropenia. *(Rudolph:1527; Hathaway:382–383,604)*

27. (A) The clinical features described—muscle weakness, erythematous, scaly rash, and heliotropic (reddish-purple) patches on the eyelids—are characteristic of dermatomyositis, a disease of presumed autoimmune etiology. The rash is most frequent over the dorsum of the hand. The rash and facial heliotrope are almost pathognomonic of dermatomyositis. Muscle weakness is not a feature of eczema, Henoch-Schönlein purpura, or juvenile rheumatoid arthritis. Rash is not a feature of trichinosis. *(Rudolph:485; Hathaway:535)*

28. (C) Brain abscess is an infrequent but not rare disorder of childhood. It has been estimated that almost one-third of all brain abscesses occur in pediatric-age patients. Recognized predisposing conditions include penetrating head injury, brain surgery, immunodeficiency, cystic fibrosis, and infection of the middle ear, mastoid, or facial sinuses. Right-to-left intracardiac shunts in children with cyanotic congenital heart disease bypass the macrophage-filtering mechanism of the lung and increase the access of bacteria to the brain. In these children, cerebral hypoxia and focal encephalomalacia also may predispose to infection. *(Rudolph:1845,705)*

29. (C) There are three classic clinic presentations of juvenile rheumatoid arthritis (JRA)—acute systemic, pauciarticular, and polyarticular. A positive rheumatoid factor (RF) is uncommon in JRA, occurring only in some patients, usually females, with the polyarticular form. Those patients with polyarticular JRA who are RF positive tend to be older and to have more severe joint involvement than those who are RF negative. Neither ankylosing spondylitis nor psoriatic arthritis is associated with RF. *(Rudolph:478–481)*

30. (D) Acute rheumatic fever (ARF) is a nonsuppurative complication of group A beta-hemolytic streptococcal pharyngitis. Following an initial bout, recurrent episodes are most effectively prevented by continuous penicillin prophylaxis against group A beta-hemolytic streptococcal infection. This is most reliably accomplished by injections of benzathine penicillin every 4 weeks. Daily oral penicillin can be effective, but compliance is a problem. Since streptococcal pharyngitis can occur with only minimal symptoms, treatment of symptomatic pharyngitis with either antibiotics or corticosteroids is inadequate to insure prevention of recurrence. Treatment with prophylactic antibiotics at the time of dental and surgical procedures is designed to prevent *bacterial endocarditis* rather than to prevent recurrences of rheumatic fever and would be indicated, in addition to continuous penicillin, in patients with rheumatic heart disease. *(Rudolph:494)*

31. (D) The child described has the classic hand-foot syndrome seen in infants and toddlers with sickle cell disease. Dactylitis, presumably secondary to infarction of the small bones, causes painful swelling of the hands and feet. *(Rudolph:1124)*

32. (C) The interval between the streptococcal infection and the onset of manifestation is much greater for chorea (months) than for any of the other signs or symptoms of acute rheumatic fever (1 to 2 weeks). As a result, rheumatic chorea often occurs in the absence of any other clinical or laboratory manifestations of acute rheumatic fever and frequently in the absence of evidence of recent streptococcal infection. [*Note:* The key word in this question, of course, is *isolated.*] *(Rudolph:494)*

33. (E) Inadequate dietary iron is the leading cause of iron deficiency anemia in children. Milk has a low iron content, and the iron in cow milk is not well absorbed. If a large percentage of dietary calories comes from milk, the diet is apt to be low in iron. Additionally, microscopic gastrointestinal blood loss associated with the intake of unmodified cow milk is an important contributing factor to iron deficiency. *(Rudolph:1100–1101)*

34. (A) Cystic hygroma is a benign lymphangioma of infancy and early childhood. About three-quarters of cases arise or present in the head and neck region. The mass feels soft and rubbery, compressible, and cystic to palpation, a characteristic that permits quite accurate diagnosis on physical examination. Although benign, the lesion does tend to grow, and excision can be difficult. Unlike hemangiomas, spontaneous regression is rare, and surgical removal is the treatment of choice. *(Rudolph:172; Hathaway:354)*

35. (D) The two most common solid malignant tumors of the abdomen in the first few years of life are Wilms's tumor and neuroblastoma. These usually can be distinguished by intravenous pyelography or abdominal ultrasound examination. Wilms' tumor distorts the renal image, whereas neuroblastoma displaces the kidney downward without intrinsic distortion. Adrenal hemorrhage is rare beyond the newborn period. Adrenal carcinoma is rare and usually occurs in the older child, presenting as an abdominal mass or, if functioning, as Cushing's syndrome. *(Rudolph:1202)*

36. (B) Although rhabdomyosarcoma and, infrequently, hepatoblastoma can metastasize to bone, few solid cancers of childhood spread to bone as regularly as neuroblastoma. Additionally, whereas bone metastases of other tumors tend to be focal, involvement by neuroblastoma frequently is diffuse. In some series of neuroblastoma, bone *marrow* involvement has exceeded 50% of cases. Thus, bone marrow aspiration, even in the absence of radiographic evidence of osseous involvement, is more likely to be diagnos-

tic in neuroblastoma than in any other solid cancer of childhood. *(Pediatr Clin North Am 32:755–763,1985; Rudolph:1202)*

37. (E) This child most likely has otitis externa (OE). Swimming is a common etiologic factor in OE because the water tends to macerate the skin of the canal and because the water often contains *Pseudomonas* and other pathogenic bacteria. The clinical findings are absolutely classic for OE. There is nothing to suggest mastoiditis—the child is afebrile, and there is no swelling or tenderness over the region of the mastoid. Cholesteatoma is rare, usually results from very chronic otitis media (OM), and does not present with swelling of the canal. Although it is possible that the child has a draining purulent OM with a *secondary* OE, it is unlikely. *(Feigin:172–173)*

38. (A) Intestinal lactase deficiency in infancy may be either genetic (rare) or acquired (common) secondary to damage to the intestinal mucosa. Watery diarrhea is a prominent feature of these disorders. The stool is strongly acidic because of lactic and other acids produced by the action of bowel bacteria on the undigested sugars. Neither pancreatitis nor intestinal obstruction has been reported as associated with disaccharidase deficiency. There is also a late-onset lactase deficiency that occurs secondary to a regulatory gene that turns off lactase activity after lactation. This is most common in nonwhite individuals. *(Rudolph:1009)*

39. (E) For most types of childhood cancer, the risk of malignancy in a sibling is quite small. For all tumors combined, the risk of malignancy in a sibling of an index case is about three times that of the general pediatric population. The chance of leukemia developing in the *identical twin* of an index case is about 1 in 20. Retinoblastoma, however, clearly has a genetic basis in about 40% of cases. Most hereditary retinoblastomas are bilateral. It is recommended that siblings of a new case of retinoblastoma undergo periodic ophthalmologic examination under general anesthesia up to the age of 7 years. *(Rudolph:1909; Pediatr Clin North Am 32:541–556,1985)*

40. (E) Anaphylactoid purpura (Henoch-Schönlein purpura) is an acute vasculitis of undetermined origin involving the arterioles and capillaries and characterized by the deposition of IgA in skin, kidneys, and other tissues. Tests of bleeding function are normal, and the purpura is a manifestation of the vasculitis rather than a bleeding disorder. *(Rudolph:1158)*

41. (C) The McCune-Albright syndrome consists of fibrous dysplasia of bone, multiple large pigmented nevi (generally on only one side of the trunk), and precocious puberty, which is more common in females than in males. Other endocrine disorders occur less frequently and include hyperthyroidism and hyperadrenalism (Cushing's syndrome). *(Rudolph:1673)*

42. **(A)** Congenital hypoplastic anemia (Diamond-Blackfan syndrome) is a disorder of unknown etiology in which hypoplastic anemia appears at, or within a few months of, birth. The response of many patients to corticosteroids suggests that the cause is not simply the absence of a cell line. Approximately one-third of patients have associated congenital abnormalities, most commonly the Turner syndrome phenotype and abnormalities of the thumbs. Urinary, cardiac, and skeletal anomalies also are seen occasionally. There is no evidence of intrauterine infection or intrauterine twin-to-twin transfusion. The anemia is macrocytic, and hepatosplenomegaly is not a feature. *(Rudolph:1109)*

43. **(B)** Since aortic pressure is significantly greater than pulmonary artery pressure throughout the cardiac cycle, a patent ductus arteriosus (PDA) characteristically results in a continuous left-to-right shunt and a continuous murmur. The increased left ventricular output, coupled with runoff from the aorta through the ductus, produces a widened pulse pressure and a bounding or collapsing pulse. The increased flow to the lungs and back to the left ventricle causes hypertrophy of that chamber rather than of the right ventricle. Manifestations of a PDA in a premature infant would be quite different from those in a 6-month-old. These infants are relatively intolerant of left-to-right shunts and are more likely to develop congestive heart failure. Also, the high pulmonary vascular resistance results in a systolic-only murmur rather than the classical continuous murmur. *(Rudolph:1361–1362)*

44. **(E)** Clinical features of tetralogy of Fallot include evidence of a right-to-left shunt: cyanosis, clubbing, and polycythemia. Episodes of sudden increase in right-to-left shunting of blood typically result in anoxic spells ("blue spells," "tet spells"). The systolic murmur reflects the ventricular septal defect. Children with tetralogy often will squat during or after physical exertion. Presumably, this position increases system vascular resistance and decreases the magnitude of the intracardiac right-to-left shunt. *(Rudolph:1397–1398)*

45. **(B)** Endocardial fibroelastosis commonly results in congestive heart failure in the first year of life. In patients with Marfan's syndrome, cardiac symptoms rarely begin before the fifth year of life. In Friedreich's ataxia, symptoms rarely begin in infancy, and cardiac failure at any age is uncommon, arrhythmias and electrocardiographic abnormalities being the more common cardiac manifestations. Uncomplicated and isolated atrial septal defects rarely cause symptoms during infancy, chiefly because the pressure gradient between the two atria is small.

[*Note:* If the student fails to note that the question specifies heart failure *in infancy*, he or she would find the question confusing and might choose **(E)**, all of the above.] *(Rudolph:1368,1416–1417,1886)*

46. **(C)** Congenital megacolon (Hirschsprung's disease) is the result of congenital absence of ganglion cells in a segment of large bowel. Absent or deficient peristalsis in the affected segment results in functional obstruction, which causes constipation and distention of bowel *proximal* to the aganglionic area. It is this chronically distended bowel that has led to the name *megacolon*. Severe cases present as neonatal intestinal obstruction. Enterocolitis with diarrhea is a well-recognized complication, especially in older, undiagnosed, and untreated infants, but certainly is not the most common presentation. *(Rudolph:1039)*

47. **(B)** Transient erythroblastopenia of childhood is a disorder of unknown etiology characterized by transient suppression of erythropoiesis. The condition is seen most commonly in children between the ages of 6 months and 4 years. Severe anemia requiring transfusion is not uncommon. The red cells are not macrocytic and do not contain increased amounts of fetal hemoglobin, and it is unusual for individuals to experience more than one episode in a lifetime. The prognosis is excellent. *(Rudolph:1109–1110)*

48. **(C)** Complex partial seizures is the current name for what had previously been termed temporal lobe or psychomotor seizures. Complex partial seizures are characterized by alterations of mental status, consciousness, or responsiveness. During the seizure, there may be confusion, emotional reactions, feelings of detachment, and hallucinations. Automatisms (semipurposeful but inappropriate motor acts) are frequent. There is no tonic or clonic component. Postictal confusion is common. The usual EEG finding is spike-wave activity over one or both temporal lobe regions. A three-per-second spike-and-wave pattern on EEG is characteristic of *absence seizures*. *(Rudolph:1772)*

49. **(D)** Infantile spasms are characterized by brief, sudden jerks of various muscle groups, for example, sudden flexion of the head and trunk with simultaneous adduction of the arms and legs. These massive flexor spasms have been referred to as *salaam attacks*. Consciousness is not lost during these episodes. The attacks may be repeated a few to several hundred times a day. *(Rudolph:1773)*

50. **(C)** The most common presenting sign in children with Hodgkin's disease is painless enlargement of a single group of superficial lymph nodes, most frequently in the cervical region. Hepatosplenomegaly and anemia are infrequent presenting complaints. Pruritus is unusual in children. Although weight loss is an occasional early complaint, failure to

thrive is not a feature, especially since the disease is rare before the age of 5 years. *(Rudolph:1196–1197)*

51. **(A)** Infantile spasms represent a type of seizure disorder that presents almost exclusively in the child less than 2 years of age. The prognosis regarding neurologic and intellectual outcome in general is poor. Seizures are resistant to the usual anticonvulsant agents but can be controlled by ACTH, although there are no convincing data that such treatment improves ultimate neurologic or intellectual outcome. The classical electroencephalographic finding in this disorder is a rather gross abnormality that has been referred to as *hypsarrhythmia*. Infantile spasms are not related to hypocalcemia or any other electrolyte disturbance. *(Rudolph:1773)*

52. **(A)** The electrocardiogram shown (Figure 9–1) is indicative of right ventricular hypertrophy. The findings are: a right electrical axis (about 110°), tall R waves over the right precordial leads, and deep S waves over the left precordial leads. There also is an rsR′ pattern in V_1. These findings are most compatible with an atrial septal defect. Coarctation of the aorta and ventricular septal defect produce *left* ventricular hypertrophy. *(Rudolph:1368–1369)*

53. **(A)** The roentgenograms shown in this question (Figure 9–2) reveal old fractures of the humerus, femurs, and tibias. There also are two linear skull fractures and a separation fracture of the coronal suture. The bones appear metabolically normal. These findings are classic for the battered child syndrome. *(Rudolph:842)*

54. **(B)** Although all mammalian milks are relatively poor sources of folate, both human milk and cow milk contain sufficient amounts to prevent anemia in the nursing infant. Goat milk, however, is markedly deficient in this vitamin. None of the currently available liquid infant multivitamin preparations contain folate or folic acid. Megaloblastic anemia has been noted frequently in infants being fed goat milk. Folate is not fat soluble, and deficiency has not been a problem in infants with cystic fibrosis. *(Rudolph:237,1103–1104)*

55. **(B)** Familial dysautonomia is an autosomal recessive disease occurring predominantly in children of Ashkenazi (European) Jewish ancestry. It affects sensory and autonomic functions in many organ systems. Findings include failure to thrive, irritability, insensitivity to pain, and hypoactive deep tendon reflexes. Crying without tears and absence of fungiform papillae on the tongue are striking features. Chronic respiratory disease is presumed to result primarily from repeated bouts of pulmonary aspiration. *(Rudolph:1798)*

56. **(A)** The head is large in achondroplasia, not just relative to the small body. Although this is not associ-

ated directly with increased intracranial pressure, achondroplasia also is associated with platybasia of the skull, which often results in obstructive hydrocephalus and increased intracranial pressure. Overdoses of *vitamin A* have been associated with pseudotumor cerebri, but overdoses of *vitamin C* do not have this effect. *(Rudolph:399)*

57. **(D)** Werdnig-Hoffman disease is an autosomal recessive disorder characterized by progressive degenerative changes in the anterior horn cells of the spinal cord. Characteristic clinical findings include hypotonia, weakness, and decreased to absent deep tendon reflexes. Muscle fasciculations, usually visible only in the tongue, are almost pathognomonic. Recurrent respiratory infections, the result of muscle weakness with impaired suck, cough, and swallowing, is the usual cause of death. *(Rudolph:1794)*

58. **(E)** Iridocyclitis (anterior uveitis) is the only ophthalmologic complication seen in children with juvenile rheumatoid arthritis (JRA). It usually occurs in those with the ANA-positive, pauciarticular form of the disease. Iridocyclitis may be insidious yet severe, resulting in permanent blindness. Corneal ulcerations, ptosis, glaucoma, and cataracts are not recognized complications of JRA. *(Rudolph:478,1906)*

59. **(D)** Pseudotumor cerebri, also referred to as benign intracranial hypertension, is a condition characterized by increased intracranial pressure in the absence of an intracranial mass, hemorrhage, or injury and associated with normal or small ventricles. Headache, visual disturbance, and papilledema are present in many cases. Palsy of cranial nerve VI, presumably caused by stretching of the nerve, is common, but true focal findings and alterations of consciousness are absent. *(Rudolph:1747)*

60. **(B)** Spasmus nutans is an unusual condition seen in early childhood. Its etiology is unknown. Onset most frequently is during the first year of life. Recovery is complete, although symptoms may persist for months to years. The major features of this peculiar condition are nystagmus and head nodding. A deviation of the head or head tilt is seen occasionally. Trismus is not a feature. Differential diagnosis includes brain tumor (especially an optic glioma), brainstem encephalitis, and ophthalmologic problems. *(Rudolph:1915)*

61. **(E)** In the pediatric age group, non-Hodgkin's lymphoma is several times more frequent than is Hodgkin's disease. Intussusception secondary to involvement of the ileum or other region of bowel is a well-recognized presentation of intraabdominal non-Hodgkin's lymphoma. Central nervous system and bone marrow involvement are common. Chemotherapy is the main aspect of treatment. Radiotherapy has a limited role in the treatment of this tumor, and

radiotherapy alone rarely is curative. Appropriate treatment always includes chemotherapy. *(Rudolph: 1195)*

62. **(B)** Leukemia is the most common form of childhood cancer, and acute lymphoblastic is the most common type of leukemia in childhood. The peak incidence in the pediatric age group is between 2 and 6 years of age. The incidence is almost twice as great in white as in black children. There is an increased incidence of leukemia in children with Down's syndrome as well as in children with Bloom's syndrome (facial erythema and telangiectasia and dwarfism; chromosomal breaks and rearrangements are common). *(Rudolph:1184–1185)*

63. **(D)** Central nervous system relapse is a common and important problem in children with acute leukemia, either as part of a generalized relapse or as an isolated finding even while the bone marrow remains in remission. Routine, periodic lumbar puncture and examination of the cerebrospinal fluid, even during bone marrow remission, permit early detection of CNS relapse, before the advent of symptoms such as headache, vomiting, and papilledema. Most systemic chemotherapeutic agents do not cross the blood-brain barrier and penetrate the cerebrospinal fluid poorly. Both prevention and treatment of CNS involvement require specific therapy—either intrathecal medication, such as methotrexate, or craniospinal irradiation. Systemic chemotherapy alone is not effective. *(Rudolph:1188)*

64. **(A)** Between acute episodes or crises, the hemoglobin concentration in children with uncomplicated sickle cell disease varies between 7 and 10 g/dL. A value of 5.0 g/dL or less should suggest a secondary problem such as folic acid deficiency or an associated G6PD deficiency. The total WBC count is elevated as the result of bone marrow stimulation and usually is about 15,000 to 20,000/mm³, even in the absence of infection or acute crises. Reticulocytosis is regularly present except during an aplastic crisis. Sickle cells are regularly noted on peripheral blood smear. The predominance of young red blood cells in the circulation results in macrocytosis. *(Hathaway:487)*

65. **(C)** G6PD deficiency is inherited as an X-linked recessive disorder and is worldwide in distribution. Differences in the kinetics of the disorder in different races and ethnic groups result in different clinical pictures. In blacks, G6PD deficiency is associated with neonatal hemolysis and jaundice in the premature but usually not in the full-term newborn. In blacks with G6PD deficiency, young red blood cells have significantly greater enzyme activity than older cells and therefore are not susceptible to drug-induced hemolysis. The significance of this is that acute hemolytic episodes in blacks tend to spare the young cells, and consequently the hematocrit level

does not fall as low as in patients with the Mediterranean variant of G6PD deficiency. *(Hathaway:486)*

66. **(B)** Periorbital (or preseptal) cellulitis usually occurs in an infant or young child and usually is not associated with an underlying sinusitis. Orbital cellulitis, a more serious, deeper infection, occurs in older children and usually is associated with an underlying ethmoid sinusitis. Other features that distinguish orbital from periorbital cellulitis include proptosis, edema of the eyelids and bulbar conjunctiva (chemosis), involvement of extraocular muscles, and decreased visual acuity. *(Rudolph:1922)*

67. **(C)** Wilson's disease is an autosomal recessive disorder resulting in excessive accumulation of copper in liver, brain, kidneys, and cornea. The major clinical abnormalities are hepatic (cirrhosis) and neurologic (hypertonia, rigidity, tremors, dysarthria, and clumsiness). Pigmented corneal rings (Kayser-Fleischer rings) are characteristic. Renal involvement presents as hematuria and tubular dysfunction, including glycosuria. Hemolytic anemia is noted occasionally. There is no involvement of the heart, and heart failure is not a feature. *(Rudolph:1079)*

68. **(C)** Intracranial arteriovenous malformations (AVMs) may present in a variety of ways, including neurologic findings such as convulsions, increased intracranial pressure (either because of the mass itself or of obstruction of the third ventricle), and intracranial hemorrhage. Because these AVMs often are comprised of very large vessels, high-output congestive heart failure is another common form of presentation. The AVMs do not predispose to meningitis. *(Rudolph:1753)*

69. **(C)** Hepatoblastoma is a malignant tumor of the liver that is most common in the first 3 years of life (60% in the first year). In most cases, an enlarged liver is the presenting sign. Often the parent notices abdominal enlargement. Elevated serum levels of alpha-fetoprotein and alkaline phosphatase are common. Associated abnormalities in some cases include hemihypertrophy, Beckwith-Wiederman syndrome, and diaphragmatic and umbilical hernias. *(Rudolph:1213)*

70. **(D)** The modified Jones criteria for the diagnosis of acute rheumatic fever consist of five major and five minor manifestations. The major criteria are carditis, polyarthritis, chorea, erythema marginatum, and subcutaneous nodules. The minor manifestations are fever, elevated acute-phase reactants (white blood cell count, erythrocyte sedimentation rate, or C-reactive protein), past history of acute rheumatic fever, prolonged PR or QT interval on ECG, and *arthralgia*. Thus, arthralgia is a minor rather than a major criterion. In general, there is a high probability of acute rheumatic fever in the pres-

ence of two major or one major and two minor manifestations *and* (in either case) evidence of a recent streptococcal infection—scarlet fever, positive throat culture, rapid strep test, or elevated antistreptococcal antibodies. *(Rudolph:493)*

71. (D) Letterer-Siwe disease (acute disseminated histiocytosis X; Langerhans's cell histiocytoses) is usually rapidly progressive and fatal before 2 years of age. Involvement of lymph nodes, liver, and spleen as well as lungs and skin is common. The rash, however, is greasy and scaly, hemorrhagic or petechial and maculopapular; it is *not* urticarial. Lytic lesions in the skull and long bones are common. *(Rudolph:912,1218–1219)*

72. (C) Sudden infant death syndrome (SIDS) is the leading cause of death between 1 and 12 months of age, accounting for about two deaths per 1,000 live births. The peak incidence occurs between 2 and 4 months of age. For unknown reasons, the frequency of SIDS is higher among patients of lower socioeconomic status and among nonwhites. There does appear to be clustering in families, and the risk for a sibling of a SIDS victim is four to seven times greater than the risk among the general population. There also is an increased frequency among infants who were of low birth weight, especially those who were premature. The cause of SIDS remains unknown. The most prevalent hypothesis involves an abnormality of central control of ventilation. *(Rudolph:850–856)*

73. (D) The prognosis in children with systemic lupus erythematosus is determined primarily by the extent of renal involvement. The major causes of death are renal failure and opportunistic infection. The latter usually is secondary to immunosuppressive therapy of kidney disease. None of the other items listed (fever, leukocytosis, anti-DNA antibodies, polyserositis, or seizures) is prognostic of a fatal outcome. (Rudolph:484)

74. (C) The clinical course and natural history of ventricular septal defects that are not surgically corrected are quite varied. Large defects can lead to congestive heart failure early in life, whereas small defects frequently close spontaneously. The mechanism of such closure may include hypertrophy of muscle at the edge of the defect or growth of a membrane across the defect. Bacterial endocarditis is a small but definite risk. Progressive increase in pulmonary vascular resistance is an ominous event that can eventually lead to a right-to-left shunt (Eisenmenger's syndrome). In such a situation, pulmonary vascular disease is irreversible, and surgical closure of the defect is no longer helpful. Today, no child should reach this stage. Although progressive *aortic* insufficiency, secondary to prolapse of an aortic valve leaflet, has been noted in a number of infants with ventricular septal defects, *pulmonary* valvular obstruction is not a recognized complication. *(Rudolph:1367)*

75. (D) Prader-Willi syndrome is characterized by hypotonia, hypogonadism, mental retardation, and undescended testis in males. Although there may be feeding difficulties in infancy, these children eventually develop excessive appetites and obesity. The obesity accentuates the appearance of a micropenis. Hypotonia becomes less marked with time. Seizures are not a feature of the Prader-Willi syndrome. This disorder is now recognized as a difficult-to-detect chromosomal deletion. *(Rudolph:420,1812;* Clin Genet *30:241–248,1986)*

76. (C) Tetralogy of Fallot is not associated with either increased pulmonary blood flow or obstruction or impairment of left ventricular output, so congestive heart failure is not a problem in patients with this disorder. The right-to-left shunt results in hypoxemia and cyanosis, and poor growth is proportionate to the severity of the hypoxemia. Acute episodes of increased hypoxemia, with or without dyspnea or loss of consciousness, are a major feature of tetralogy after the first few months of life. These episodes, which have been referred to as blue spells, cyanotic spells, anoxic spells, and "tet" spells, represent an acute increase in right-to-left shunting. Spells can be triggered by a reduction in systemic arterial resistance or an increase in right ventricular outflow obstruction as by constriction of the infundibular region. Brain abscess is a recognized complication of cyanotic congenital heart disease. *(Rudolph:1397–1398)*

77. (D) Localized coarctation of the aorta is distinguished from hypoplasia or interruption of the aortic arch. The former is a localized narrowing of the aorta, whereas the latter is a diffuse narrowing or total interruption of the arch. Localized coarctation is always closely related to the area of insertion of the ductus arteriosus into the aorta. In most cases the shelf of narrowing is directly opposite the orifice of the ductus. Under these circumstances, aortic blood flow can bypass the coarctation by flowing through the orifice or proximal portion of the ductus, around the protruding aortic shelf. When the ductus closes, this is no longer possible, and obstruction becomes more severe. Thus, closure of the ductus arteriosus will be associated with worsening rather than improvement of symptoms. Symptoms such as congestive heart failure may develop early (usually between 3 and 6 months) or be delayed until adulthood. Although the great majority of children with hypoplasia or interruption of the arch have associated major intracardiac defects, this is true for only a few patients with coarctation. However, coarctation does have an association with Turner's syndrome and with bicuspid aortic valve. There also is an increased incidence of aberrant subclavian artery, patent ductus arteriosus, ventricular septal defect, parachute mitral valve, and berry aneurysm of the circle of Willis. Hypertension secondary to an untreated coarctation may increase the risk of rupture of a berry aneurysm. (Rudolph:1383–1384)

78. **(A)** Tetralogy of Fallot is a form of cyanotic congenital heart disease characterized by four cardinal features: (1) stenosis and obstruction of the outflow tract of the right ventricle; (2) a ventricular septal defect; (3) dextroposition of the aorta; and (4) right ventricular hypertrophy. This combination of features results in diminished pulmonary blood flow and a right-to-left shunt at the ventricular level. (Rudolph:1397)

79. **(D)** Mucocutaneous lymph node syndrome (Kawasaki syndrome) is an acute vasculitis of undetermined origin occurring primarily during the first half decade of life. Clinical features include prolonged fever, conjunctivitis, erythema of the lips and other oral tissues, cervical lymphadenopathy (usually unilateral), swelling and/or erythema of the hands and feet, and desquamation of skin, especially of the hands and feet and often starting in the subungual regions. Involvement of coronary vessels occurs in up to 20% of children and can lead to aneurysm formation. An erythematous pleomorphic or morbilliform rash is common; the rash is neither violaceous nor purpuric. (Rudolph:491; Hathaway:463–464)

80. **(C)** Retinoblastoma, neuroblastoma, and Wilms's tumor all are most common in the first few years of life. The peak incidence of childhood leukemia is between 2 and 6 years of age. Hodgkin's disease, in contrast, is quite rare in the first half-decade of life. (Rudolph:1196)

81. **(D)** Congenital abnormalities of the spleen (asplenia and polysplenia) often are associated with abnormalities of situs. Asplenia is associated with bilateral right-sidedness (each lung has a middle lobe), and polysplenia is associated with bilateral left-sidedness. Dextrocardia, atrial septal defects, and cyanotic congenital heart disease are also frequently associated. Congenital malformations of the gastrointestinal and urinary systems have been reported. The spleen plays a vital role in immunologic defense, especially the filtering of bacteria from the blood. Patients without spleens (whether on a congenital or a surgical basis) are very susceptible to overwhelming, fatal septicemia with encapsulated bacteria such as *S. pneumoniae*. Anemia is not a feature of asplenia, but the presence of red cell inclusions such as Howell-Jolly bodies is. (Rudolph:1152,1316; J Pediatr 81:1130–1133,1972)

82. **(A)** Thrombocytopenia is a regular feature of the hemolytic uremic syndrome, an acute microangiopathy of undetermined origin. Hemolytic uremic syndrome usually follows a gastrointestinal infection and is characterized by hemolytic anemia, acute renal failure, and thrombocytopenia. Thrombocytopenia also can be seen as the result of platelet trapping in a giant hemangioma. There is an association of congenital thrombocytopenia and absence of radius bilaterally, the TAR (thrombocytopenia, absent radius) syndrome. Hypersplenism can result in decreased numbers of platelets as well as erythrocytes and leukocytes. Lead poisoning is not associated with thrombocytopenia. (Rudolph:420,1160)

83. **(A)** Neurofibromatosis is associated with a variety of malignant tumors, including fibrosarcoma, Schwannoma, and pheochromocytoma. There is an increased incidence of leukemia in children with Down's syndrome. Like many other immunodeficiency disorders, Wiskott-Aldrich syndrome is associated with an increased risk of malignancy, primarily lymphoma. Hemihypertrophy is associated with Wilms's tumor. Cystic fibrosis is not associated with an increased risk of cancer of any type. (Rudolph:296, 467,1199)

84. **(C)** Medulloblastoma is the most common posterior fossa tumor in children, accounting for almost half of the tumors in this region. Most cases present in the first decade of life, with a peak incidence between 3 and 5 years of age. Obstruction of the ventricular system, with resultant increased intracranial pressure, occurs frequently and early. Spread along the meninges and neuraxis is common. Complete surgical removal of the tumor is rarely feasible, and, although the tumor is very sensitive to irradiation, the prognosis for cure is unfavorable. [*Note:* At first glance it might appear that choices **(D)** and **(E)** are incompatible; that is, they cannot both be true. However, this is not the case. The fact that a tumor is radiosensitive means only that it *regresses* in response to such therapy, not necessarily that it can be *cured* in this manner.] (Rudolph:1735–1736)

85. **(B)** In idiopathic thrombocytopenia (ITP) the platelet count is decreased, usually below 60,000/mm^3, while the remainder of the blood count is normal unless there has been significant bleeding, in which case the Hb may be decreased and the reticulocyte count increased. Most pediatric cases of ITP occur in the first 5 to 6 years of life, when the mean hemoglobin value ranges from 12 to 13 g/dL. (Rudolph:1159)

86. **(A)** A Hb concentration of 12 g/dL and a WBC count of 11,500/mm^3 are within statistical "normal" limits for a 2-year-old child (mean 12.5; 10th percentile 11.5). Whether or not a hemoglobin of 12 g/dL might be increased by the administration of iron therapy is a moot point not relevant to this question, as all of the other choices have at least one clearly *abnormal* value. (Rudolph:1092–1093; Hathaway:471)

87. **(E)** In children with sickle cell disease the Hb is usually between 7 and 10 g/dL, and the white blood cell count is between 15,000 and 25,000/mm³. The reticulocyte count is increased except in the presence of an aplastic crisis, which usually does not involve the platelets. [*Note:* The values in choice **(D)** are compatible with sickle cell disease during an aplastic crisis. The question, however, clearly stipulates that the patient is not having a crisis.] *(Hathaway:487)*

88. **(D)** In the presence of iron deficiency anemia, the reticulocyte count typically is low. Hemoglobin values of 5 g/dL are common, and values as low as 2 g/dL are seen occasionally in very severe cases. Striking increases in platelet counts have been noted in children with iron deficiency anemia. *(Rudolph:1101–1102; Hathaway:472–473)*

89. **(C)** Acute lymphoblastic leukemia often presents with anemia and thrombocytopenia. The total white blood cell count may be increased, normal, or decreased. In about 10% of cases the peripheral WBC is below 3,000/mm³ at the time of presentation. [*Note:* Although leukemia can present with a completely normal peripheral blood count and manifestations such as fever, bone pain, hepatosplenomegaly, and lymphadenopathy, or with isolated depression of a single blood element, answer **(C)** should be considered the *best* choice since it is characteristic and *most* suggestive of leukemia.] *(Rudolph:1186–1187)*

90. **(C)** As the name implies, in pancytopenia, *all* blood elements are quantitatively diminished. Answer **(C)** is the only choice in which the erythrocytes (hemoglobin), leukocytes (WBC), and platelets are abnormally low. The low reticulocyte count reflects failure of the bone marrow, which is the usual cause of pancytopenia. Occasionally, pancytopenia with a *normal* or *elevated* reticulocyte count can be seen with hypersplenism. *(Hathaway: 471)*

91. **(E)** Meconium ileus is intestinal obstruction in the newborn caused by impacted meconium in the small bowel, usually the ileum. The condition is essentially always associated with cystic fibrosis. In this disease, meconium is abnormally thick and sticky, partly because of abnormal glycoproteins and partly because of pancreatic insufficiency, and accumulates in the intestinal lumen, producing bowel obstruction even before birth. About 10 to 15% of infants with cystic fibrosis have meconium ileus at birth. *(Rudolph:1033)*

92. **(D)** Malrotation of the intestines is an abnormality that results from a failure of counterclockwise rotation of the fetal intestine as it returns to the abdominal cavity at about week 10 of gestation. The condition often is associated with duodenal obstruction secondary to constricting peritoneal bands. However, in a small percentage of cases obstruction results from a midgut volvulus. This is a potentially devastating complication in which the mobile, malrotated bowel twists about the superior mesenteric artery. Infarction and necrosis of major segments of bowel may occur. Midgut volvulus is a surgical emergency. *(Rudolph:1032)*

93. **(A)** Enterocolitis is a well-recognized complication of congenital aganglionic megacolon (Hirschsprung's disease) that occurs primarily in undiagnosed or inadequately managed patients. Severe recurrent diarrhea secondary to enterocolitis may be the presenting complaint in a young infant with congenital megacolon. Recognition of the underlying abnormality is important, as the mortality rate of secondary enterocolitis ("toxic megacolon") can be quite high. *(Rudolph:1039)*

94. **(C)** Both Friedreich's ataxia and Huntington's chorea are genetically determined, degenerative neurologic diseases. Friedreich's ataxia is inherited by an autosomal recessive pattern, although related spinocerebellar degenerative syndromes follow an autosomal dominant pattern. Huntington's chorea is transmitted as an autosomal dominant trait. *(Rudolph:1867–1868,1886)*

95. **(A)** Interstitial myocarditis and myocardial fibrosis eventually develop in many patients with classic Friedreich's ataxia. There is no cardiac involvement in Huntington's chorea. *(Rudolph:1867–1868,1886)*

96. **(C)** Both Friedreich's ataxia and Huntington's chorea are progressive disorders with a relentless, downhill course. *(Rudolph:1867–1868,1886)*

97. **(A)** Kyphoscoliosis is seen commonly in patients with Friedreich's ataxia but not in those with Huntington's chorea. *(Rudolph:1867–1868,1886)*

98. **(D)** Neither Friedreich's ataxia nor Huntington's chorea is associated with immunodeficiency. *(Rudolph:1867–1868,1886)*

99. **(B)** Absence seizures (petit mal seizures) are rarely evident before 3 years of age and usually disappear by puberty. Grand mal seizures, in contrast, may occur at any age, including the newborn period. *(Rudolph:1770–1775)*

100. **(A)** Absence seizures are a type of primary epilepsy with a strong genetic basis and are not seen as a result of acquired central nervous system injury or lesions. Grand mal seizures, on the other hand, may be either primary or secondary to a variety of insults (such as hypoglycemia or anoxia) or specific intracranial lesions. *(Rudolph:1770–1775)*

101. **(B)** A three-per-second spike-and-wave pattern on an electroencephalogram is characteristic of absence seizures. *(Rudolph:1770–1775)*

102. (A) Grand mal seizures almost always cause the patient to fall to the ground. In contrast, patients rarely lose muscle tone or fall during an absence seizure. *(Rudolph: 1770–1775)*

103. (A) A grand mal seizure occasionally is preceded by an aura. Absence seizures are not associated with auras. *(Rudolph:1770–1775)*

104. (D) Death during any type of seizure is rare unless the underlying cause (hypoxia, head trauma, metabolic disorder) is itself lethal. *(Rudolph:1770–1775)*

105. (B) Absence seizures are more frequent in girls than in boys. Grand mal seizures occur with approximately equal frequency in males and females. *(Rudolph:1770–1775)*

106. (A) The normal electrocardiogram of an infant is quite different from that of an older child or adult. An Rs pattern over the right precordium of an infant or child less than 2 years is a reflection of the normal right ventricular predominance at that age. *(Rudolph:1322–1328)*

107. (C) The T waves are inverted in V_{3r} through V_3 in most infants and may remain inverted in V_{3r} and V_1 up to 15 years of age. *(Rudolph:1322–1328)*

108. (D) For reasons that are not clear, in the first few days of life T waves over V_{3r} and V_1 usually are upright, while the T waves in V_5 and V_6 are inverted. After that time, inverted T waves in leads V_5 and V_6 always are abnormal. *(Rudolph:1322–1328)*

109. (D) Inverted P waves in lead I are never normal. In a child, a negative P wave in lead I usually indicates dextrocardia. *(Rudolph:1322–1328)*

110. (A) Large ventricular septal defects can produce left-to-right shunting with markedly increased pulmonary blood flow and congestive heart failure. However, the relatively high pulmonary vascular resistance present at birth usually prevents a large left-to-right shunt at that time, and congestive heart failure does not appear until a few months later, when pulmonary arterial resistance has fallen. Cyanosis is not a feature of ventricular septal defects per se, although mild cyanosis may be noted in infants with very severe congestive heart failure. *(Rudolph:1365–1368)*

111. (B) Tetralogy of Fallot is characterized by a right-to-left shunt at the ventricular level. This results in persistent cyanosis, which can be quite severe and often is associated with striking clubbing of the fingers and toes. Pulmonary blood flow is decreased (because of right ventricular outflow obstruction), there is no obstruction to left ventricular outflow, and no abnormal recirculation of blood flow. There-

fore, congestive heart failure is not a feature of this cardiac abnormality. *(Rudolph:1397–1398)*

112. (C) In transposition of the great arteries, the output of the right ventricle enters the aorta and returns to the right atrium. The output of the left ventricle flows to the lungs and from there to the left atrium. These two independent circulations would be incompatible with life unless an avenue of mixing such as a foramen ovale, ductus arteriosus, or ventricular septal defect were available. Both cyanosis (from the right-to-left component of the mixing) and congestive heart failure (from left ventricular output flowing to the lungs) are clinical features of this abnormality. *(Rudolph:1404–1406)*

113. (D) Ostium secundum defects usually are isolated lesions that cause a left-to-right shunt at the atrial level. Since the shunt is exclusively left to right, cyanosis is not present. The pressure gradient between the atria is small, and the increased volume load to the right ventricle is well tolerated. Congestive heart failure rarely develops in infants or young children with uncomplicated ostium-secundum-type atrial septal defects. *(Rudolph: 1368–1369)*

114. (D) Double aortic arch is a congenital malformation of the aorta resulting in a "vascular ring" that encircles the trachea. Symptoms result from compression of the trachea and include primarily inspiratory stridor and, to a lesser extent, expiratory wheezing. Neither congestive heart failure nor cyanosis is a clinical feature of this abnormality. *(Rudolph:1390–1392)*

115. (C) Congestive heart failure is seen in both bacterial endocarditis (BE) and acute rheumatic fever (ARF). In BE heart failure usually is caused by valvular destruction and resultant mitral or aortic insufficiency, whereas in ARF heart failure usually is related to myocarditis. *(Rudolph:492–494,1417–1419)*

116. (C) Although noted in fewer than half the cases, the appearance of a new murmur is a characteristic and important finding in both BE and ARF. In BE the murmurs are created by the presence of vegetations on the valves or by erosion of valve leaflets. Occasionally, rupture of the chordae tendineae may produce valvular insufficiency. In ARF, new murmurs result from inflammation and edema of valve leaflets. *(Rudolph:492–494,1417–1419)*

117. (B) Subcutaneous nodules (painless nodules about 1 cm in diameter, primarily over the spine and the extensor surfaces of the extremities) are seen in a small number of children with ARF but are not seen in patients with BE. These nodules are very different from the cutaneous and subcutaneous manifestations of infective carditis: Osler nodes, which are painful, erythematous swellings on the dorsum of the fingers or toes, and Janeway lesions, which are painless hemorrhagic lesions on the palms and soles. *(Rudolph:492–494,1417–1419)*

118. **(A)** Petechiae are common manifestations of embolic phenomena in BE but are not a finding in ARF. *(Rudolph:492–494,1417–1419)*

119. **(B)** Erythema marginatum, like subcutaneous nodules, is an infrequent but characteristic finding in ARF. This rash is macular, erythematous, and migratory, appearing in one area as it disappears from another. The name derives from the tendency of lesions to have serpiginous, erythematous edges and clear centers. Erythema marginatum does not occur in association with BE. *(Rudolph:492–494,1417–1419)*

120. **(D)** Anemia, usually mild to moderate, is common in both BE and ARF. The anemia, however, is normocytic and normochromic. *(Rudolph:492–494,1417–1419)*

121. **(B)** Both duodenal atresia and congenital hypertrophic pyloric stenosis are causes of high intestinal obstruction early in life. However, despite its name, *congenital* hypertrophic pyloric stenosis is not a true congenital malformation as is duodenal atresia. Rather, pyloric stenosis develops during the first weeks of life. Hypertrophic pyloric stenosis is essentially never found in stillborns or in infants dying in the first few days of life. Therefore, duodenal atresia, since it causes complete high intestinal obstruction present at birth, is associated with vomiting in the first 24 hours of life, whereas hypertrophic pyloric stenosis is a progressive disorder in which vomiting rarely appears before 7 to 10 days of age. *(Rudolph:1001–1002; Hathaway:540–541,543)*

122. **(B)** In the great majority of cases of duodenal atresia, the obstruction is distal to the ampulla of Vater, and the vomitus is bile stained, whereas in pyloric stenosis the obstruction always is proximal to the ampulla, and the vomitus is free of bile. *(Rudolph:1001–1002; Hathaway:540–541,543)*

123. **(A)** The diagnosis of pyloric stenosis usually is made only after a week or more of vomiting. The prolonged vomiting of pure gastric contents (acid) commonly leads to a metabolic alkalosis, which is characteristic of this disorder. In contrast, the newborn with duodenal atresia is also losing bicarbonate-rich pancreatic secretion in the vomitus. Additionally, the diagnosis of duodenal atresia usually is made fairly rapidly. For these reasons, infants with duodenal atresia do not develop metabolic alkalosis. *(Rudolph:1001–1002; Hathaway:540–541,543)*

124. **(B)** There is a well-recognized association of duodenal atresia and Down's syndrome (about one-third of infants with duodenal atresia have Down's syndrome), but there is no association between pyloric stenosis and Down's syndrome. *(Rudolph:1001–1002; Hathaway:540–541, 543)*

125. **(C)** Surgical correction (duodenoduodenostomy or duodenojejunostomy) offers the only hope for survival in cases of duodenal atresia. Although nonsurgical management of hypertrophic pyloric stenosis with eventual remission has been reported, such an approach has been virtually abandoned in the developed countries of the world. Surgical pylorotomy is safe and effective and is the treatment of choice. *(Rudolph:1001–1002; Hathaway:540–541,543)*

126. **(D)** Factor VIII deficiency (hemophilia A) is inherited as an X-linked defect. Idiopathic thrombocytopenic purpura (ITP) is an acquired, usually temporary, condition associated with antiplatelet autoantibodies. Thus, neither condition is associated with autosomal transmission. *(Rudolph:1159–1160; 1162–1164)*

127. **(B)** Petechiae are characteristically seen in platelet disorders but not in other coagulopathies that do not involve the platelets. Petechiae are not noted in patients with hemophilia. *(Rudolph:1159–1160; 1162–1164)*

128. **(A)** Hemarthrosis is very common in hemophilia but not in thrombocytopenia. *(Rudolph:1159–1160; 1162–1164)*

129. **(D)** Bleeding disorders do not predispose to infection. Neither hemophilia nor ITP is associated with an increased risk of systemic infection or sepsis. *(Rudolph:1159–1160; 1162–1164)*

130. **(B)** Splenectomy has no effect on the course of hemophilia. Since the spleen is a major site of removal and destruction of antibody-coated platelets, it is not surprising that splenectomy is associated with prolonged platelet survival and improvement in platelet counts in ITP. However, since the majority of cases of ITP in children resolve completely, and since splenectomy predisposes to overwhelming sepsis, splenectomy is indicated only in a very few selected children with chronic ITP. *(Rudolph:1159–1160; 1162–1164)*

131. **(D)** Neither hemophilia nor ITP responds to aspirin. As a matter of fact, since aspirin interferes with platelet aggregation and prolongs the bleeding time, it should be avoided in all patients with disorders of coagulation. *(Rudolph:1159–1160; 1162–1164)*

132. **(B)** Many cases of ITP appear to follow an acute viral infection such as rubella or varicella. Hemophilia, being a genetically determined coagulopathy, is unrelated to viral infections. *(Rudolph:1159–1160; 1162–1164)*

133. (C) Autosomal recessive polycystic kidney disease (PKD) was formerly known as infantile PKD, and autosomal dominant PKD was known as adult PKD. It is now recognized that neither disorder is completely age specific, both forms can affect infants and children, and both forms have considerable clinical variation. *(Rudolph:1256–1257)*

134. (A) The autosomal recessive form of PKD is usually accompanied by hepatic involvement with cystic (Caroli disease) and/or fibrotic (congenital hepatic fibrosis) changes. The liver involvement usually presents as hepatomegaly and/or portal hypertension rather than jaundice and hepatic failure. *(Rudolph:1074,1256–1257)*

135. (D) Neither the autosomal recessive nor the autosomal dominant form of PKD is associated with pulmonary emphysema or lung cysts. *(Rudolph:1256–1257)*

136. (C) Both autosomal recessive and autosomal dominant PKD can progress to renal failure, and both can do so in childhood. Occasionally an infant or child with autosomal dominant PKD may present as renal failure while the disease is still mild and undiagnosed in the parent. *(Rudolph:1256–1257)*

BIBLIOGRAPHY

Feigin RD, Cherry JD. *Textbook of Pediatric Infectious Diseases.* 3rd ed. Philadelphia, Pa: Saunders; 1992.

Freedom RM. The asplenia syndrome. *J Pediatr.* 1972;81: 1130–1133.

Hathaway WE, Groothius JR, Hay WW, et al. *Current Pediatric Diagnosis & Treatment.* 10th ed. Norwalk, Conn: Appleton & Lange; 1991.

Lopez-Ibor B, Schwartz AD. Neuroblastoma. *Pediatr Clin North Am.* 1985;32:755–778.

Lum LG, Jones MD. The effect of cuff width on systolic blood pressure measurements in neonates. *J Pediatr.* 1977;91:963–966.

Pratt CB. Some aspects of childhood cancer epidemiology. *Pediatr Clin North Am.* 1985;32:541–556.

Rudolph AM, Hoffman JIE, Rudolph CD. *Pediatrics.* 19th ed. Norwalk, Conn: Appleton & Lange; 1991.

Takano T, Nakagome Y. High-resolution cytogenetic studies in Prader-Willi syndrome. *Clin Genet.* 1986;30:241–248.

Steinfield L, Dimich I, Redev R. Sphygmomanometry in the pediatric patient. *J Pediatr.* 1978;92:934–938.

CHAPTER 10

Case Diagnosis—Management Problems
Questions

Case diagnosis and management problems are common in national examinations. The basic format is a case description followed by two or more questions about the case. These questions are designed to assess the examinee's clinical judgment and thinking ability as well as his or her fund of knowledge.

To maximize your learning experience in this chapter, it is important to try to answer all questions about a case before looking at the answers. Only if absolutely unable to proceed with a problem should you seek help from the answers before completing the case. Refrain from looking ahead at the next question in hopes of obtaining additional information for the question at hand. Not only would this negate the learning-testing experience, but it might actually lead to an incorrect answer! For example, diagnostic or therapeutic steps that might be correct later in the case might be considered incorrect earlier when certain information was not available. Covering the next question with a piece of paper will be helpful in preventing accidental preview.

DIRECTIONS: This part of the test consists of a series of cases followed by a group of related questions. For each question, study the case and select the ONE best answer to complete each statement that follows. [*Note:* The student should try to complete all questions about a case before looking at the answers.]

Questions 1 through 5

An 8-year-old white male child was hospitalized because of generalized seizures. The child had been well until 10 days prior to admission, when he developed fever and a sore throat, which resolved without medical attention. He was then well again until 2 days prior to admission, when he developed nausea and vomiting, headache, and facial puffiness. On the day of admission, the child experienced a generalized tonic-clonic seizure lasting about 5 minutes. Vital signs were T 38.5°C, HR 96, RR 22, BP 155/125. On examination, the child was found to be disoriented, confused, combative, and lethargic. There was moderate pitting edema of the hands and feet. A grade II/VI systolic murmur was audible over the left sternal border. The liver was palpable 2 cm below the right costal margin. There were no focal neurologic signs, and the fundi were normal.

1. The most likely diagnosis in this patient is

   (A) a brain tumor
   (B) a cerebral vascular accident
   (C) bacterial meningitis
   (D) epilepsy
   (E) hypertensive encephalopathy

2. The most likely cause of the elevated blood pressure is

   (A) essential hypertension
   (B) a ventricular septal defect
   (C) a pheochromocytoma
   (D) renal disease
   (E) drug ingestion

3. Diagnostically, at this time you should order

   (A) a blood culture
   (B) a head CT scan
   (C) a lumbar puncture
   (D) an electroencephalograph
   (E) serum electrolytes and BUN

4. Therapeutically, at this time you should

   (A) administer an anticonvulsant agent
   (B) administer an antihypertensive agent
   (C) intubate and ventilate the patient
   (D) start an intravenous infusion of saline

5. You anticipate that this patient also may need

(A) a blood transfusion
(B) an exchange transfusion
(C) dialysis
(D) neurosurgical intervention

Questions 6 through 10

Remember to answer all the questions in this group before looking at any of the answers.

A 12-year-old child with asthma is brought to the emergency room because of wheezing. On arrival he is noted to be in severe respiratory distress and is given a treatment of aerosolized albuterol, without any apparent improvement. T 37.5°C, RR 46, HR 140, BP 140/80. There is slight, generalized cyanosis. Examination of the chest reveals bilateral inspiratory and expiratory wheezes and coarse inspiratory and expiratory rales. The child appears agitated, and the liver edge is palpable 3 cm below the right costal margin.

6. Which of the following would be the most appropriate next step in the care of this child?

(A) Administer a diuretic agent
(B) Repeat the aerosolized albuterol
(C) Administer oxygen by mask
(D) Obtain a chest roentgenogram
(E) Obtain an arterial blood gas measurement on room air

7. Arterial blood gases obtained while the patient is receiving oxygen reveal the following values: pH 7.30; PCO_2 39; bicarbonate 18 mEq/L; oxygen saturation 85%. The patient has a

(A) respiratory acidosis
(B) combined metabolic and respiratory acidosis
(C) metabolic acidosis
(D) compensated metabolic acidosis
(E) metabolic alkalosis and respiratory acidosis

8. Despite therapy with humidified oxygen and intravenous aminophylline, the child looks more uncomfortable, with increasing distress and wheezing. Therapy with corticosteroids should be

(A) initiated at this time
(B) initiated if the arterial PCO_2 reaches 60 mm Hg
(C) initiated if the arterial PO_2 falls to 60 mm Hg or less
(D) initiated as soon as the chest roentgenograph has been confirmed as not showing evidence of pneumonia
(E) withheld

9. The child's condition continues to deteriorate despite appropriate pharmacotherapy, and within a few hours he has been intubated and is being ventilated with a volume-controlled ventilator and an inspired oxygen concentration of 60%. Arterial blood gases reveal: pH 7.25; PCO_2 75; bicarbonate 32 mEq/L; PO_2 95. At this time the best course of action would be to

(A) cautiously increase the concentration of inspired oxygen
(B) change to a pressure-controlled ventilator
(C) attempt to adjust the ventilator so as to increase net alveolar ventilation
(D) administer 2 mEq/kg of sodium bicarbonate intravenously
(E) discontinue all bronchodilators

10. On the second hospital day, while still intubated and receiving assisted ventilation, the child suddenly develops cyanosis, a fall in blood pressure, and a displacement of the cardiac impulse to the right. The most likely explanation of these findings is that the

(A) patient has developed cor pulmonale
(B) patient has developed a tension pneumothorax
(C) patient has developed pneumonia
(D) tidal volume of the ventilator has been set too low
(E) endotracheal tube has slipped into the right mainstem bronchus

Questions 11 through 16

Remember to answer all the questions in this group before looking at any of the answers.

A 12-year-old girl is seen with complaints of fever and sore throat. Physical examination revealed an inflamed pharynx, enlarged and inflamed tonsils, and moderately enlarged and tender bilateral cervical lymph nodes. The child is given 600,000 units of procaine penicillin intramuscularly and then 400,000 units of penicillin G orally four times a day. The fever and sore throat persist, and the child is reexamined on the sixth day of illness, at which time she is found to have a severe exudative tonsillitis and bilateral, large tender cervical lymph nodes, including posterior cervical nodes. The oral penicillin G is discontinued, and ampicillin, 250 mg four times a day, is prescribed. Two days later the child is still febrile, and an erythematous, maculopapular rash is noted.

11. Which of the following would have been most appropriate in the initial management of this patient when she was first seen?

(A) Blood culture
(B) Throat culture or rapid strep test
(C) Complete blood count
(D) PA and lateral chest roentgenograms
(E) Tuberculin skin test

12. When the patient was seen the second time, the attending physician should have

(A) prescribed 500 mg of ampicillin four times a day
(B) prescribed 500 mg of oxacillin four times a day
(C) hospitalized the child
(D) obtained a CBC and a monospot test
(E) obtained a CBC and a throat and blood culture

13. The most likely cause of this child's illness is

(A) penicillin-resistant group A beta-hemolytic strep-tococcal infection
(B) T-cell leukemia
(C) EBV infectious mononucleosis
(D) measles
(E) peritonsillitis or peritonsillar abscess

14. The patient is found to have a positive monospot test. At this time the physician should

(A) repeat the monospot test
(B) order a bone marrow examination
(C) assume that this represents a false-positive test
(D) assume that the patient has infectious mononucleosis
(E) realize that the monospot test can be positive many months following EB virus infection and in this case probably represents past infection

15. This patient developed a rash on the eighth day of illness, 2 days after starting ampicillin therapy. Such a rash

(A) probably represents penicillin allergy
(B) probably represents modified scarlet fever
(C) is probably the rash of infectious mononucleosis
(D) suggests that the illness is modified or atypical measles
(E) is common in patients with infectious mononucleosis treated with ampicillin

16. The physician now prescribes a 7-day course of corti-costeroids for this patient. It is expected that the steroids would

(A) have no effect
(B) increase the length of the illness
(C) decrease the period of symptomatology
(D) cause resolution of the rash but have no other effect
(E) cause the monospot test to revert to negative but have no effect on the clinical course of the illness

Questions 17 through 21

Remember to answer all the questions in this group before looking at any of the answers.

A 5-month-old male infant, previously well, is admitted following 2 days of severe diarrhea. During this time, the infant has been fed unmodified cow milk, orange juice, tea, rice water, and plain water. There has been no vomiting. On admission, the child is noted to be lethargic and appears dehydrated with sunken eyes, depressed fontanel, dry mucous membranes, and poor skin turgor. Pulses are adequate, and capillary refill time is 2 seconds. BP is 70/30, HR 160, T 38°C, wt. 6.3 kg. The remainder of the examination is within normal limits.

17. This patient's fluid deficit is probably about

(A) 100 mL
(B) 300 mL

(C) 500 mL
(D) 700 mL
(E) 900 mL

18. The child should immediately be given a rapid intra-venous infusion (bolus) of

(A) 1 to 2 mL/kg
(B) 3 to 5 mL/kg
(C) 10 to 20 mL/kg
(D) 50 mL/kg
(E) 100 mL/kg

19. The initial intravenous hydrating fluid (bolus) given to this child should contain

(A) 140 mEq/L of sodium
(B) 100 mEq/L of sodium
(C) 75 mEq/L of sodium
(D) 35 mEq/L of sodium
(E) no sodium

20. This initial hydrating solution should contain

(A) 60 mEq/L of potassium
(B) 40 mEq/L of potassium
(C) 20 mEq/L of potassium
(D) 10 mEq/L of potassium
(E) no potassium

21. Assuming a desire to replace the child's total fluid deficit in 24 hours, and assuming that all diarrhea ceases when the child is ordered NPO, the total fluid requirement for this child for the first 24 hours would be in the order of

(A) 300 mL
(B) 500 mL
(C) 750 mL
(D) 1,000 mL
(E) 1,500 mL

Questions 22 through 25

Remember to answer all the questions in this group before looking at any of the answers.

A 12-year-old black boy, previously well, presents with fever and jaundice. He has had headaches and nausea for 3 days. Today, the parents noted that his eyes and skin are yellow. His urine was noted to be dark. On examination, the child is alert and does not appear very ill. He is icteric. The liver is enlarged and tender. There is no adenopathy and no pallor. There is no history of recent injections or blood transfusion and no history of contact with other jaundiced individuals. There is no history of drug ingestion or abuse.

22. The most likely diagnosis is

(A) sickle cell anemia
(B) viral hepatitis
(C) cholecystitis
(D) G6PD deficiency
(E) choledochal cyst

23. The child has a hemoglobin of 14 g/dL. Of the following tests, which would be most useful?

(A) Serum haptoglobin
(B) Abdominal ultrasound
(C) Serum electrolytes
(D) Monospot test
(E) AST (SGOT) and ALT (SGPT) levels

24. Hepatitis B surface antigen is demonstrated in the child's blood. This suggests that the child

(A) has hepatitis B viral infection
(B) has an acute exacerbation of chronic hepatitis
(C) is developing autoantibodies to hepatic tissue
(D) is immunodeficient
(E) will develop hepatic necrosis

25. Mental confusion, emotional instability, and restlessness develop and progress rapidly to coma. The most likely cause of these findings is

(A) a cerebral vascular accident
(B) viral encephalitis
(C) adrenal insufficiency
(D) hepatic failure
(E) bilirubin encephalopathy

Questions 26 through 30

Remember to answer all the questions in this group before looking at any of the answers.

An 8-month-old child is seen because of vomiting for 24 hours. The child passed one soft stool at the onset and has had no bowel movements since. The infant has had recurrent episodes of screaming and agitation lasting about 4 or 5 minutes since the onset of the vomiting. On examination, the child is found to be listless and apathetic. T 39°C. The child appears moderately dehydrated. The abdomen is soft and nontender. There is a palpable mass, about 2 by 5 cm, deep in the right upper quadrant. Rectal examination is unremarkable.

26. The appropriate first step in the management of this patient would be to

(A) perform a barium enema
(B) start an intravenous infusion
(C) obtain blood and stool cultures
(D) perform an exploratory laparotomy
(E) administer a broad-spectrum antibiotic

27. Appropriate diagnostic tests to be performed promptly include all of the following EXCEPT

(A) flat and upright abdominal roentgenogram
(B) serum electrolytes
(C) blood count
(D) liver-spleen scan
(E) serum creatinine and blood urea nitrogen

28. The above tests are obtained and are all either normal or nondiagnostic. You should now

(A) observe the child
(B) perform a barium enema
(C) order an abdominal CT scan
(D) perform an exploratory laparotomy
(E) administer ampicillin and clindamycin

29. The condition is successfully treated. The risk of recurrence is

(A) essentially zero
(B) about 5%
(C) about 25%
(D) about 50%
(E) close to 100%

Questions 30 through 32

Remember to answer all the questions in this group before looking at any of the answers.

A 1-month-old female infant is admitted with a 1-week history of not moving the right arm. The parents are undocumented aliens, and the infant had been born at home. Neonatal course was said to have been uncomplicated. One week prior to admission, the mother noted that the infant did not clench her right fist or move her right arm as well as the left. Physical examination at the time of admission reveals a well-nourished infant in no distress. Temperature is 38°C. The only abnormalities are decreased tone and decreased spontaneous movement of the right arm.

30. The differential diagnosis ought to include all of the following EXCEPT

(A) congenital syphilis
(B) craniopharyngioma
(C) congenital hemiparesis
(D) battered child
(E) osteomyelitis

31. Roentgenograms reveal osteochondritis of the right humerus with destructive changes and periosteal reaction. One should now order

(A) psychosocial examination of the parents
(B) an abdominal ultrasound
(C) an erythrocyte sedimentation rate
(D) a serologic test for syphilis
(E) serum calcium and phosphorus levels

32. The test obtained above is positive. One should now order

(A) a bone marrow examination
(B) referral to a child protection agency
(C) a lumbar puncture
(D) a hematology-oncology consultation
(E) a technetium bone scan

Questions 33 through 35

Remember to answer all the questions in this group before looking at any of the answers.

A 5-month-old child develops a cold and cough. The cough fails to clear and, over a 2-week period, worsens to the point of severe paroxysms associated with cyanosis. The paroxysms occasionally end with vomiting. The child is afebrile, and physical examination is within normal limits.

33. At this time it would be most important to obtain a history regarding

   (A) birth weight
   (B) immunizations
   (C) consanguinity of parents
   (D) early infant deaths in relatives
   (E) family members with reactive airway disease

34. The most appropriate method to try to culture the responsible organism from this child would be

   (A) throat swab
   (B) nasopharyngeal swab
   (C) blood culture
   (D) lung puncture
   (E) bronchoscopy

35. The white blood cell count is 32,000/mm³, with 80% lymphocytes, 18% polymorphonuclear cells, and 2% eosinophils. At this time it would be appropriate to

   (A) order a bone marrow examination
   (B) prescribe oral erythromycin
   (C) prescribe intravenous gamma-globulin
   (D) perform a lumbar puncture
   (E) repeat the blood count in 24 hours

Questions 36 through 38

Remember to answer all the questions in this group before looking at any of the answers.

An 8-year-old child returns from a camping trip with malaise and headache. The next day he develops chills and a temperature of 40°C. Two days later, a maculopapular eruption begins on the wrists and ankles and spreads to the arms, legs, and trunk. There is generalized arthralgia. Two days after the appearance of the rash, it becomes purpuric. Spiking fevers continue, and on the eighth day of illness, the child has a brief generalized convulsion. Physical examination reveals a semicomatose child, toxic, and acutely ill. The neck is supple, the fundi are normal, and there are no focal neurologic signs. The spleen is moderately enlarged. T 40.2°C, RR 18, HR 112, BP 110/75.

36. In the diagnostic workup of this patient, which of the following should be done first?

   (A) Skull roentgenogram
   (B) CT scan of the brain
   (C) Lumbar puncture
   (D) Electroencephalogram
   (E) Neurology consultation

37. You anticipate that this child is likely to have a history of preceding

   (A) diarrhea
   (B) tick bite
   (C) travel to Mexico
   (D) contact with a sick cat
   (E) contact with a 10-year-old with meningitis

38. Cerebrospinal fluid is normal. One should

   (A) withhold all therapy
   (B) treat with antibiotics
   (C) treat with corticosteroids
   (D) treat with fresh frozen plasma
   (E) treat with both antibiotics and corticosteroids

Questions 39 through 42

Remember to answer all the questions in this group before looking at any of the answers.

A white female infant had a normal birth and neonatal period. Development had been normal until about 6 months of life, when her progress appeared to halt. Soon thereafter, she developed apathy, weakness, and the loss of previously acquired functions. At 9 months, she cannot sit without assistance and sits poorly even with support; she cannot roll over; the parents think that she no longer can see. She frequently has coarse, jerking movements of her limbs.

39. This child most likely has

   (A) anterior horn cell disease
   (B) cerebral palsy
   (C) degenerative brain disease
   (D) emotional deprivation syndrome
   (E) toxic encephalopathy

40. Which of the following disorders is LEAST likely in this child?

   (A) Fabry's disease
   (B) Niemann-Pick disease
   (C) Tay-Sachs disease
   (D) Infantile Gaucher's disease
   (E) Juvenile G_{M1} gangliosidosis

41. Examination of the child reveals normal-size liver and spleen and a "cherry-red" spot in the macula. The most likely diagnosis is

   (A) Fabry's disease
   (B) Niemann-Pick disease
   (C) Tay-Sachs disease
   (D) Infantile Gaucher's disease
   (E) Juvenile G_{M1} gangliosidosis

42. Specific therapy of the disorder afflicting this child

(A) is not available

(B) consists of periodic infusions of fresh plasma

(C) consists of intravenous injections of hexosaminidase A

(D) consists of intrathecal injections of hexosaminidase A

(E) is effective only if started prior to the onset of neurologic symptoms

Questions 43 through 48

Remember to answer all the questions in this group before looking at any of the answers.

A 14-year-old girl is admitted with the chief complaint of weakness and tingling of the extremities. She had been in her usual state of good health until 2 weeks prior to admission, when she developed fever, nasal congestion, and a sore throat, all of which cleared without therapy. Five days prior to admission, she developed weakness in her lower extremities, difficulty walking, calf pain, and tingling in her toes and fingers. Weakness progressed until the child was unable to walk. Physical examination revealed decreased muscle strength in all extremities, lower more than upper, and absent deep tendon reflexes in the legs. Cranial nerves were within normal limits, and there was no papilledema. T 37.8°C, RR 16, PR 102, BP 110/65.

43. The most likely pathophysiologic process in this patient is

(A) an intracranial lesion

(B) a spinal cord lesion

(C) a polyneuropathy

(D) myositis

(E) arthritis

44. An especially important and high-priority item on the physical examination of this patient would be

(A) the rectal examination

(B) inspection of hairy areas of the body

(C) inspection of the fingernails

(D) palpation of the breasts

(E) an estimate of visual acuity

45. Examination of the cerebrospinal fluid in this patient reveals protein 75 mg/dL, glucose 62 mg/dL, 6 WBC (5 mononuclear) per mm^3. The most likely diagnosis now is

(A) viral encephalitis

(B) bacterial meningitis

(C) spinal cord tumor

(D) postinfectious polyradiculopathy

(E) an epidural spinal abscess

46. By the second hospital day, peripheral motor weakness had progressed. Cough and gag reflexes were present but slightly diminished. Vital capacity was 75% of predicted. Involvement of cranial nerves VII,

IX, and X was noted. The respiratory rate was 20. Arterial PCO$_2$ was 34 mm Hg, and oxygen saturation 97%. The child's most immediate danger is

(A) aspiration pneumonia

(B) cardiovascular collapse

(C) hypoventilation

(D) brain herniation

(E) cardiac arrhythmia

47. At this point the most appropriate course of action would be to

(A) restrict the child's diet to liquids and observe her closely

(B) order the child NPO and transfer her to the ICU for close monitoring

(C) insert an endotracheal tube and institute intermittent mandatory ventilation

(D) perform a tracheostomy

(E) put the child in a negative-pressure ventilator

48. Without treatment, one would expect the weakness or paralysis to

(A) improve rapidly

(B) progress for 1 to 7 days

(C) progress for 1 to 3 months

(D) progress for 1 to 2 years

(E) remain unchanged

Questions 49 through 54

Remember to answer all the questions in this group before looking at any of the answers.

A 14-month-old white male child is hospitalized because of "failure to thrive." The child had been full term and weighed 7 lb at birth. The child's current diet and feeding habits appear normal by history. He had been growing well until about 11 months of age, when he began to have frequent large and greasy stools and lost weight. There is no history of vomiting. Physical examination reveals a thin child, somewhat apathetic, in no distress. Weight is below the third percentile, length at the 10th percentile, and head circumference between the 10th and 25th percentiles. There is a mild erythematous rash with a few small areas of denudation in the diaper region. The remainder of the physical examination is within normal limits.

49. The most appropriate diet to order for this child on admission would be a

(A) regular diet for age

(B) milk-free diet

(C) gluten-free diet

(D) high-calorie, low-fat diet

(E) clear liquid diet

50. All of the following tests would be appropriately ordered at the time of admission EXCEPT

  (A) urine analysis
  (B) urine culture and colony count
  (C) barium enema
  (D) blood urea nitrogen
  (E) serum albumin

51. The urine analysis is within normal limits. Urine culture, collected by the bag method, reveals 25,000 colonies of *E. coli* per milliliter. The most appropriate next step would be to

  (A) look elsewhere than the urinary system
  (B) repeat the urine culture by the bag method
  (C) collect another urine specimen by catheterization or suprapubic aspiration
  (D) institute appropriate antimicrobial therapy
  (E) order a renal ultrasound examination

52. On a regular diet in the hospital the child is noted to eat well. The stools are soft and greasy but not watery. They are bulky but are passed only once or twice a day. Appropriate diagnostic tests at that time would include all of the following EXCEPT

  (A) sweat test
  (B) examination of peripheral blood smear for acanthocytes
  (C) determination of stool pH
  (D) lumbar puncture
  (E) chest roentgenogram

53. Examination of the stool would be most appropriate for which of the following organisms?

  (A) *Candida*
  (B) *Giardia*
  (C) Rotavirus
  (D) *Shigella*
  (E) *Salmonella*

54. A 2-day fecal fat collection reveals about 12 g of fat per day (about 25% of the fat intake). A peroral jejunal biopsy reveals loss of villi and obliteration of intervillous spaces. The most likely diagnosis is

  (A) gluten-induced enteropathy
  (B) lymphosarcoma
  (C) protein-losing enteropathy
  (D) sucrase-isomaltose deficiency
  (E) Whipple's disease

Questions 55 through 57

Remember to answer all the questions in this group before looking at any of the answers.

A 1-week-old infant is admitted because of vomiting and lethargy. History reveals that vomiting began in the newborn nursery. The infant has been fed a cow milk formula. There has been no diarrhea. Physical examination reveals a lethargic white male infant in no acute distress. The infant is not dehydrated. Skin and sclera appear jaundiced. The liver edge is palpable 4 cm below the right costal margin; the spleen tip is palpable. The abdomen is otherwise normal. Rectal temperature is 96.5°F. Peripheral pulses are good. Except for marked lethargy, the neurologic examination is within normal limits. A lumbar puncture reveals clear fluid with 2 white blood cells per cubic millimeter, no red cells, protein 26 mg/dL; and glucose 5 mg/dL. No organisms are seen on Gram's stain. The following values are reported from the laboratory: serum Na 137 mEq/L, K 3.9 mEq/L, bicarbonate 18 mEq/L, BUN 22 mg/dL; arterial pH 7.36; serum glucose 10 mg/dL; urine analysis, 2+ sugar (reducing substance), trace albumin, zero acetone, 2 to 3 WBC, and 1 to 2 RBC per HPF.

55. This infant most likely has

  (A) diabetic ketoacidosis
  (B) galactosemia
  (C) glycogen storage disease
  (D) ketotic hypoglycemia
  (E) primary renal glycosuria

56. The diagnosis might be established by careful examination of the

  (A) genitalia
  (B) eyes
  (C) nails
  (D) umbilicus
  (E) palmar skin creases

57. Treatment of this child should include a

  (A) normal diet
  (B) glucose-free diet
  (C) high-glucose diet
  (D) galactose-free diet
  (E) high-galactose diet

Questions 58 through 60

Remember to answer all the questions in this group before looking at any of the answers.

A 9-month-old child presents to the emergency room with a 2-day history of a cold followed today by the onset of fever. Physical examination reveals an alert infant in no distress and with no obvious focus of infection. T 40.0°C, HR 160, RR 22. While being examined, the infant suddenly becomes stiff, his eyes roll up, and he displays tonic-clonic movements of all four extremities.

58. The examining physician should first

  (A) perform a spinal tap
  (B) check and maintain the patient's airway
  (C) complete the history and physical examination
  (D) administer an anticonvulsant drug intravenously
  (E) check blood glucose by an appropriate fingerstick method

59. The convulsion ceases spontaneously, before any treatment can be given. The child is unresponsive, but the neurologic examination is otherwise unremarkable. Optic disks are normal. An estimate of blood sugar by a finger-stick method is within normal limits. An acetaminophen rectal suppository has been administered. At this time the physician should order

(A) a CT scan of the head
(B) an EEG
(C) a lumbar puncture
(D) skull roentgenograms
(E) a urinalysis and serum electrolytes

60. All indicated diagnostic tests are normal. The child awakens, and the neurologic examination is normal. At this time it would be appropriate to initiate

(A) a 10-day course of amoxicillin
(B) daily administration of amoxicillin for the next 1 to 2 years
(C) a 14-day course of phenobarbital
(D) daily administration of phenobarbital for the next 1 to 2 years
(E) daily administration of acetaminophen for the next 1 to 2 years

Questions 61 through 65

Remember to answer all the questions in this group before looking at any of the answers.

The patient is a 2,400-g male infant born to a type 0, Rh-positive woman after an uneventful 40 week pregnancy. It was the mother's first pregnancy. The infant is normal at birth but is noted to be jaundiced at about 48 hours of age. The infant is feeding and acting well, and physical examination is entirely within normal limits except for the presence of jaundice of the skin and sclera. Serum bilirubin at 48 hours is found to be 15.5 mg/dL.

61. The serum bilirubin concentration in this child is

(A) within physiologic limits and requires neither investigation nor monitoring
(B) within physiologic limits and requires no investigation but should be monitored
(C) within physiologic limits and should be investigated but requires no monitoring at this time
(D) above physiologic limits and requires both investigation and monitoring
(E) above physiologic limits and should be monitored but requires no diagnostic investigation at this time

62. All of the following tests should be included in the first battery of investigation EXCEPT

(A) determination of the infant's blood type
(B) examination of a peripheral blood smear
(C) hemoglobin electrophoresis
(D) determination of hemoglobin and hematocrit
(E) count of nucleated red blood cells and/or reticulocyte count

63. Of the following additional tests, which would be most important at this time?

(A) Sickle prep
(B) Coombs's test
(C) Glucose-6-phosphate dehydrogenase level
(D) Liver biopsy
(E) Serum AST, ALT

64. The results of the tests ordered above are all negative or within normal limits. Repeat bilirubin at 54 hours of life is 16.5 mg/dL with a conjugated fraction of 1.1 mg/dL. At this time it would be advisable to

(A) perform an exchange transfusion
(B) initiate phototherapy
(C) order an abdominal ultrasound
(D) administer ampicillin and gentamicin
(E) wait for a repeat bilirubin in 6 hours

65. The appropriate action suggested above is accomplished. At 72 hours of age the total serum bilirubin is 11 mg/dL, with a conjugated fraction of less than 1 mg/dL. Of the entities listed below, which would best explain this infant's findings?

(A) Crigler-Najjar syndrome
(B) Rotor syndrome
(C) Extrahepatic biliary atresia
(D) Intrahepatic biliary atresia
(E) Neonatal hepatitis

Questions 66 through 72

Remember to answer all the questions in this group before looking at any of the answers.

A 3,780-g term male infant is born at a large medical center with a major pediatric department. Pregnancy and delivery had been unremarkable. Shortly after birth, physical examination reveals severe generalized cyanosis and tachypnea but no signs of respiratory distress. RR 60, HR 180, T 37°C. There are no cardiac murmurs audible, and the liver is not enlarged. The remainder of the physical examination is within normal limits.

66. Which of the following tests should be performed LAST, if at all?

(A) Electrocardiogram
(B) Chest x-ray examination
(C) Methemoglobin level
(D) Arterial PO_2
(E) Echocardiogram

67. The infant is placed in 60% oxygen by hood without significant improvement in his color. This suggests that the infant has

(A) methemoglobinemia
(B) hypoventilation
(C) cyanotic congenital heart disease
(D) an arteriovenous fistula
(E) pneumonia

68. The chest roentgenogram reveals normal lung fields and a generous, but not definitely enlarged, heart. The upper mediastinum appears narrow on AP view. The most likely diagnosis at this time would be

(A) transposition of the great vessels
(B) ventricular septal defect
(C) tetralogy of Fallot
(D) endocardial fibroelastosis

69. Arterial blood gases in 60% oxygen reveal pH 7.15, PCO_2 32, HCO_3^- 14 mEq/L, PO_2 20 mm Hg. The most likely cause of the acidosis is

(A) hypoxemia
(B) an inborn metabolic error
(C) prerenal azotemia
(D) intrauterine asphyxia
(E) sepsis

70. The child appears worse, and cyanosis is severe even in 100% oxygen. The appropriate next step would be to administer intravenously

(A) bicarbonate
(B) bicarbonate and furosemide
(C) bicarbonate and PGE_1
(D) ampicillin and gentamicin

71. Echocardiogram reveals transposition of the great arteries. Cardiac catheterization

(A) is unnecessary
(B) should be performed as an emergency
(C) should be deferred until the operating room is prepared and the open heart team is scrubbed and ready
(D) should be deferred for 24 to 48 hours while the child is stabilized
(E) should be deferred for 3 to 7 days

72. At cardiac catheterization one should

(A) insert an umbrella device to close the ductus
(B) insert an umbrella device to close the foramen ovale
(C) ablate the AV node
(D) perform a balloon atrial septostomy
(E) perform a balloon dilation of the pulmonary artery

Questions 73 through 75

Remember to answer all the questions in this group before looking at any of the answers.

A 3-year-old girl is brought to the hospital because of "black and blue marks." The child had been well until 2 days prior to admission, when the mother noted several black and blue marks on the child's legs. On the day of admission, similar marks appeared on her trunk and arms. Physical examination revealed a well-nourished child in no distress and not appearing ill. There are fresh ecchymoses on the legs and trunk and petechiae on the face, trunk, and extremities. There is no fever, pallor, hepatosplenomegaly, or lymphadenopathy. Blood count reveals Hb 13 g/dL, WBC 8,200/mm³, 55% lymphocytes, and 45% polymorphonuclear cells. The platelet count is 20,000/mm³. Prothrombin time and partial thromboplastin time are normal.

73. The most likely diagnosis is

(A) acute leukemia
(B) idiopathic thrombocytopenia
(C) hypersplenism
(D) subacute bacterial endocarditis
(E) aspirin poisoning

74. Bone marrow examination reveals an increased number of megakaryocytes, many of which are immature. Of the following, which would be most appropriate for this child?

(A) A single transfusion of platelets
(B) Daily transfusion of platelets
(C) Daily transfusion of fresh frozen plasma
(D) Administration of corticosteroids
(E) Administration of epsilon-aminocaproic acid (EACA)

75. An indication for splenectomy in this patient would be

(A) platelet count below 10,000/mm³
(B) severe mucous membrane bleeding
(C) persistence of thrombocytopenia for more than 30 days
(D) persistence of thrombocytopenia for more than 1 or 2 years
(E) anemia

Questions 76 through 80

Remember to answer all the questions in this group before looking at any of the answers.

A 9-year-old girl is seen for an annual examination. She has no complaints and is very active in sports. Physical examination reveals a grade 3/6 systolic ejection murmur, loudest at the upper left sternal border. The second heart sound is widely split and does not vary with respiration. The remainder of the examination is within normal limits.

76. The child most likely has

(A) acute rheumatic fever
(B) an innocent heart murmur
(C) cardiomyopathy
(D) congenital heart disease
(E) rheumatic heart disease

77. To ascertain if the murmur is innocent or organic in this child, it would be most useful to auscultate the murmur

(A) after exercise
(B) during the Valsalva maneuver
(C) with the patient squatting
(D) with the patient supine and 15° head down

78. Chest roentgenogram reveals a slightly enlarged heart and increased pulmonary vasculature. The electrocardiogram reveals incomplete right bundle branch block and right ventricular hypertrophy. The most likely diagnosis is

(A) atrial septal defect
(B) obstructive cardiomyopathy
(C) patent ductus arteriosus
(D) pulmonic stenosis
(E) ventricular septal defect

79. While awaiting echocardiographic studies and possible cardiac catheterization, the wisest course of action would be to

(A) restrict the child to bed rest
(B) restrict the child to home activity
(C) permit the child to attend school but restrict physical activity
(D) permit full activity
(E) permit full activity but start monthly bicillin prophylaxis

80. Repair or correction of this child's defect

(A) is not indicated
(B) should be done as soon as possible
(C) should be done within the next 1 to 2 years
(D) should be done only if signs of heart failure appear
(E) should be done soon after puberty

Questions 81 through 86

Remember to answer all the questions in this group before looking at any of the answers.

A white male infant was born after the uneventful 40 week pregnancy of a 20-year-old primigravida. Birth weight was 3,210 g. The infant was well, but jaundice was noted on the third day of life. Physical examination was otherwise entirely normal. The infant was acting normally and feeding well on a standard commercial formula. The mother is blood type A, Rh positive. The infant is found to be type O, Rh negative.

81. The available laboratory data

(A) suggest an ABO incompatibility as the cause of the jaundice
(B) suggest an Rh incompatibility as the cause of the jaundice
(C) suggest a minor blood group incompatibility as the cause of the jaundice

(D) rule out a major blood group incompatibility as the cause of the jaundice
(E) rule out any blood group incompatibility as the cause of the jaundice

82. The serum total bilirubin level is found to be 15 mg/dL. At this point, the physician should

(A) obtain further diagnostic studies
(B) wait and repeat the bilirubin level in 6 hours
(C) institute phototherapy
(D) perform an exchange transfusion
(E) start antibiotics

83. The serum bilirubin is repeated in 12 hours and found to be 17 mg/dL. Phototherapy is begun. Over the ensuing 3 days, with continuous phototherapy, the total serum bilirubin remains in the range of 15 to 17 mg/dL. At this time, the most important consideration would be to

(A) obtain further diagnostic studies
(B) continue the phototherapy
(C) decrease the phototherapy to 12 hours out of 24 hours
(D) perform an exchange transfusion
(E) discontinue the phototherapy

84. On the fourth day of phototherapy, a bronze discoloration to the skin is noticed, and it also is noted that the urine is brown. These findings are related to

(A) dehydration
(B) hemolysis
(C) meconium aspiration
(D) phototherapy
(E) sepsis

85. The major error in the management of this case was the

(A) delay of 12 hours in instituting phototherapy
(B) use of continuous rather than intermittent phototherapy
(C) use of phototherapy without adequate prior diagnostic investigation
(D) use of phototherapy rather than exchange transfusion
(E) failure to administer antibiotics

86. The bronze discoloration probably will

(A) be permanent
(B) resolve eventually but cause permanent neurologic damage
(C) resolve eventually but cause permanent renal damage
(D) resolve eventually but cause permanent hepatic damage
(E) resolve eventually without permanent sequelae

Questions 87 through 89

Remember to answer all the questions in this group before looking at any of the answers.

A 12-year-old boy has been complaining of pain in the left hip for 4 days. He recalls falling from his bike 2 days prior to the onset of the pain. Past history has been unremarkable. Physical examination reveals an obese child in no distress. He walks with a limp. There is pain with motion of the left hip and limitation of flexion. There is no swelling, local heat, or tenderness. The temperature is 98.6°F, and the remainder of the examination is within normal limits. CBC and ESR are normal.

87. Which of the following is the most likely cause of the pain and limp?

(A) Acute rheumatic fever
(B) Juvenile rheumatoid arthritis
(C) Legg-Calvé-Perthes disease
(D) Pyogenic arthritis
(E) Slipped capital femoral epiphysis

88. Results of x-ray examination are compatible with the expected diagnosis. Appropriate management would be

(A) massive doses of vitamin D
(B) surgical intervention
(C) prolonged bed rest
(D) corticosteroids
(E) antibiotics

89. The chance of the right hip being afflicted by a similar process is

(A) almost zero
(B) about 5%
(C) between 10% and 30%
(D) between 50% and 80%
(E) almost 100%

Questions 90 through 93

Remember to answer all the questions in this group before looking at any of the answers.

A 10-month-old child is admitted because of fever and tachypnea. Although weight gain has been slow, the parents had considered the child to have been well until 2 months prior to admission, when he developed intermittent, low-grade fever. Physical examination at that time was unrevealing except for a greasy, maculopapular rash on the trunk, face, and scalp. One month prior to admission he developed a dry cough. On the day of admission, he was seen in clinic and noted to be pale and tachypneic, with hepatosplenomegaly and generalized lymphadenopathy. The rash was still present.

90. Which of the following is LEAST likely to be helpful in the workup of this child?

(A) Bone marrow aspiration
(B) Renal ultrasound
(C) Skin biopsy
(D) Complete blood count
(E) Chest roentgenogram

91. Diagnoses to be considered in this child include all of the following EXCEPT

(A) Langerhans cell histiocytosis (Letterer-Siwe syndrome)
(B) Farquhar's syndrome (familial hemophagocytic reticulocytosis)
(C) disseminated neuroblastoma
(D) leukemia
(E) acquired immunodeficiency syndrome (HIV infection)

92. Chest roentgenogram reveals bilateral, numerous small nodules and diffuse honeycombing. The most likely diagnosis is

(A) Langerhans cell histiocytosis (Letterer-Siwe syndrome)
(B) Farquhar's syndrome (familial hemophagocytic reticulocytosis)
(C) disseminated neuroblastoma
(D) leukemia
(E) acquired immunodeficiency syndrome (HIV infection)

93. If he remains untreated, you expect this patient to

(A) die in a few weeks
(B) die in a few months
(C) die in a few years
(D) survive with chronic disease
(E) eventually recover completely

Questions 94 through 96

Remember to answer all the questions in this group before looking at any of the answers.

An 8-year-old child recently immigrated from Asia is seen because of swelling of the side of the face. The day prior he noted fever and pain on opening his mouth. Today he noted a painful and tender swelling on the right, at about the angle of the jaw. Examination confirms a mass anterior to the ear and pushing the ear upward and outward. The remainder of the examination is unremarkable except for a temperature of 38.5°C.

94. The most likely diagnosis is

(A) onchocerciasis
(B) bacterial adenitis
(C) a dental abscess
(D) mumps
(E) mycobacterial adenitis

95. Appropriate management would include

(A) a chest roentgenogram and a tuberculin test
(B) excisional biopsy
(C) dental x-rays
(D) oral antibiotics
(E) fluids and acetaminophen

96. The child is treated appropriately. He returns the following day with headache and vomiting. Temperature is now 40.1°C. He is alert, oriented, and cooperative. There is marked nuchal rigidity. The mass is unchanged, but a similar swelling has appeared on the left side of the face. The most useful test at this time would be

(A) a lumbar puncture
(B) serum amylase
(C) dental x-rays
(D) cervical spine roentgenograms
(E) a blood count

Questions 97 through 100

Remember to answer all the questions in this group before looking at any of the answers.

A 6-month-old child was seen for a well-baby examination. History was unremarkable, and physical examination entirely normal. The child was given his third DPT immunization, 0.5 mL intramuscularly, and his second trivalent polio vaccine orally. That night, about 8 hours after the immunizations, the child developed a high fever followed shortly by a brief, generalized convulsion. Examination in the emergency room reveals an irritable and lethargic child with a temperature of 40°C. The remainder of the examination is within normal limits.

97. The most likely explanation for the fever is that the child

(A) is teething
(B) had a reaction to the DPT
(C) had a reaction to the oral polio vaccine
(D) has an infection unrelated to the office visit or the immunization
(E) contracted an infection while in the doctor's waiting room that afternoon

98. The physician should

(A) not have administered the DPT and polio vaccines simultaneously
(B) have given the DPT subcutaneously rather than intramuscularly
(C) have prescribed acetaminophen and phenobarbital prophylactically for 24 to 48 hours following the immunization
(D) have administered intramuscular phenobarbital at the same time as the DPT
(E) have administered the DPT and TOP as was done

99. Lumbar puncture reveals clear spinal fluid with 4 mononuclear cells per cubic millimeter. The protein content is 26 mg/dL, and glucose 82 mg/dL. The most likely diagnosis is

(A) bacterial meningitis
(B) viral meningitis
(C) febrile reaction to the immunization and a febrile seizure
(D) postimmunization encephalitis
(E) viral encephalitis

100. When the child is due for his booster immunization at 18 months, he should be given

(A) DPT and oral polio
(B) DT and oral polio
(C) DPT alone
(D) oral polio alone
(E) DT alone

Questions 101 through 106

Remember to answer all the questions in this group before looking at any of the answers.

A 6-year-old black child had been well until 5 days prior to admission, when his mother noted signs of an upper respiratory infection and a cough. On the day of admission he developed jaundice and pallor. Past medical history was unremarkable. A sickle cell test at 3 years of age was said to have been negative. Physical examination reveals pallor and scleral icterus. T 38°C, HR 138, RR 18, BP 105/70. The remainder of the examination is within normal limits. Laboratory data reveal Hb 7.0 g/dL, WBC 8,000/mm^3, bilirubin 4.0 mg/dL.

101. Which of the following is NOT indicated initially?

(A) Bone marrow examination
(B) Examination of a peripheral blood smear for RBC morphology
(C) Careful history of all medicines taken for the URI
(D) Fractionation of the serum bilirubin into conjugated and unconjugated components
(E) Reticulocyte count

102. Bone marrow aspiration is performed and reveals erythroid hyperplasia but is otherwise normal. Red cell morphology on smear is normal. Further questioning reveals that the child had been given several unidentified cold remedies by a grandparent. Bilirubin fractionation reveals conjugated 0.4 mg/dL, unconjugated 3.2 mg/dL. Reticulocyte count is 12%. Which of the following diagnoses is most likely?

(A) Sickle cell anemia
(B) Hereditary spherocytic hemolytic anemia
(C) Infectious hepatitis
(D) G6PD deficiency
(E) Preleukemia

103. The erythrocyte content of G6PD is found to be nearly normal. This

(A) is a common finding in acute hemolysis regardless of cause
(B) rules out acute hemolysis regardless of cause
(C) rules out G6PD deficiency
(D) is compatible with a diagnosis of G6PD deficiency
(E) indicates that the hemolysis has been chronic

104. Of the following additional tests, which would be most important at this time?

(A) Erythrocyte sedimentation rate
(B) Coombs's test
(C) AST, ALT levels
(D) Serum haptoglobin level
(E) Abdominal ultrasound

105. The most appropriate management at this time would be

(A) immediate transfusion to raise the patient's hemoglobin concentration to 14 g/dL
(B) immediate transfusion to raise the patient's hemoglobin concentration to 10 g/dL
(C) withhold transfusion and follow vital signs and hemoglobin concentration
(D) withhold transfusion and begin therapy with 2 mg/kg of prednisone per day
(E) immediate transfusion of 10 cc/kg of packed red blood cells and initiation of 2 mg/kg of prednisone per day

106. If the child responds to therapy (or improves without therapy), appropriate follow-up should include

(A) repeat bone marrow examination
(B) repeat measurement of G6PD levels
(C) a spleen scan
(D) a challenging dose of aspirin
(E) a serologic test for HIV

Questions 107 through 110

Remember to answer all the questions in this group before looking at any of the answers.

A 2-week-old female infant was admitted because of vomiting and failure to thrive. The infant weighed 2.8 kg at birth. Vomiting and poor feeding were noted at 6 days of age, and loose stools at 9 days. The infant had been fed only a standard prepared cow milk formula. On examination, the child is found to be poorly nourished and mildly dehydrated. Weight is 2.5 kg. The clitoris is large, and the posterior aspects of the labia are fused. The remainder of the physical examination is normal. Serum electrolytes reveal Na 110 mEq/L; Cl 82 mEq/L; K 7.2 mEq/L; BUN 32 mg/dL.

107. The most likely cause of the hyponatremia and hyperkalemia is

(A) prerenal azotemia
(B) obstructive uropathy

(C) adrenal insufficiency
(D) inappropriate secretion of ADH
(E) inappropriate feeding

108. Chromosomal analysis of this patient probably would reveal

(A) XX
(B) XY
(C) XXY
(D) XO
(E) XYY

109. Therapy for this child will include

(A) peritoneal or hemodialysis
(B) low protein diet
(C) daily intranasal DDAVP
(D) glucocorticoid and mineralocorticoid replacement
(E) low salt diet

110. Therapy probably will need to be maintained

(A) until the patient is stable
(B) until the electrolytes are normal
(C) until the patient is stable and the electrolytes are normal
(D) for 10 days
(E) for life

Questions 111 through 116

Remember to answer all the questions in this group before looking at any of the answers.

A 12-year-old girl is brought to the clinic because of changing behavior and difficulty controlling her body movements. The problem began gradually about 4 weeks ago and has been getting more severe in all respects. The child has become clumsy and has difficulty with writing and holding objects. She stumbles frequently. She appears nervous, fidgety, irritable, and emotionally labile. The parents have noted irregular, coarse, spasmodic movements of the extremities and peculiar grimacing, all of which disappear when the child is asleep. Physical examination is entirely within normal limits except for coarse, spasmodic, and writhing movements, which get worse when the child is agitated or upset. Her palmar grasp seems to reflect the same changes, with intermittent spasm and weakness.

111. The most probable diagnosis is

(A) cerebellar tumor
(B) hysteria
(C) lead poisoning
(D) LSD ingestion
(E) rheumatic chorea

112. Which of the following would be especially relevant in this case?

(A) Audiometric examination
(B) Dental examination
(C) Ophthalmologic examination
(D) Pelvic examination
(E) Psychometric testing

113. The following laboratory data all are reported as negative or within normal limits: throat culture, CBC, ESR, ASO titer, urinalysis, rheumatoid factor, ANA, chest roentgenogram, ECG, VDRL, AST, and ALT. The most likely diagnosis now is

(A) cerebellar tumor
(B) hysteria
(C) lead poisoning
(D) LSD ingestion
(E) rheumatic chorea

114. Abnormal movements such as these also have been observed in children with

(A) polymyositis
(B) lupus erythematosus
(C) hepatic failure
(D) endocardial fibroelastosis
(E) subdural effusions

115. Long-term management ought to include

(A) zinc
(B) pencillinamine
(C) formal psychotherapy
(D) continuous penicillin prophylaxis
(E) continuous phenobarbital administration

116. Most likely the abnormal movements will

(A) clear completely within a few days
(B) clear completely within 2 to 12 months
(C) improve but never clear completely
(D) remain the same or become progressively worse
(E) remit and recur over the next 5 to 25 years

Questions 117 through 119

Remember to answer all the questions in this group before looking at any of the answers.

An 18-month-old child is admitted for evaluation of persistent diarrhea and weight loss of several months' duration. According to the mother, the child has always had frequent colds and a poor appetite. The child has been kept on a diet of table foods and regular cow milk. Physical examination reveals only a lack of subcutaneous fat. Length is at the 25th percentile for age, weight below the 5th percentile, and head circumference between the 50th and 25th percentiles.

117. In obtaining a history, which of the following would be LEAST relevant to this child?

(A) Family history of diabetes
(B) History of HIV risk factors in both parents
(C) Family history of cystic fibrosis
(D) Family history of celiac disease
(E) History of travel, pets, and other animal exposures in patient

118. Which of the following laboratory tests would be LEAST useful in determining the cause of this infant's problem?

(A) Sweat test
(B) Stool examination for ova and parasites
(C) Blood glucose
(D) Screening test for HIV
(E) CBC

119. On admission you should order

(A) a regular diet for age
(B) a low-fat diet
(C) an elemental formula such as pregestimil
(D) a carbohydrate-free formula
(E) the child NPO and begin parenteral nutrition

Answers and Explanations

1. (E) The most likely cause of this patient's clinical symptoms is hypertensive encephalopathy. The markedly elevated blood pressure and the seizure are compatible with this diagnosis. Although the hypertension could be secondary to increased intracranial pressure, such hypertension rarely is of this severity, and one would have expected other signs of increased intracranial pressure such as papilledema or bradycardia. Although blood pressure can be elevated during a seizure, it is usually not as high as in this patient, and epilepsy would not explain the peripheral edema. [*Reminder:* You should be trying to answer all questions in the series *before* looking at any of the answers!] *(Rudolph:1439–1443;* Pediatr Clin North Am *23:751–758,1976)*

2. (D) Essential hypertension would be exceedingly rare in an 8-year-old child, as would be a pheochromocytoma. Ventricular septal defects are not associated with hypertension. Renal disease is the most common cause of hypertension in this age group and is the most likely diagnosis in this child. Although ingestion of drugs such as amphetamines or phenylpropanolamine can cause hypertension, this is seen most frequently in the adolescent age group. Accidental ingestion might have occurred, but this most often is in the toddler or preschooler. At any rate, drug ingestion is *less likely* than renal disease. The presence of generalized pitting edema also is suggestive of renal disease. *(Pediatr Clin North Am 23:751–758,1976)*

3. (E) Determining serum electrolytes, creatinine, and BUN is the first diagnostic priority in this youngster with hypertension and edema. The lack of preceding neurologic symptoms and the absence of papilledema and of focal neurologic signs make an intracranial cause of the hypertension unlikely. There is no urgent need for a head CT. *(Rudolph:1439–1443;* Pediatr Clin North Am *23:751–758,1976)*

4. (B) The most important aspect of management at this point is to reduce the blood pressure by the administration of a rapidly acting antihypertensive drug such as diazoxide. In view of the child's age and the fact that it is unlikely he has been chronically hypertensive, there is essentially no risk associated with rapid reduction of blood pressure. *(Rudolph: 1442–1443,1261)*

5. (C) The history of a sore throat about 10 days prior to the onset of the seizure suggests acute poststreptococcal glomerulonephritis as the cause for the child's edema and hypertension. He may be in acute renal failure, and it would be prudent to anticipate the need for either peritoneal or hemodialysis. *(Rudolph:1439–1443;* Pediatr Clin North Am *23:751–758,1976)*

6. (C) The child is cyanotic and in respiratory distress. Cyanosis indicates *significant hypoxemia,* and oxygen should be administered promptly. It is unnecessary to determine the blood oxygen content *before* administering oxygen to this patient. A transcutaneous measurement of arterial oxygen saturation (pulse oximetry), which gives no information about arterial PCO_2, usually can be obtained more rapidly than an arterial blood gas, but it is not necessary to wait for any confirmatory measure of the patient's oxygen status before administering oxygen. *(Rudolph:508–510;* J Pediatr *96:1–12,1980)*

7. (C) The serum bicarbonate is somewhat low (normal is 22 to 24 mEq/L); therefore, the patient has a moderate metabolic acidosis. The arterial PCO_2 of 39 is within normal limits; therefore, the patient has neither a respiratory acidosis nor a compensating respiratory alkalosis. However, the absence of a respiratory alkalosis is worrisome. Early in an attack of asthma, hyperventilation in response to hypoxia leads to a fall in arterial PCO_2. The "normal" PCO_2 suggests that this patient is no longer able to hyperventilate effectively and compensate for the abnormalities of ventilation-perfusion ratios in his lungs. Metabolic acidosis is common in patients with status asthmaticus and probably reflects tissue hypoxia. *(Rudolph:508–510;* J Pediatr *96:1–12,1980)*

8. (A) Therapy with corticosteroids is indicated for the treatment of status asthmaticus, especially those cases that fail to respond to appropriate doses of bronchodilators. The continued wheezing and increasing respiratory distress in this patient demand prompt intervention, and one should not await an arbitrary rise in the arterial PCO_2 or a fall in the PO_2. Even if the roentgenogram were to reveal an infiltrate (which would be unlikely in this afebrile child), corticosteroids still would be indicated for treatment of the status asthmaticus. *(Rudolph:508–510; J Pediatr 96:1–12,1980)*

9. **(C)** The patient is in ventilatory failure (PCO_2 75 mm Hg) with respiratory acidosis (pH 7.25). Effective alveolar ventilation needs to be increased by increasing minute ventilation so as to lower arterial PCO_2. This is best accomplished by continuing measures to reduce airway resistance and by optimizing ventilator settings. Sometimes a faster inspiratory flow rate coupled with an increase in the expiratory/inspiratory time ratio is helpful. Also, it is important to check for leaks or obstructions in the mechanical system of the ventilator and tubes. Serum bicarbonate already is elevated (32 mEq/L) and oxygenation is adequate (PO_2 95). *(Rudolph:508–510; J Pediatr 96:1–12,1980)*

10. **(B)** The findings described suggest a left tension pneumothorax. Pneumothorax is a relatively common complication in asthmatic patients on assisted ventilation. If the endotracheal tube had slipped into the right mainstem bronchus, one would expect collapse of the *left* lung and a shift of the mediastinum and cardiac impulse to the *left*. *(Rudolph:508–510; J Pediatr 96:1–12,1980)*

11. **(B)** Appropriate management of pharyngitis or tonsillitis in a child should include a throat culture to look for group A beta-hemolytic streptococci. Equally acceptable is the use of one of the rapid throat swab tests for streptococcal antigen. If the rapid strep test is negative and suspicion of streptococcal pharyngitis is high, a throat culture should be done. If the rapid strep test is positive, culture need not be performed. [*Note:* It would not have been inappropriate *also* to have obtained a blood count at the initial visit. However, the *most* helpful and *most* appropriate test would be a specific test for streptococcal infection. Therefore, **(B)** is the *best* answer.] *(Rudolph:1569–1574)*

12. **(D)** Most cases of bacterial tonsillitis, excluding diphtheria, are caused by group A beta-hemolytic streptococci and therefore are quite susceptible to penicillin. The lack of response to adequate penicillin therapy should have suggested a nonbacterial etiology. The fact that penicillin was administered parenterally as well as orally makes it unlikely that the problem is one of compliance. It would have been better to obtain a CBC and a monospot test. Blood culture is unlikely to have been positive in this child. *(Rudolph:1569–1574)*

13. **(C)** The illness clearly is not measles. There is no mention of cough, rhinorrhea, conjunctivitis, or Koplik's spots, and exudative tonsillitis and cervical adenitis are not features of measles. There is nothing to indicate that this patient has peritonsillitis or a peritonsillar abscess: there is no mention of trismus, drooling, or fullness or bulging in the peritonsillar area. Of the remaining choices, infectious mononucleosis is the most common and the most likely. The clinical picture is entirely compatible with infectious mononucleosis. *(Rudolph:1569–1574)*

14. **(D)** Although it is true that the monospot test may remain positive for several months following EBV infectious mononucleosis, it would be most reasonable in the presence of a clinical picture so highly suggestive of infectious mononucleosis to assume that the positive test does represent current infection. It is not necessary in *routine* cases to verify a positive monotest with specific EBV antibodies. *(Rudolph:1569–1574)*

15. **(E)** Rash occurs in 10 to 15% of all cases of infectious mononucleosis, usually appearing within the first week. Nonurticarial rashes also are common in patients receiving ampicillin and frequently do not represent drug allergy in the usual sense, the rash often clearing despite continuance of the drug. Such nonallergic rashes are especially common in patients with EBV infectious mononucleosis who are treated with ampicillin. *(Rudolph:1569–1574)*

16. **(C)** It has been shown that steroids do hasten resolution of fever, pharyngitis, and other symptoms in patients with mononucleosis. These drugs probably are prescribed more frequently in adolescents and adults than in children. The fact that steroids offer effective symptomatic relief does not necessarily imply that they should be prescribed in the routine situation. Recognition of chronic EBV infection and the association of EBV with Burkitt's lymphoma and with a severe and fatal lymphoproliferative illness in some patients with a specific X-linked immunologic deficit raises *theoretical* concern about the use of an immunosuppressant agent during EBV infection. [*Note:* The question did not ask whether corticosteroids were indicated. The question only addressed the anticipated effect of these agents.] *(Rudolph:1569–1574)*

17. **(D)** Moderate dehydration of a young infant generally means a loss of about 10% of body weight as water. For an older child or adult, moderate dehydration corresponds to a loss of only 8% of body weight. For this child a *rough estimate* of deficit would be 0.10 times 6.3 kg, which equals 630 mL. However, to be more precise, the deficit should be calculated not on the basis of the current weight but rather on the basis of the premorbid or "true" weight. Since the child has lost 10% of his normal weight,

current weight equals premorbid weight times 0.90. Solving for premorbid weight (6.3/0.9), one gets 7 kg. The deficit then is calculated as 7 kg times 0.10 = 700 mL. Also; 7.0 minus 6.3 = 700 mL. [Note: The question asked for the fluid *deficit,* not for the fluid *requirement,* which would be deficit *plus* maintenance *plus* ongoing abnormal losses, if any.] *(Hathaway:1069–1070)*

18. **(C)** The child should be given a rapid intravenous push (bolus) of 10 to 20 mL/kg to restore intravascular volume and protect perfusion. This volume is administered as rapidly as the vein and infusion apparatus will permit, usually over a 5- or 10-minute period. If the patient's clinical status does not improve, a second or third bolus may be required. *(Hathaway:1069–1070)*

19. **(A)** The initial hydrating solution should contain 135 to 150 mEq/L of sodium for two reasons. First, since sodium does not enter the intracellular space readily, saline will expand the intravascular volume more efficiently and more rapidly than an equal osmolar load of glucose. Second, it is safer than a lower-sodium-content solution in the event the patient turns out to be hypernatremic, in which case a rapid decrease in serum sodium might result in convulsions or intracranial hemorrhage. Saline also would be most appropriate should the patient be hyponatremic. *(Hathaway:1069–1070)*

20. **(E)** Concern about renal impairment or actual renal damage secondary to dehydration and hypoperfusion dictates that potassium should not be administered until it is known that renal function is adequate and that the serum potassium concentration is not elevated. The former is documented either by a normal BUN or by the patient voiding. The latter is documented by direct laboratory measurement. *(Hathaway:1069–1070)*

21. **(E)** Assuming that the diarrhea stops when the child is not fed, total fluid requirement would be equal to maintenance plus deficit. If the diarrhea were to persist, then the abnormal stool losses would need to be measured or estimated and calculated in the replacement figures. Deficit is estimated at 700 mL. Maintenance for a child weighing less than 10 kg is 100 mL/kg, which in this case would equal 700 mL. Maintenance plus deficit then is estimated as 700 mL plus 700 mL, or a total of 1,400 mL. *(Hathaway: 1069–1070)*

22. **(B)** Viral hepatitis is certainly the most likely diagnosis in the child described. Sickle cell anemia probably would have presented earlier and is unlikely (not impossible) to have gone undiagnosed to this age. Acute hemolysis secondary to G6PD deficiency is a possibility but would not explain the tender hepatomegaly. Cholecystitis does occur in children but is rather uncommon, and one would expect right upper quadrant pain rather than abdominal cramps. Choledochal cysts usually present in infancy. [Note: The examinee should not be misled into assuming that the fact that this child is black is relevant. It certainly should not lead to a premature diagnosis of sickle cell disease.] *(Feigin:678–688)*

23. **(E)** If the child were anemic, determination of serum haptoglobin might point to a hemolytic etiology for the anemia. However, in the absence of anemia, the serum haptoglobin determination would be of little value. Although serum haptoglobin concentration can be decreased as a nonspecific reflection of hepatic damage, it is not very useful in this regard. Determination of AST and ALT levels can help confirm and quantitate hepatocellular injury. Epstein-Barr virus infectious mononucleosis can be associated with hepatitis, but jaundice is uncommon. A monospot test might be useful in the workup of this child, but at this time it is much more important to first document hepatocellular injury. *(Feigin:678–688)*

24. **(A)** The finding of hepatitis B surface antigen (HBsAg) in the blood indicates that the child has type B hepatitis but does not indicate chronic disease. It also does not mean a poor prognosis. Although hepatitis B infection is more serious than hepatitis A, most children recover fully. *(Feigin:680–683)*

25. **(D)** A very small percentage of children with hepatitis B virus infection develop fulminant hepatitis and hepatic failure. Encephalopathy and coma are the most characteristic features of this disturbance. The central nervous system dysfunction is caused by a variety of metabolic products (such as ammonia) that usually are detoxified by the liver. Bilirubin encephalopathy occurs when unconjugated bilirubin exceeds the binding capacity of albumin and enters the brain. This occurs at a serum concentration of about 20 mg/dL of unconjugated bilirubin, a condition rarely seen beyond the newborn period. *(Feigin:682–683,668)*

26. **(B)** The first priority in this child, *who is described as moderately dehydrated,* is to start an intravenous infusion to restore intravascular volume. Appropriate diagnostic workup can then be undertaken while the child is being rehydrated. *(Rudolph:1034)*

27. **(D)** Serum electrolytes and BUN should be measured to assess the results of the vomiting and dehydration. A blood count is indicated to check the white cell count in regard to possible infection. The clinical picture described is classic for intussusception: a child in the second half of the first year of life with vomiting and abdominal colic, the passage of a single stool followed by no further stools, listlessness, and a sausage-shaped abdominal mass. Although a flat

and upright film of the abdomen usually will neither confirm nor rule out intussusception, it can suggest that diagnosis. More important, the abdominal film might show free air or signs of severe intestinal obstruction, both of which might lead to immediate surgical intervention. A liver-spleen scan is not indicated. *(Rudolph:1034)*

28. **(B)** Hydrostatic reduction of the intussusception by barium enema is the treatment of choice. This is successful in the majority of cases and obviates the need for surgery. It is important to limit the hydrostatic pressure used in the enema to avoid perforation or reduction of gangrenous bowel. *(Rudolph:1034)*

29. **(B)** The rate of recurrence after hydrostatic reduction is between 2% and 6%. In some series this is about the same as that after operative reduction; in other series it is somewhat higher. A few children have repeated bouts of intussusception. *(Rudolph:1034)*

30. **(B)** Craniopharyngioma is not a tumor of infancy. Even when the tumor does occur in older children, initial manifestations do not include hemiparesis. Congenital hemiparesis, as a form of cerebral palsy, may be noted at birth or weeks to months later. Both congenital syphilis and the battered child syndrome may present with pseudoparesis secondary to pain in the involved bone. Osteomyelitis can present in a similar fashion. Young infants with osteomyelitis may be afebrile. [*Note:* The student cannot assume a priori that the history regarding the parents being illegal aliens and the child being born at home is necessarily a valid clue. However, it clearly makes untreated congenital syphilis a more plausible diagnosis.] (Pediatr Clin North Am *26:377–386,1979; Rudolph: 619)*

31. **(D)** The changes described on the roentgenograph (osteochondritis and periosteal reaction) are most suggestive of congenital syphilis. The radiographic appearance of neuroblastoma metastases to bone would be localized, lytic lesions. Therefore, an abdominal ultrasound examination is not indicated. The radiographic appearance of child abuse would be a fracture. Therefore, there is no indication for psychosocial evaluation of the parents. Erythrocyte sedimentation rate and serum calcium and phosphorus levels would be of little diagnostic help. (Pediatr Clin North Am *26:377–386,1979; Rudolph:619)*

32. **(C)** A lumbar puncture is an important part of the diagnostic evaluation of infants suspected of having congenital syphilis. Although initial treatment of infants with CSF pleocytosis is not different from that for those without pleocytosis, the follow-up is. Infants with CSF pleocytosis should be followed until the CSF is normal, and retreatment may be necessary. (Pediatr Clin North Am *26:377–386,1979; Rudolph: 622)*

33. **(B)** The history in this infant is most suggestive of pertussis, with progression from the catarrhal to the paroxysmal stage. In young infants with pertussis, the whoop often is absent despite severe and frequent paroxysms. Posttussive emesis is common. A normal physical examination between paroxysms of cough also is characteristic of pertussis. A history indicating whether or not the child had received any diphtheria-pertussis-tetanus immunizations would be helpful and important. [*Note:* All the items listed are valid and important. However, the history of immunizations would be most likely to be helpful and would be considered the *most* important item. Again, remember, the rules call for the one *best* answer and do not imply that all other choices are totally incorrect.] *(Feigin:1208–1213)*

34. **(B)** *Bordetella pertussis* most often is recovered from the nasopharynx. Cultures are more likely to be positive early in the course of infection. The organism is difficult to grow on ordinary media, and special medium is required. *(Feigin:1212)*

35. **(B)** A very high total white blood cell count with a marked lymphocytosis is characteristic of pertussis. It would be reasonable, at this time, to begin therapy with erythromycin while awaiting the results of culture or fluorescent antibody staining of pharyngeal secretions. Treatment with antibiotics will not affect the clinical course of the disease unless given prior to the onset of the paroxysmal stage. Such treatment, however, will hasten eradication of the organism and decrease spread of the infection both in the hospital and, after discharge, at home. [*Note:* Although such treatment is not mandatory, it would be "appropriate" and preferable to any of the other choices, all of which would be inappropriate.] *(Feigin:1212)*

36. **(C)** The highest priority in this patient is the need to diagnose or rule out bacterial meningitis. The high fever, toxic appearance, convulsion, and semicomatose state all are compatible with bacterial meningitis. Although a maculopapular rash is not characteristic of bacterial infection, the rash has become purpuric and could represent disseminated intravascular coagulation. There are no signs of increased intracranial pressure, and the rash suggests a systemic illness rather than a brain abscess or other intracranial mass. Therefore, there is no indication for a head CT scan prior to the lumbar puncture. Even though bacterial meningitis is not the most likely diagnosis, it is the most urgent to investigate and treat. *(Rudolph:1829–1830)*

37. **(B)** The history of a camping trip, the clinical picture, and especially the rash are most suggestive of Rocky Mountain spotted fever, which has been reported from at least 44 states. You therefore anticipate a history of the child having been bitten by a tick, although the tick bite can go unnoticed. *(Rudolph:696–697)*

38. (B) Although the finding of normal cerebrospinal fluid argues against meningitis, it does not rule out bacteremia or sepsis. The high fever, the toxicity, the convulsion, and the semicomatose state warrant presumptive therapy for the possibility of bacterial sepsis. In addition, the hemorrhagic rash raises the question of disseminated intravascular coagulation, which may be associated with bacterial sepsis or with Rocky Mountain spotted fever as well as a variety of other infections. Of course, Rocky Mountain spotted fever also is treated with antibiotics, and this is another reason why such therapy should be instituted promptly. Although there are a number of antibiotics or combinations of antibiotics that would be appropriate for this child, chloramphenicol alone would cover Rocky Mountain spotted fever as well as the usual causes of pyogenic meningitis. The role of corticosteroids both in treating septic shock and in treating Rocky Mountain spotted fever is controversial and uncertain at best. There is no clear indication for their use in this child, who is not in shock and in whom the diagnosis of Rocky Mountain spotted fever has not been confirmed. Incidentally, if the child were in shock, chloramphenicol would be contraindicated because of decreased hepatic clearance and possible myocardial toxicity. *(Feigin:1852; Rudolph:696–697,1841)*

39. (C) The loss of previously acquired developmental landmarks in an infant or young child strongly suggests degenerative brain disease. This term encompasses the progressive genetic metabolic diseases as well as a variety of progressive neurologic disorders of unknown etiology. Cerebral palsy is a static encephalopathy characterized by a failure of development rather than the loss of already acquired abilities. Neither anterior horn cell disease nor emotional deprivation would explain the apparent blindness or the jerking movements. Although physical abuse with traumatic brain injury could explain the findings, it is not one of the listed choices. A toxic encephalopathy such as lead poisoning is a possibility but is unlikely to start at 6 months of age. *(Rudolph: 1720–1723,1849–1877)*

40. (A) Fabry's disease is associated with minimal, if any, central nervous system manifestations. Neurologic manifestations in this disorder involve primarily the peripheral nervous system. Additionally, Fabry's disease is X-linked, and this patient is a girl. Niemann-Pick, Tay-Sachs, and infantile Gaucher's disease, as well as juvenile G_{M1} gangliosidosis, all are associated with significant central nervous system involvement and symptomatology. *(Rudolph: 1855–1857)*

41. (C) Of the diseases listed, only Niemann-Pick disease and Tay-Sachs disease are associated with a "cherry-red" spot in the macula. The former, however, is regularly associated with hepatosplenomegaly, which is not present in this patient. Therefore,

Tay-Sachs disease is the only diagnosis that fits. *(Rudolph:1855–1856)*

42. (A) Tay-Sachs disease is associated with decreased serum and tissue levels of hexosaminidase A. At this time, specific therapy of Tay-Sachs disease is not available. Genetic counseling can be offered regarding future pregnancies. Antenatal diagnosis by amniocentesis is available. *(Rudolph:1855–1856)*

43. (C) The most likely pathophysiologic process in this child with tingling of the hands and feet, diffuse weakness, and absent reflexes in both lower extremities is peripheral polyneuropathy. With an intracranial lesion, one might expect focal neurologic signs or signs of increased intracranial pressure. It is difficult to explain diffuse weakness and loss of reflexes in both lower extremities on the basis of a central process. With a spinal cord lesion, one would expect a motor or sensory level, which is not present in this patient. There is no evidence of either arthritis or myositis. *(Rudolph:1681–1685,1795–1798)*

44. (B) Although a complete and careful physical examination is always important, inspection of the scalp and other hairy areas would be especially important in this patient; the object of the search is a female tick, the bite of which can be associated with progressive ascending paralysis. The mechanism involves a neurotoxin elaborated by the tick. Improvement usually is evident within a few days of removal of the tick; hence, the obvious importance of making the correct diagnosis. *(Rudolph:1797)*

45. (D) Acute polyneuritis is still the most likely diagnosis. Although the cerebrospinal fluid findings are compatible with viral encephalitis, there are no clinical signs of encephalitis. Nor is there anything to suggest bacterial meningitis. As mentioned above (answer 43), with a spinal lesion one would expect to find a motor or sensory level. An elevated CSF protein with few mononuclear cells is a common finding in polyneuritis. The most common cause of polyneuritis in a child of this age with evidence of an ascending paralysis is infectious or postinfectious polyradiculopathy, the Guillain-Barré syndrome. *(Rudolph: 1796–1798)*

46. (A) Cranial nerve involvement is common in Guillain-Barré syndrome. Involvement of cranial nerves IX and X means impaired gag and swallow mechanisms and the danger of aspiration pneumonia. A vital capacity of 75% is quite adequate for ventilation and presents no *immediate* danger. The child is at no special risk of cardiovascular collapse, cardiac arrhythmia, or brain herniation. *(Rudolph:1796–1798)*

47. (B) It would be dangerous for the child to continue to take even liquids while the gag and swallow mechanisms were impaired. Neither a tracheostomy nor endotracheal intubation is indicated at this time, since there is no mention of the patient being unable to handle secretions, and the gag reflex is not totally absent. In view of the adequate vital capacity and normal blood gases, there is no need for ventilatory support at this time. However, progression of involvement of cranial nerves and/or the muscles of respiration might occur. The wisest course would be to discontinue all oral intake and transfer the patient to an intensive care unit or other appropriate setting for close monitoring of her airway and serial measurement of vital capacity or other measure of ventilatory ability. (Rudolph:1796–1798)

48. (B) In Guillain-Barré syndrome, weakness or paralysis generally reaches its peak by 7 to 15 days, and clinical improvement begins at about that time in most cases. This child has been symptomatic with weakness for 7 days, so one would expect that progression of weakness might continue for as much as another 5 to 7 days before improvement begins. (Rudolph:1796–1798)

49. (A) The patient described is best begun on a regular diet for age so that his eating habits and stool pattern can be observed before any special diet is initiated. Since there is no history of watery diarrhea, and since the patient does not appear dehydrated on physical examination, there is no immediate danger and no need to restrict his intake to clear fluids. (Rudolph:245–247; Hathaway:773–775)

50. (C) In the management of a patient with nonacute illnesses, the physician must strike a balance between the need to complete the diagnostic workup without undue delay or prolonged hospitalization and, on the other hand, the need to avoid unnecessary invasive, dangerous, or expensive tests. The barium enema involves discomfort, expense, and exposure to radiation. Also, in this patient it is not likely to be diagnostic. It ought to be deferred until less-invasive diagnostic maneuvers have proven negative. (Hathaway:773–775)

51. (C) A negative urine analysis does not rule out chronic urinary tract infection. A colony count of 25,000/mL collected by the bag method in an infant is inconclusive and might represent either infection or contamination. A repeat specimen obtained by suprapubic bladder aspiration or by catheterization will answer the question appropriately. Antimicrobial therapy and/or radiographic or ultrasound investigation of the urinary system at this time would be premature. (Rudolph:1288–1289)

52. (D) There is no indication in this patient for a lumbar puncture. A sweat test to rule out cystic fibrosis should be performed promptly. Although a beta-lipoproteinemia is a rare cause of steatorrhea, it is easily ruled in or out by examination of the periph-

eral blood smear for acanthocytes. Determination of stool pH may give a clue to the presence of a primary or secondary disaccharidase problem. Chest roentgenogram might reveal evidence of cystic fibrosis, immunodeficiency, or heart disease, all of which can cause failure to thrive. (Rudolph:245–247; Hathaway: 773–775)

53. (B) Although all the organisms listed can cause diarrhea, only *Giardia* clearly has been associated with *chronic* diarrhea or steatorrhea and with failure to thrive. Infection with this organism is quite common. (Rudolph:748–749)

54. (A) A normal child will excrete less than 10% of ingested fat. The lesions described on biopsy are characteristic of gluten-induced enteropathy. Some authors feel that these changes are specific for gluten enteropathy, but others point out their similarity to the changes resulting from a variety of noxious agents. Absolute proof would depend on demonstrating a return to a normal mucosa by repeat biopsy after a time on a gluten-free diet and then relapse clinically and histologically after reintroduction of wheat into the diet. Such vigorous criteria are not always pursued, and the rechallenge is often omitted or deferred. (Rudolph:1017)

55. (B) In this infant who is lethargic and jaundiced, it is very important to rule out serious bacterial infection, including meningitis. The CSF is normal except for the low glucose, which reflects the hypoglycemia. Primary renal glycosuria as an isolated renal defect is an extremely rare condition that usually is not associated with hypoglycemia, does not present in infancy, and would not explain the jaundice and hepatomegaly. Besides, the urinary sugar has not been identified as glucose. Diabetes is exceedingly rare in early infancy, and the infant is not hyperglycemic. The presence of only minimal acidosis and the absence of ketonuria rule out diabetic ketoacidosis and ketotic hypoglycemia. Glycogen storage disease is associated with hypoglycemia but not with glycosuria. Of the conditions listed, only galactosemia can explain vomiting from early infancy, hepatomegaly, jaundice, positive reducing substance in the urine (galactose), and hypoglycemia. (Rudolph:321–322,329, 1831)

56. (B) Cataracts are a common feature in patients with galactosemia. Although not present at birth, they may be noted in some patients as early as a few days of life. In other infants, they may take months to develop. (Rudolph:321)

57. (D) Galactosemia results from a deficiency of galactose-1-phosphate uridyl transferase, which catalyzes the conversion of galactose to glucose. Galactose is not an essential nutrient. This child should be treated with a galactose-free diet. Since galactose

derives only from lactose, a sugar found exclusively in mammalian milk, provision of a galactose-free diet is not difficult. Incidentally, children with galactosemia are at increased risk of overwhelming sepsis, so the diagnosis of galactosemia does not obviate the need to carefully and vigorously evaluate this child for serious infection. *(Rudolph:321–322)*

58. **(B)** The first priority in managing a convulsion is to ascertain that the airway is patent and the patient is ventilating adequately or else to secure the airway and establish effective ventilation. Be prepared to suction the airway if the patient should vomit. Treating the seizure itself is addressed after the A, B, C of life support: airway, breathing, circulation. *(Hathaway:673)*

59. **(C)** The clinical picture and laboratory findings are fully compatible with a febrile seizure, which is the most likely diagnosis in this patient. He is the right age (most febrile seizures occur between 6 months and 2 years of age) and has a high fever. The most pressing need in this child, however, is to rule out meningitis. In the absence of focal neurologic findings or evidence of increased intracranial pressure, there is no need to obtain a CT scan or any other diagnostic test prior to the lumbar puncture. The low yield on skull roentgenograms, urinalysis, and serum electrolytes (especially since hypoglycemia has already been excluded) in children with febrile seizures makes these tests not cost effective. Although it is not universally accepted that *all* children with an apparent febrile seizure must have a lumbar puncture to rule out meningitis, it is frequently recommended. Certainly, a lumbar puncture would be appropriate for this infant who is less than a year of age, has no obvious source for the fever, and who is now unresponsive (even though this is likely to turn out to be postictal depression). [*Note:* Even though a lumbar puncture is not unequivocally necessary, **(C)** is the *best* answer, as all other choices are incorrect.] *(Pediatr Emerg Care 2:191–196,1986;* Am J Dis Child *137:1153–1156,1983;* Am J Dis Child *135:431–433,1981)*

60. **(D)** Although *all* children with febrile seizures do not require long-term prophylaxis with phenobarbital, several factors indicate a high risk of recurrence and generally are accepted as relative indications for the administration of continuous, prophylactic phenobarbital for 1 to 2 years. These indications include age less than 12 months at the time of the first febrile seizure, an abnormal neurologic examination, a focal or prolonged seizure, and a family history of epilepsy. This child meets the first of these criteria. [*Note:* Again, although the use of prophylactic phenobarbital in this child would be considered optional rather than mandatory, **(D)** is the best answer, as all other listed choices are inappropriate.] *(Rudolph:*

1793; Pediatrics:*59:378–384,1977;* J Pediatr *94:177–184,1979)*

61. **(D)** In general, 10 to 12 mg/dL is accepted as the upper limit of physiologic hyperbilirubinemia for a term infant, and 15 mg/dL for a premature infant. Although many infants with values above these levels ultimately turn out to have no discernible disease, both diagnostic investigation and monitoring of the bilirubin level are indicated. Also, these maximum levels usually are reached on the fourth or fifth day rather than at 48 hours. *(Rudolph:1055; Schaffer:754–756)*

62. **(C)** Most of the common hemoglobinopathies, such as sickle cell disease or thalassemia, do not cause symptoms in the newborn period, and, therefore, a hemoglobin electrophoresis generally would not be included in the first battery of tests for this patient. Determination of the infant's blood group is important because ABO disease may occur in the absence of a positive Coombs's test, and the Coombs's test may be positive in cases of minor group incompatibility. The peripheral blood smear should be examined for spherocytes (which usually are evident in cases of ABO disease as well as in congenital spherocytosis) and evidence of other congenital red cell defects such as elliptocytosis or stomatocytosis. Measurement of hemoglobin and hematocrit, nucleated red blood cell count, and reticulocyte count can be helpful in diagnosing hemolytic disease. *(Rudolph:1056; Schaffer:754–756)*

63. **(B)** A Coombs's test would be most important in this infant born to a type O mother. An ABO incompatibility with jaundice is not uncommon, even in a first pregnancy. Sickle cell anemia does not cause neonatal jaundice. Although glucose-6-phosphate dehydrogenase (G6PD) deficiency occurs in about 10% of black males, its association with hyperbilirubinemia appears restricted to premature infants. Liver enzymes need not be ordered at this time, and liver biopsy should not even be considered. *(Rudolph:1056; Schaffer:754–756)*

64. **(B)** The serum bilirubin at 54 hours of age is 16 mg/dL, which is considerably beyond normal limits and approaching 20 mg/dL, at which point neurologic damage (kernicterus) would be possible. This must be avoided. Phototherapy should be initiated at this time, and the serum bilirubin level should be monitored closely. Generally, in a preterm infant, phototherapy is indicated for *nonhemolytic* hyperbilirubinemia exceeding 12 mg/dL. Exchange transfusion would be indicated only if phototherapy failed to keep the unconjugated bilirubin level within the safe range for a term infant (less than 20 mg/dL). With the hyperbilirubinemia being essentially all unconjugated, there is no concern about biliary obstruction, and no indication for abdominal ultrasound. *(Rudolph:1057; Schaffer:754–756)*

65. (A) *Of the disorders listed in this question*, only Crigler-Najjar syndrome, a rare congenital deficiency of glucuronyl transferase in the liver, can explain this infant's persistent unconjugated hyperbilirubinemia. Rotor syndrome causes primarily conjugated hyperbilirubinemia. Biliary atresia, both intrahepatic and extrahepatic, and neonatal hepatitis cause elevation of conjugated as well as unconjugated bilirubin. [*Note:* Crigler-Najjar syndrome is extremely rare and most likely is *not* what this baby has. However, of the list of possible choices given, it is the only one that can explain all the findings and therefore is the correct answer *to this question.* Most infants like this actually recover without a specific diagnosis and probably have extreme physiologic hyperbilirubinemia.] *(Rudolph:1056; Schaffer: 754–756)*

66. (C) Determination of the methemoglobin level would be the lowest priority of the items listed. Although congenital methemoglobinemia does occur, it is among the rarest causes of neonatal cyanosis. Measurement of arterial PO_2 would indicate or obviate the need for a methemoglobin determination. Demonstration of a low arterial PO_2 would document true hypoxemia as the cause of the cyanosis, whereas a normal PO_2 would suggest methemoglobinemia. Incidentally, a simple test to screen for methemoglobinemia is to observe the color of a drop of heel-prick blood on a piece of filter paper. In methemoglobinemia the blood fails to become pink or red. *(Rudolph:1140–1141)*

67. (C) The lack of response to increased ambient oxygen suggests a right-to-left shunt, most likely because of cyanotic congenital heart disease. Hypoventilation would respond to increased ambient oxygen. An arteriovenous fistula is a left-to-right shunt that may be associated with congestive heart failure, the cyanosis of which, like the cyanosis of pneumonia, usually will improve when oxygen is administered. Although the cyanosis associated with methemoglobinemia also will fail to respond to increased ambient oxygen, methemoglobinemia is much rarer than cyanotic congenital heart disease and therefore less likely in this patient. [*Note:* Remember the *best* choice is not always the only possible correct answer to the question.] *(Rudolph:1395–1396)*

68. (A) Transposition of the great vessels is the most likely diagnosis in this child. Isolated ventricular septal defect is associated with a left-to-right rather than a right-to-left shunt. Transposition is a much more common cause of cyanosis in the *immediate* neonatal period than is tetralogy of Fallot. Also, in tetralogy one would expect to find diminished pulmonary circulation on chest roentgenogram. The narrow mediastinum on AP roentgenogram of the chest described in this patient is very characteristic

of transposition, as is the absence of a significant murmur. *(Rudolph:1404–1406)*

69. (A) The acidosis clearly is metabolic in origin (low HCO_3^- and low PCO_2). It almost certainly is secondary to hypoxemia and tissue hypoxia. Metabolic acidosis secondary to tissue hypoxia is frequent in infants with severe cyanotic heart disease. *(Rudolph: 1407)*

70. (C) Intravenous bicarbonate to correct the metabolic acidosis would be appropriate. Furosemide would be of little help in this infant, who has no signs of congestive heart failure. The most likely reason for this child's worsening condition is closure of the ductus arteriosus. An infusion of PGE_1 should be started immediately to reopen and maintain the ductus, affording some opportunity for mixing of blood between the two circulations. *(Rudolph: 1407)*

71. (B) This infant is critically ill, and immediate intervention is required. The extreme hypoxia and associated metabolic acidosis make urgent cardiac catheterization mandatory, more for therapy (palliation) than diagnosis. Such infants are in very precarious condition and may deteriorate or die suddenly. The operating room and open heart team are unnecessary. *(Rudolph:1407)*

72. (D) Transposition of the great arteries results in two separate circulations, which would be incompatible with life without some shunting or mixing of blood between the two circulations. Those infants who are most severely hypoxic early generally are those with an intact ventricular septum. Since, in this condition, right atrial pressure is higher than left atrial pressure, the foramen ovale usually remains patent. A balloon catheter is passed through the foramen, and an atrial balloon septostomy performed. This safe and relatively simple procedure usually will increase intracardiac mixing sufficiently to permit waiting several months before undertaking more extensive surgical procedures or total correction. *(Rudolph:1407)*

73. (B) Idiopathic thrombocytopenic purpura (ITP) is the most likely cause of a seemingly isolated platelet problem in an otherwise well child of this age. Although thrombocytopenia is a common feature of acute leukemia, it usually is seen in conjunction with other signs of bone marrow invasion such as anemia. One cannot entertain the diagnosis of hypersplenism in the absence of splenomegaly. Aspirin causes platelet dysfunction, not thrombocytopenia. *(Rudolph:1159)*

74. (D) Appropriate treatment for ITP includes either corticosteroids or intravenous immunoglobulin. Since most children recover spontaneously, there is some controversy regarding the need for treatment in all cases. Many authors suggest treatment only for children with major bleeding, very low platelet counts, or persistent thrombocytopenia. Because platelet survival time is so brief, platelet transfusions generally are used only to control major bleeding manifestations. Epsilon-aminocaproic acid (EACA) is an inhibitor of the fibrinolytic enzyme system of mucosal tissue and is occasionally used to control oral bleeding in factor VIII deficiency. It has no role in the management of ITP. [*Note:* Even though the use of corticosteroids is controversial and might not be prescribed for this patient by some physicians, it is clearly the *best* answer because all the other choices would be inappropriate for this patient.] *(Rudolph:1159–1160)*

75. (D) Splenectomy is not necessary for most cases of ITP and usually is reserved for chronic cases. Low platelet counts, severe bleeding, and anemia are not in themselves indications for splenectomy. The usual indication is persistence of thrombocytopenia for several *years*. Occasionally splenectomy is required to control CNS bleeding. *(Rudolph:1159–1160)*

76. (D) Although an innocent murmur cannot be ruled out at this time, the loudness of the murmur and the fact that the second sound is widely split and fixed suggests organic heart disease. Acute rheumatic fever is very unlikely in this asymptomatic girl, and she is rather young for rheumatic heart disease, which also is statistically uncommon. The lesion most likely is congenital. *(Rudolph:1368–1369)*

77. (B) The response to a Valsalva maneuver is very helpful in distinguishing an innocent pulmonary flow murmur from certain organic lesions. During the maneuver, which increases intrathoracic pressure, systemic venous return falls, as does right ventricular stroke volume, and the innocent pulmonary flow murmur suddenly decreases in intensity. With certain organic lesions such as an atrial septal defect (ASD), enough blood enters the right ventricle via the defect to maintain pulmonary flow and the murmur. *(Rudolph:1368–1369)*

78. (A) The findings on physical examination, chest roentgenogram, and electrocardiogram are best explained by an ASD. The usual murmur associated with an ASD is caused not by the flow of blood across the atrial defect, but by the increased flow through the right ventricle outflow tract and therefore is a systolic ejection murmur. The murmur of a *ventricular* septal defect would be maximal at the lower sternal border and associated with left, or combined, ventricular hypertrophy on ECG rather than right ventricular hypertrophy. Pulmonic stenosis would cause decreased rather than increased pulmonary vascularity on chest roentgenogram. The classical murmur of a patent ductus arteriosus is continuous and is heard best under the left clavicle; one would

expect LVH rather than RVH on ECG. Since an atrial septal defect is associated with a left-to-right shunt at the atrial level, the right side of the circulation is overloaded, resulting in a pulmonic murmur, increased pulmonary vascularity radiographically, and right ventricular hypertrophy. *(Rudolph:1368–1369)*

79. (D) The child is asymptomatic. There are no signs of congestive heart failure, impaired cardiac output, or myocardial ischemia. There is no need to restrict her activity. Since it is most unlikely that the child has rheumatic heart disease, there is no reason for monthly bicillin prophylaxis. *(Rudolph:1279–1280)*

80. (C) With current surgical techniques and the resultant ease and relative safety of surgical repair, operative correction generally is recommended for any atrial defect large enough to cause cardiomegaly and increased pulmonary vascularity. There is no urgency for surgery, but there also is no reason for undue delay. Although bacterial endocarditis is seen only rarely with atrial defects, atrial fibrillation, pulmonary vascular disease, and congestive heart failure all are seen with increasing frequency in later life. Some centers now are investigating nonsurgical closure by insertion of an umbrella-like device via cardiac catheterization. *(Rudolph:1369)*

81. (D) ABO incompatibility is seen most commonly when the mother is type O and the infant is type A or occasionally type B or AB. An ABO incompatibility problem is not possible if the infant is type O. Similarly, Rh problems arise when the mother is Rh negative (negative for D) and the infant is Rh positive (positive for D). Thus, the data rule out a *major* blood group incompatibility but do not permit one to rule out a *minor* blood group incompatibility, for example, Kell, Kidd, or Duffy antigens. *(Oski:404–406)*

82. (A) A serum bilirubin level of greater than 12 mg/dL in a term infant is an indication for investigation to determine the etiology. There is no indication, at this time, for exchange transfusion, as the bilirubin level is safely much less than 20 mg/dL. Although phototherapy probably will be needed, it ought not to be initiated until one is certain that the hyperbilirubinemia is of the unconjugated type. *(Oski:402–408)*

83. (A) Again, the crucial issue is the need for adequate investigation of the nature of the hyperbilirubinemia. Fractionation of the bilirubin into conjugated and unconjugated reacting portions as well as Coombs's test and other laboratory investigations *that should have been done before starting phototherapy* certainly must be done now that jaundice has persisted for another 3 days. For example, if the infant had hepatitis, a good portion of the hyperbilirubinemia might be conjugated, which carries no risk of neurologic damage and no need for phototherapy. *(Oski:400–407)*

84. (D) The "bronze baby syndrome" (a bronze discoloration of the skin and urine) has been noted occasionally in infants with liver disease and conjugated hyperbilirubinemia who are treated (inappropriately) with phototherapy. Although sepsis has been associated with elevation of both direct and unconjugated bilirubin, it is not associated with the bronze discoloration syndrome. *(Rudolph:1057)*

85. (C) The major error in the management of this infant was the initiation of phototherapy without adequate investigation to determine the cause of the jaundice and to be certain that it resulted from elevated *unconjugated* bilirubin. Choice **(D)**, use of phototherapy rather than exchange transfusion, is incorrect because there are not sufficient data to indicate that *either* exchange transfusion or phototherapy was indicated. Since neurologic damage is associated only with elevated serum levels of unconjugated bilirubin, neither modality is indicated until it has been demonstrated that the hyperbilirubinemia is of the unconjugated variety. *(Oski:400–407)*

86. (E) There appear to be no permanent sequelae to the bronze baby syndrome. The abnormal pigments may persist for several months even after phototherapy is discontinued but have not been shown to be harmful. *(Rudolph:1057)*

87. (E) The history and physical findings are classical for slipped capital femoral epiphysis (SFE). Both pyogenic arthritis and acute rheumatic fever would be unlikely in an afebrile child. Legg-Calvé-Perthes disease is uncommon at this age, usually occurring in children between 4 and 8 years old. Juvenile rheumatoid arthritis is a possibility but is unlikely in the absence of fever and local signs of inflammation. Slipped capital femoral epiphysis is especially frequent among obese adolescent or preadolescent males. *(Rudolph:1941–1942; Oski:943–944)*

88. (B) The diagnosis of slipped capital femoral epiphysis usually is easily confirmed by x-ray examination, which reveals the head of the femur to be displaced medially and posteriorly relative to the neck. Treatment consists of prompt repositioning of the femoral head by traction, followed by surgical introduction of a nail or pin to maintain the alignment. However, overzealous repositioning may increase the risk of avascular necrosis of the femoral head, and in some cases it is wisest to pin the hip directly in the slipped position. *(Rudolph:1941–1942; Oski:943–944)*

89. (C) The etiology of SFE is unknown. Its occurrence most frequently in obese males just before or around the time of puberty has led to suggestions that both

mechanical and hormonal factors may be involved. Occasionally, the slip appears to be precipitated by trauma, as might be the case in this child. Bilateral involvement occurs in 10 to 30% of cases. *(Rudolph:1941–1942; Oski:943–944)*

90. (B) The persistent rash and diffuse involvement of the reticuloendothelial system demonstrated by enlargement of lymph nodes, liver, and spleen makes hydronephrosis, Wilms's tumor, or neuroblastoma rather unlikely diagnoses. A renal ultrasound, therefore, is not likely to be diagnostic, although it might disclose retroperitoneal enlarged lymph nodes. The pallor (probable anemia) and diffuse RE system involvement strongly suggest the possibility of leukemia or another bone marrow invasive disease. The tachypnea warrants a chest roentgenogram. *(Rudolph:1096–1099,1129–1131)*

91. (C) Langerhans cell histiocytosis (Letterer-Siwe disease, histiocytosis X), Farquhar's syndrome (familial hemophagocytic reticulocytosis), leukemia, and acquired immunodeficiency syndrome (AIDS, HIV infection) all are characterized by multisystem involvement including lung, skin, lymph nodes, liver, and spleen. Organ involvement may be primary or secondary to infection. Neuroblastoma is not really a multisystem disease. Lymph node metastases tend to be regional or localized rather than diffuse. Metastases to skin do occur, but these take the form of nodules, often purpuric, rather than a diffuse, greasy rash. *(Rudolph:1218–1219)*

92. (A) Radiographic changes such as those described in the lungs of this child are seen commonly in patients with Langerhans cell histiocytosis. These findings represent direct pulmonary involvement by the disease process. The diffuse honeycomb appearance is especially characteristic of this disorder. *(Rudolph:1219–1220)*

93. (B) Letterer-Siwe syndrome is the most rapidly progressive form of this disease. Although not malignant in a neoplastic sense, it often behaves in a malignant fashion, and many cases respond, at least temporarily, to chemotherapeutic agents such as vincristine and methotrexate. Without treatment, the usual course is progressively downhill, with death occurring in a few months. *(Rudolph:1219–1221)*

94. (D) The mass described is almost certainly the parotid gland. Most cases of cervical adenitis do not extend to the angle of the jaw, nor do they push the ear upward and outward. Although onchocerciasis does produce subcutaneous nodules, especially around the head, these are fibrotic rather than inflammatory. Also, *Onchocerca volvulus*, the responsible organism, is endemic in Africa and South America rather than Asia. The most likely cause of acute parotitis in a child who may be unimmunized (recent immigration from Asia) is mumps virus infection. [*Note:* In current texts, journals, and examinations, body temperature often is given only in centigrade. Learn the centigrade scale. 38.5°C equals 101°F.] *(Rudolph:680–681; Feigin:1610–1612)*

95. **(E)** No laboratory investigation is required. The diagnosis of mumps is easily established on the basis of the clinical findings alone. There are few other causes of acute parotitis in a previously well child. *(Rudolph:680–681; Feigin: 1610–1612)*

96. **(A)** The appearance of the swelling on the opposite side of the face virtually confirms the diagnosis of viral parotitis, almost certainly mumps. Serum amylase probably would be elevated but would be of little diagnostic significance, since the diagnosis already is assured. Although aseptic meningitis is very common with mumps infection, in view of the headache, high fever, and marked nuchal rigidity, a lumbar puncture to rule out bacterial meningitis would be advisable. [*Note:* 40.1°C = 104.2°F.] *(Rudolph:680–681; Feigin:1611)*

97. **(B)** The onset of the fever within a few hours of immunization suggests that it is a reaction to the DPT injection, a fairly common occurrence. Febrile reactions to oral polio vaccine, in contrast, are decidedly uncommon and would not be expected to occur so quickly. It is unlikely that the fever represents an infection contracted in the waiting room, as this would imply an incubation period of less than 12 hours. Although a coincidental, unrelated infection is a possibility, it is statistically less likely than a reaction to the DPT immunization. *(Rudolph:559)*

98. **(E)** There is no evidence of error in the physician's initial handling of this case. DPT and oral polio vaccines are routinely administered simultaneously, and it is appropriate to administer the DPT intramuscularly rather than subcutaneously. The prophylactic prescription of acetaminophen has been recommended by some, but its use is not mandatory. Usually, this is done only if there is a history of febrile reactions to prior DPT injections or a family or personal history of convulsions. There is no indication for prophylactic phenobarbital. *(Oski:559)*

99. **(C)** The findings of the cerebrospinal fluid examination are entirely within normal limits. This suggests that the child had a febrile reaction to the DPT and a seizure secondary to the fever. There is considerable doubt about the existence of post–pertussis immunization encephalopathy and no evidence for it in this infant, whose seizure occurred only 8 hours after the injection. *(Oski:559; Feigin:1214)*

100. **(B)** It is generally believed that almost all reactions to DPT are caused by the pertussis antigen. It is recommended that children who have severe reactions

to DPT, including convulsions, should subsequently receive only DT. There is no reason not to administer the booster dose of oral polio vaccine. *(Oski:559–560)*

101. **(A)** The combination of anemia and jaundice suggests a hemolytic or hepatic problem rather than a bone marrow disorder. Bone marrow aspiration is relatively invasive as well as expensive and is not indicated at this moment. A reticulocyte count should be obtained. An elevated reticulocyte count would indicate that the marrow is functional and strengthen the decision not to perform a bone marrow examination at this time. The peripheral blood smear should be examined for spherocytes, sickle cells, and other abnormal red cell forms. A history of drug ingestion or medicines taken might point to an enzyme defect of the erythrocytes. *(Rudolph:394; Oski:1520–1521)*

102. **(D)** Although not indicated, a bone marrow aspiration was performed in this patient. The results are compatible with a hemolytic anemia. Sickle cell disease is unlikely in view of the absence of sickle cells on smear and the history of a negative sickle test. The absence of spherocytes on peripheral blood smear argues against spherocytosis. In infectious hepatitis, one would expect more of a conjugated or mixed hyperbilirubinemia. A variety of drugs have been incriminated as precipitating hemolytic episodes in G6PD-deficient patients. *(Rudolph:394; Oski: 1520–1521)*

103. **(D)** Intraerythrocyte levels of G6PD usually decrease with cell age. In patients with hereditary G6PD "deficiency" (of which there are many variants), the activity level falls more rapidly than normal. In hemolytic episodes associated with G6PD deficiency in blacks, only older cells with the lowest G6PD levels are destroyed, while younger erythrocytes with higher enzyme levels survive. At such times, the assay of enzyme activity may reveal almost normal G6PD activity despite the deficiency state. In persons of Mediterranean ancestry the enzyme defect is more severe, and even young erythrocytes are G6PD deficient and subject to hemolysis. *(Rudolph:394; Oski:1520–1521)*

104. **(B)** Since the cause of the hemolysis in this patient has not yet been firmly established, a Coombs's test would be important to identify or rule out an autoimmune hemolytic anemia. A decreased serum haptoglobin level could confirm that hemolysis had occurred, but there is already so little doubt about this from the available data that the test would not be very helpful. *(Rudolph:394; Oski:1520–1521)*

105. **(C)** In the presence of a hemoglobin concentration of 7 g/dL, no distress, and stable vital signs, there is no need for immediate transfusion with all its associated risks. Transfusion also would depress the bone

marrow as well as complicate diagnostic endeavors. Many hemolytic episodes, especially those associated with G6PD deficiency in blacks, stabilize at a reasonably safe hemoglobin level. *(Rudolph:394; Oski:1520–1521)*

106. (B) For reasons explained in answer 103, the G6PD level might be only normal or slightly below normal at this time but might be clearly abnormal when the child has recovered. If the child is demonstrated to have a G6PD deficiency, it is best to avoid potentially aggravating drugs rather than to attempt a challenge. *(Rudolph:394; Oski:1520–1521)*

107. (C) The history of vomiting and diarrhea, the failure to thrive, the low serum concentration of sodium, and the high concentration of potassium suggest adrenal insufficiency. The finding of an enlarged clitoris and fused labia suggest that this infant has been virilized. The most likely diagnosis to explain all these findings is congenital adrenal hyperplasion (CAH), a condition resulting from an inherited defect in the synthesis of cortisol. Most forms of the disorder are associated with virilization from the excessive accumulation of androgenic steroid precursors. Neither the dehydration nor the prerenal azotemia (BUN 32) is severe enough to explain the markedly elevated serum potassium. In situations of inappropriate ADH secretion, all serum electrolytes would be low (diluted). *(Rudolph:1579–1599)*

108. (A) Congenital adrenal hyperplasia is a genetic but not a chromosomal disorder. The patient almost certainly is a partially virilized female (XX), most likely with the 21-hydroxylase deficiency form of the disorder. There is also an exceedingly rare nonvirilizing form (impaired conversion of cholesterol to pregnenolone) in which males may be partially feminized. [*Note:* The question asked which pattern was "probable," not certain.] *(Rudolph:1597–1598)*

109. (D) Therapy of the salt-losing form of adrenal hyperplasia requires replacement with both a glucocorticoid and a mineralocorticoid. A high salt intake is important. For infants, NaCl is added to the formula. *(Rudolph:1596–1598)*

110. (E) Replacement therapy with one or another form of cortisone is required for life. In some children mineralocorticoid therapy can be discontinued after infancy, and the child successfully maintained on cortisol and salt only. *(Rudolph:1596–1598)*

111. (E) The picture described is quite typical for Sydenham's chorea (rheumatic chorea). Although a posterior fossa brain tumor certainly needs to be considered, the absence of other cerebellar or neurological signs, as well as the absence of evidence of increased intracranial pressure, would be against this diagnosis. The emotional upset and lability are characteristic of chorea and need not suggest a conversion reaction (hysteria). The same is true of the tendency for the movements to worsen with agitation and to disappear during sleep; this is exactly the pattern seen in rheumatic chorea. Ingestion of LSD produces visual hallucinations and psychotic symptoms rather than a movement disorder. The usual neurologic manifestations of lead poisoning are ataxia and seizures. *(Rudolph:494)*

112. (C) A careful ophthalmologic examination should be performed to look for evidence of hepatolenticular degeneration (Wilson's disease), which can present with abnormal movements, grimacing, emotional lability, and agitation. The characteristic eye finding in this disorder is the Kayser-Fleisher ring. *(Rudolph:387–388)*

113. (E) The negative acute-phase reactants (CBC and ESR) and other normal laboratory data do not rule against a diagnosis of Sydenham's (rheumatic) chorea. Although the disorder is believed to be a manifestation of rheumatic fever following a group A streptococcal infection, the length of time between the infection and the onset of symptoms is so long that usually the laboratory parameters, including ASO titer, have returned to normal by the time the patient comes to medical attention. *(Rudolph:494)*

114. (B) Choreiform movements also have been noted as a presenting manifestation of systemic lupus erythematosus. The abnormal movements noted in patients with hepatic failure generally are tremors rather than choreiform movements. None of the other conditions listed is associated with abnormal movements. *(Rudolph:494; Am J Med 62:99–115,1977)*

115. (D) Since rheumatic chorea may be followed by subsequent attacks of acute rheumatic fever with carditis and the development of rheumatic heart disease, continuous prophylactic penicillin therapy to prevent streptococcal infection is indicated and is the most important aspect of management. Sympathetic understanding and a quiet environment with restricted activity may well be the most important aspects of symptomatic treatment. For *short*-term management, barbiturates and chlorpromazine have been found useful. Clonazepam (Clonopin) and haloperidol (Haldol) also have been used to control the abnormal movements. Most authorities believe that adrenocorticosteroids have no beneficial effect in this disorder. *(Rudolph:494)*

116. (B) The abnormal movements and other manifestations associated with rheumatic chorea eventually resolve completely. In most cases this takes several months; occasionally, it may take up to 2 years. Recurrences are rare. *(Rudolph:494)*

117. (A) Even a strong family history of diabetes mellitus would have little relevance to this child's current problem. Although juvenile diabetes mellitus (JDM) does occur this young, it is uncommon. More importantly, in children the interval between the onset of symptoms (glycosuria, polyuria, and weight loss) and diabetic ketoacidosis is very brief, and so JDM does not present as weight loss over several months. Finally, of course, JDM would not explain the diarrhea. *(Rudolph:989–990)*

118. (C) For the reason discussed above, serum glucose is very unlikely to be helpful in determining the cause of the diarrhea and weight loss. Although it is true that infants with diarrhea may occasionally develop hypoglycemia *secondary* to malabsorption or decreased oral intake, this is most frequent in the very young infant (less than 6 months) and, even if present, is rarely of *diagnostic* importance. *(Rudolph:989–990)*

119. (A) On admission it would be most appropriate to continue the regular diet for age that the child had been on at home. This would permit observation of the child's intake and stool pattern as well as examination of the stool for blood, glucose, pH, and fat droplets. It would be premature to place this 18-month-old on a restrictive diet or on parenteral nutrition prior to observation and examination of the stool. If, for example, the stool were positive for *Giardia*, no dietary manipulation would be needed. *(Rudolph:989–990)*

BIBLIOGRAPHY

Feigin RD, Cherry JD. *Textbook of Pediatric Infectious Diseases.* 3rd ed. Philadelphia, Pa: Saunders; 1992.

Fish AJ, Blau EB, Westberg NG, et al. Systemic lupus erythematosus within the first two decades of life. *Am J Med.* 1977;62:99–115.

Fishman M. Febrile seizures: the treatment controversy. *J Pediatr.* 1979;94:177–184.

Gerber MA, Berliner BC. The child with a simple febrile seizure. *Am J Dis Child.* 1981;135:431–433.

Hathaway WE, Groothius JR, Hay WW, et al. *Current Pediatric Diagnosis & Treatment.* 10th ed. Norwalk, Conn: Appleton & Lange; 1991.

Joffe A, McCormick M, DeAngelis C. Which children with febrile seizures need lumbar puncture? A decision analysis approach. *Am J Dis Child.* 1983;137:1153–1156.

Leffert F. The management of acute severe asthma. *J Pediatr.* 1980;96:1–12.

Lewy JE. Acute poststreptococcal glomerulonephritis. *Pediatr Clin North Am.* 1976;23:751–758.

Oski FA, DeAngelis CD, Feigin RD, et al. *Principles & Practice of Pediatrics.* Philadelphia, Pa: JB Lippincott; 1990.

Rudolph Am, Hoffman JIE, Rudolph CD. *Pediatrics.* 19th ed. Norwalk, Conn: Appleton & Lange; 1991.

Schaffer R, Avery, ME. *Schaffer and Avery's Diseases of the Newborn.* 6th ed. Philadelphia, Pa: Saunders; 1991.

Taber LH, Feigin RD. Spirochetal infections. *Pediatr Clin North Am.* 1979;26:377–413.

Wears RL, Luten RC, Lyons RG. Which laboratory tests should be performed on children with apparent febrile convulsions? An analysis and review of the literature. *Pediatr Emerg Care.* 1986;2:191–196.

Wolf SW, Carr A, Davis DC, et al. The value of phenobarbital in the child who has had a single febrile seizure. *Pediatrics.* 1977;59:378–384.

CHAPTER 11

Practice Test

Carefully read the following instructions before taking the Practice Test.

1. This examination consists of 162 questions, covering the subject areas listed in the Table of Contents.
2. The Practice Test simulates an actual examination in question types and integration of subject areas.
3. You should set aside 2 hours and 10 minutes of *uninterrupted,* distraction-free time to take the Practice Test. This averages out to 50 seconds per question.
4. Be sure you have a clock (to time and pace yourself) and an adequate number of No. 2 pencils and erasers.
5. You should tear out and use the answer sheet that is provided on pages 223 and 224.
6. Be sure to answer all of the questions, and be sure the number on the answer sheet corresponds to the question number in the Practice Test.
7. Use any remaining time to review your answers.
8. After completing the Practice Test, you can check all of your answers on pages 197 to 211. A score of 75% or higher should be considered as a passing score (115 correct answers).
9. After checking your answers and your score, you can analyze your strengths and weaknesses on the Practice Test Subspeciality List on page 213. To do this, you should check off your incorrect Practice Test answers on the Subspecialty List. You may find a pattern developing. For example, you may find you do well on infectious diseases but poorly on immunopathology. In such an instance, you can go back and review the immunopathology section of this book and supplement your review with your texts and with the references cited in that section.

Questions

This chapter provides a final opportunity to increase your data base in pediatrics and to evaluate your general pediatric thinking skills and knowledge. The chapter includes all types of question formats, including case diagnosis-management problems, as well as a review of topics across the field of pediatrics. The chapter consists of 162 questions. You should be able to complete the sample examination within 3 hours. Good luck.

DIRECTIONS (Questions 1 through 106): Each of the numbered items or incomplete statements in this section is followed by answers or by completions of the statement. Select the ONE lettered answer or completion that is BEST in each case.

1. Two months after an episode of acute otitis media a 2-year-old child is noted to have decreased hearing but is otherwise well. Physical examination reveals only dull and opaque tympanic membranes with decreased mobility. The child most likely has

    (A) a recurrence of acute otitis media
    (B) bilateral cholesteatomas
    (C) chronic mastoiditis
    (D) immunodeficiency
    (E) secretary otitis media

2. Unilateral multicystic kidney in an infant usually presents as

    (A) an abdominal mass
    (B) hematuria
    (C) hypertension
    (D) nephrotic syndrome
    (E) oliguria

3. Fanconi's syndrome is characterized by

    (A) azotemia, edema, and hypertension
    (B) glycosuria, aminoaciduria, and phosphaturia
    (C) hematuria, glycosuria, and proteinuria
    (D) hypoglycemia, glycosuria, hypoglycinemia, and glycinuria
    (E) uremia, phosphaturia, and albuminuria

4. Which of the following sets of values is most suggestive of proximal renal tubular acidosis?

	Urine pH	Serum bicarbonate (mEq/L)	Serum chloride (mEq/L)
(A)	8	22	98
(B)	8	15	115
(C)	7	22	115
(D)	6	22	98
(E)	6	15	115

5. The presence of bilateral renal masses and a midline suprapubic mass in a newborn male infant is most suggestive of

    (A) bilateral Wilms's tumor
    (B) congenital neuroblastoma
    (C) congenital rubella infection
    (D) rhabdomyosarcoma of the bladder
    (E) congenital urethral or bladder neck obstruction

6. Wilms's tumor (nephroblastoma) is the most frequent malignant tumor of the genitourinary tract in childhood. The most common presenting sign of this neoplasm is

    (A) abdominal mass
    (B) abdominal pain
    (C) edema
    (D) hematuria
    (E) hypertension

7. Which of the following is most likely to be the last finding to disappear in a case of resolving post-streptococcal acute glomerulonephritis?

(A) Edema
(B) Elevated blood urea nitrogen
(C) Hypertension
(D) Hypocomplementemia
(E) Microscopic hematuria

8. The most common bacteria to cause fatal septicemia in children with acute leukemia are

(A) alpha *Streptococcus* and anaerobic organisms
(B) alpha *Streptococcus* and group B *Streptococcus*
(C) *H. influenzae, S. pneumoniae,* and group A *Streptococcus*
(D) *Staphylococcus aureus* and *S. albus*
(E) *Pseudomonas aeruginosa, E. coli,* and *S. aureus*

9. Continuous ambulatory peritoneal dialysis (CAPD) has the advantage of leaving the patient free to pursue daily activities without being restricted to a dialysis machine for long periods of time. Compared to other methods of dialysis, the major disadvantage or complication of this technique appears to be

(A) a high incidence of disequilibrium syndrome
(B) a high incidence of peritonitis
(C) a need for severe dietary restriction
(D) frequent electrolyte problems
(E) poor growth

10. Infants with congenital (autosomal recessive) nephrotic syndrome rarely

(A) have edema
(B) develop renal failure
(C) die from the disease
(D) respond to corticosteroids
(E) are symptomatic before 3 months of age

11. The peak age of onset of childhood nephrotic syndrome associated with minimal-change morphology is

(A) in the first year of life
(B) between 2 and 5 years of age
(C) between 5 and 10 years of age
(D) between 10 and 15 years of age
(E) over 15 years of age

12. The finding of a low serum concentration of C3 component of complement in a child with nephrotic syndrome

(A) indicates a high likelihood of spontaneous remission
(B) indicates a high likelihood of good response to steroid therapy
(C) suggests the presence of focal segmental sclerosis

(D) suggests the presence of membranous glomerular nephritis
(E) suggests the presence of membranoproliferative glomerular nephritis

13. Early in an attack of asthma, which of the following sets of arterial blood values is most likely?

(A) Normal PO_2 and normal PCO_2
(B) Normal PO_2 and low PCO_2
(C) Normal PO_2 and elevated PCO_2
(D) Low PO_2 and low PCO_2
(E) Low PO_2 and elevated PCO_2

14. The most common roentgenographic abnormality in a child with asthma is

(A) bronchiectasis
(B) generalized hyperinflation
(C) lower lobe infiltrates
(D) pneumomediastinum
(E) right middle lobe atelectasis

15. The pattern of inheritance of achondroplasia is

(A) autosomal recessive
(B) autosomal dominant
(C) X-linked recessive
(D) X-linked dominant
(E) polygenetic

16. The most commonly encountered bacterial pathogens in the lungs of patients with cystic fibrosis are

(A) *E. coli* and alpha *Streptococcus*
(B) *E. coli* and *Pseudomonas*
(C) *Staphylococcus* and *Proteus*
(D) *Staphylococcus* and *Pseudomonas*
(E) *Hemophilus influenzae* and pneumococcus

17. A sibling born to a child with an isolated cleft palate (normal lip) and no other congenital abnormality has

(A) an increased risk of having an isolated cleft palate
(B) an increased risk of having either a cleft lip or a cleft palate
(C) an increased risk of having both a combined cleft lip and palate
(D) no increased risk for either cleft lip or cleft palate

18. A 2-month-old infant presents with irritability and congestive heart failure. An ECG is interpreted as characteristic of myocardial infarction. Which of the following is the most likely explanation for these findings?

(A) Viral myocarditis
(B) Ventricular septal defect
(C) Endocardial fibroelastosis
(D) Anomalous origin of the left coronary artery
(E) Atherosclerotic heart disease secondary to a congenital lipid disorder

19. A 6-month-old infant is found to be lethargic and cyanotic. Blood obtained by venipuncture appears chocolate brown and does not become bright red when shaken in the presence of air. It is especially important to seek a history of exposure to

(A) automobile exhaust
(B) fava beans
(C) paint fumes
(D) undercooked meat
(E) well water

20. Serous otitis media is defined as the accumulation of fluid, usually sterile, in the middle ear. The chief symptom is

(A) fever
(B) hearing loss
(C) pain
(D) tinnitus
(E) vertigo

21. Pica refers to

(A) recurrent belching
(B) frequent head nodding
(C) small, pink, flat topped lesions
(D) the habitual ingestion of nonfood substances
(E) intermittent bursts of alpha activity on the EEG

22. The primary lesion in acne is

(A) hyperplasia of the sweat gland
(B) sterile inflammation of the sweat gland
(C) plugging of the sebaceous gland
(D) infection of the sebaceous gland
(E) increased cornification of the epidermis

23. A 7-year-old child is brought to the office because of chronic nasal obstruction. Examination reveals bilateral clear, serous discharge from the nose but is otherwise unremarkable. The most likely diagnosis is

(A) a defect in the cribriform plate
(B) allergic rhinitis
(C) choanal atresia
(D) cystic fibrosis
(E) immunodeficiency

24. Atopic dermatitis in children

(A) tends to spare the face and arms
(B) is frequently associated with uveitis
(C) rarely begins during the first 2 years of life
(D) is characterized by pruritus and lichenification
(E) is associated with elevated serum levels of IgA and IgM and decreased levels of IgE

25. A 15-year-old boy is bitten on the hand by a snake, which he then kills and brings to the emergency room. The snake is identified as a copperhead measuring 14 inches in length. The most likely complication to be expected in this child would be

(A) fever
(B) local tissue necrosis

(C) paralysis
(D) renal failure
(E) shock

26. The major concern regarding chronic serous otitis media is the development of

(A) meningitis
(B) mastoiditis
(C) permanent nerve deafness
(D) perforation of the tympanic membrane
(E) impaired speech and language development secondary to hearing loss

27. A previously well 6-year-old child suddenly develops bilateral deafness. Physical and neurologic examinations are entirely normal except for bilateral severe sensorineural hearing loss. Which of the following is the most likely cause of this condition?

(A) Bilateral acoustic neuromas
(B) Ingestion of a toxin
(C) Lupus erythematosus
(D) Neurofibromatosis
(E) Viral infection of the inner ear

28. Most nasal polyps in children usually are caused by either

(A) allergy or immunodeficiency
(B) allergy or infection
(C) allergy or cancer
(D) cystic fibrosis or cancer
(E) cystic fibrosis or allergy

29. The most common manifestation of alpha-1-antitrypsin deficiency in infancy is

(A) lung cysts
(B) myocarditis
(C) hepatic cirrhosis
(D) pancreatic insufficiency
(E) obstructive lung disease

30. The most common noniatrogenic cause of Cushing's syndrome in infancy is

(A) bilateral adrenal hyperplasia
(B) unilateral adrenal hyperplasia
(C) an adrenal cortical adenoma or carcinoma
(D) a pituitary tumor
(E) a gonadal tumor

31. A 12-year-old girl presents with panhypopituitarism. A CT scan reveals a mass lesion in the region of the anterior pituitary gland. The most likely diagnosis is a

(A) chromophobe adenoma
(B) craniopharyngioma
(C) ganglioneuroma
(D) medulloblastoma
(E) neuroblastoma

32. In children with sickle cell disease anemia, the hemoglobin level

(A) will fall to progressively lethal levels if untreated
(B) usually stabilizes between 4 and 6 g/dL
(C) usually stabilizes between 7 and 10 g/dL
(D) fluctuates between 8 and 15 g/dL
(E) rarely goes below 10 g/dL except during crisis

33. In children with sickle cell disease, splenic sequestration crises are mostly likely to occur

(A) in the neonatal period
(B) during the first 5 years of life
(C) in adolescence
(D) following transfusion
(E) in association with folic acid deficiency

34. The catheterization data shown below would indicate a diagnosis of

(A) tetralogy of Fallot
(B) Eisenmenger's syndrome
(C) ventricular septal defect
(D) primary pulmonary hypertension
(E) ventricular septal defect with aortic insufficiency

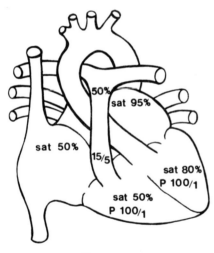

Figure 11–1

35. A 5-year-old girl has had monthly episodes of fever and aphthous stomatitis for more than a year. A CBC about 6 months ago was reportedly normal, but a CBC now reveals a total neutrophil count of less than 200/mm³. The remainder of the CBC is normal. Physical examination reveals an inflamed pharynx and oral mucosa with several aphthous lesions on the gingival and buccal mucosa. There are bilateral, tender anterior cervical lymph nodes, the largest of which is about 4 cm in diameter. The remainder of the physical examination is normal. The most likely diagnosis is

(A) Chédiak-Higashi syndrome
(B) cyclic neutropenia
(C) HIV infection
(D) leukemia
(E) Schwachman-Diamond syndrome

36. Which of the following in an 8-year-old child is most likely to indicate an underlying psychological or behavioral problem?

(A) Enuresis
(B) Encopresis
(C) Motion illness
(D) Migraine headache
(E) Recurrent pharyngitis

37. In a youngster with a history of "seizures," which of the following would be most suggestive of a nonorganic or hysterical etiology?

(A) Postictal sleep
(B) Changing pattern of the seizure
(C) Biting of the tongue during an episode
(D) Urinary incontinence during an episode
(E) Loss of memory for events during the seizure

38. The major permanent impairment resulting from pseudotumor cerebri is

(A) deafness
(B) decreased visual acuity
(C) epilepsy
(D) hemiparesis
(E) mental retardation

39. A 12-year-old child presents with fever, purulent nasal discharge, and swelling and tenderness over the area below the left eye. The remainder of the physical examination is within normal limits. The most likely diagnosis is

(A) acute sinusitis
(B) periorbital cellulitis
(C) purulent adenoiditis
(D) retropharyngeal abscess
(E) rhabdomyosarcoma

40. Chronic upper airway obstruction from enlarged tonsils and adenoids in a child may cause

(A) convulsions
(B) cor pulmonale
(C) a pneumothorax
(D) thymic hyperplasia
(E) asthma (reactive airway disease)

41. Febrile seizures occur most frequently

(A) in the first month of life
(B) in the first 6 months of life
(C) between 6 months and 5 years of age
(D) between 5 and 10 years of age
(E) around the time of puberty

42. A mother calls to inform you that her previously well 4-year-old child has been complaining of headaches for about a month. For the past 2 weeks he has been keeping his head in a tilted position, and for the past few days he has been vomiting in the morning. The most likely diagnosis is

(A) acute torticollis
(B) brain abscess
(C) brain tumor
(D) degenerative brain disease
(E) meningitis

43. Episodes of cerebellar ataxia may be seen in

(A) cystinuria
(B) Gaucher's disease
(C) Hartnup's disease
(D) oxalosis
(E) tyrosinosis

44. Which of the following is generally considered a contraindication to adenoidectomy?

(A) Recurrent otitis media
(B) Submucosal cleft palate
(C) Persistent serous otitis media
(D) Evidence of chronic or recurrent adenoiditis
(E) Midfacial hypoplasia secondary to mouth breathing

45. An 8-year-old child develops an intensely pruritic rash on the legs only. There are patches of erythematous papules and vesicles and several streaks of erythematous vesiculation. The child is afebrile and otherwise well. The most likely diagnosis is

(A) eczema
(B) Henoch-Schönlein purpura
(C) poison ivy dermatitis
(D) scabies
(E) varicella

46. Intestinal malrotation usually presents with

(A) diarrhea
(B) failure to thrive
(C) hypoglycemia
(D) necrotizing enterocolitis
(E) vomiting

47. The classic radiologic finding in duodenal atresia is

(A) a totally gasless abdomen
(B) free air below the diaphragm
(C) the double-bubble sign
(D) the anchor sign
(E) the string sign

48. Children with ketotic hypoglycemia usually

(A) are obese
(B) are hyperinsulinemic

(C) have elevated serum levels of alanine
(D) tend to become less symptomatic as they grow older
(E) have their symptoms precipitated by a high-carbohydrate diet

49. A female-appearing infant is operated on for bilateral inguinal hernias only to have the surgeon discover that the masses are undescended testes. Chromosomal analysis reveals XY constitution. The patient's adolescent sister has primary amenorrhea. Chromosomal analysis of the sister also reveals XY constitution. The most likely cause of this syndrome in the patient and sister is

(A) 20,22-desmolase deficiency complex
(B) end-organ insensitivity to androgens
(C) congenital adrenal hyperplasia
(D) true hermaphrodism
(E) Turner's syndrome

50. The most common clinical manifestation of platelet disorders is

(A) hematuria
(B) hemarthrosis
(C) gastrointestinal hemorrhage
(D) bleeding into the skin and mucous membranes
(E) spontaneous hemorrhage in brain, lung, and liver

51. The usual presentation of an annular pancreas in childhood is

(A) hypoglycemia
(B) hyperglycemic acidosis
(C) jaundice
(D) vomiting
(E) steatorrhea

52. Breath-holding spells

(A) are most common between 4 and 6 years of age
(B) are a common cause of sudden infant death
(C) are a manifestation of infantile colic
(D) represent a type of epilepsy
(E) may terminate in cyanosis and loss of consciousness

53. The most common presentation of pinworm infection is

(A) appendicitis
(B) diarrhea
(C) intussusception
(D) perianal pruritus
(E) vaginitis

54. A 10-day-old infant is evaluated for recurrent blisters and sores, mostly on the extremities at areas of friction or trauma. The child has been afebrile and well except for irritability. Examination is unremarkable except for blisters, varying in stage from fresh to ruptured and crusted, mostly on the extremities, especially the dorsal surfaces of the hands and feet. Which of the following would be highest on your differential diagnosis?

(A) Bullous impetigo
(B) Congenital syphilis
(C) Drug-induced toxic epidermal necrolysis
(D) Epidermolysis bullosa
(E) Staphylococcal scalded-skin syndrome

55. Juvenile gastrointestinal polyps

(A) occur most commonly in the ileum
(B) rarely present in the first 5 years of life
(C) usually present as blood-streaked stools
(D) often already have malignant elements when first discovered
(E) have a significant risk of malignant transformation after puberty

56. A 4-year-old child is brought to the office because of vague abdominal pain and occasional vomiting for several weeks. Physical examination reveals alopecia on one side of the head and a left upper quadrant abdominal mass. The mother notes that the child is "nervous" and frequently pulls out hairs from her head, especially when going to sleep. The most likely diagnosis is

(A) a trichobezoar
(B) hyperthyroidism
(C) gastric hypertrophy
(D) a pheochromocytoma
(E) acquired hypertrophic pyloric stenosis

57. Which of the following statements regarding appendicitis in the first 2 years of life is true?

(A) It rarely is associated with fever
(B) The mortality rate is greater than 50%
(C) The incidence of perforation at the time of diagnosis is over 50%
(D) It frequently can be treated with antibiotics without surgical intervention
(E) It usually is associated with an underlying lesion such as a Meckel's diverticulum or a hemangioma of the appendix

58. On routine examination, a 2-month-old black male infant is noted to have a moderate-size umbilical hernia. The contents of the hernia are easily reduced, and it is noted that the abdominal wall defect easily admits one examining finger but not quite two. The remainder of the examination is normal, and the infant is asymptomatic. The appropriate next step in management would be to

(A) order thyroid function tests
(B) refer the infant to a surgeon
(C) instruct the parent in how to tape the defect
(D) obtain an abdominal roentgenogram or ultrasound
(E) advise the parent that the defect will probably close spontaneously

59. Which of the following statements regarding chylous ascites in infancy is true?

(A) Congenital nephrosis is the most common cause
(B) Hypoalbuminemia and lymphopenia are common
(C) The condition usually is benign and transient
(D) Hypergammaglobulinemia is common
(E) Hepatic involvement is common

60. A 12-year-old child presents with severe abdominal pain, nausea and vomiting, abdominal distension, and epigastric tenderness. Chest roentgenogram reveals a small pleural effusion. The child is afebrile, but blood count reveals a marked leukocytosis. In this patient, one might also expect to find

(A) marked eosinophilia
(B) a positive tuberculin skin test
(C) an elevation of serum amylase
(D) a positive stool culture for *C. difficile*
(E) a prolonged QT interval on electrocardiogram

61. Idiopathic scoliosis is

(A) more common in boys than in girls
(B) rarely severe enough to warrant treatment
(C) generally associated with mental retardation
(D) most commonly noted during preadolescence or adolescence
(E) usually associated with considerable pain on motion of the back

62. A 4-year-old child presents with bleeding esophageal varices and splenomegaly. The liver is judged to be normal size by physical examination. Serum bilirubin and liver function tests are normal. Which of the following is most likely?

(A) A splenic cyst
(B) A tumor obstructing portal blood flow
(C) Hepatoma or hepatoblastoma
(D) Intrahepatic biliary atresia
(E) Thrombosis of the portal vein

63. A 2-year-old infant has a chronic cough, clubbing, and rectal prolapse; the most likely diagnosis to explain all of these findings would be

(A) agammaglobulinemia
(B) cirrhosis of the liver
(C) cystic fibrosis
(D) granulomatous colitis
(E) pinworms

64. You examine a school-age child because of itchy scalp and note minute white-gray structures firmly attached to the hair shafts. You recommend

(A) a selenium-containing shampoo
(B) a 1% permethrin cream rinse
(C) oral tetracycline
(D) oral and topical tetracycline
(E) oral griseofulvin

65. A 2-year-old child drinks some kerosene that had been left in a glass. After the first swallow, she cries and drops the glass. She is most likely to develop

(A) aplastic anemia
(B) chemical pneumonitis
(C) coma and/or convulsions
(D) hepatitis
(E) peripheral neuritis

66. Congenital hypothyroidism should be included in the differential diagnosis of a newborn with

(A) coma
(B) prolonged jaundice
(C) pulmonary edema
(D) renal failure
(E) severe anemia

67. A 2-month-old infant has had inspiratory stridor since the first month of life but has been otherwise well. Physical examination is unremarkable except for moderate inspiratory stridor and retractions, which are worse when the infant is supine or agitated and better when he is prone and quiet. The most likely cause of these findings is

(A) reactive airway disease
(B) laryngomalacia
(C) viral croup
(D) an aspirated foreign body
(E) a tracheoesophageal fistula

68. A significant number of children with otherwise unexplained recurrent gross or microscopic hematuria (normal renal ultrasound and normal tests of renal function) have

(A) hyperkaliuria
(B) hypercalciuria
(C) hypercalcemia
(D) hyperphosphatemia
(E) hemorrhagic urethritis

69. A 4-year-old child, previously well, presents with the rather sudden onset of wheezing that does not respond to treatment with aerosolized albuterol. An x-ray examination of the chest (see below) is obtained. The most likely diagnosis is

(A) asthma
(B) foreign body
(C) infantile lobar emphysema

(D) pulmonary hypoplasia
(E) right middle lobe syndrome

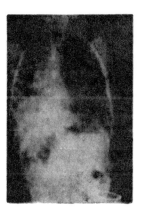

Figure 11–2

70. Physical examination of a 1-year-old child who does not walk reveals the findings shown below. The most likely diagnosis is

(A) arthrogryposis congenita
(B) congenital hip dislocation
(C) equinovarus deformity
(D) rickets
(E) tibial torsion

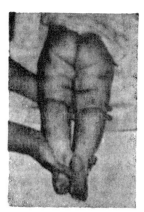

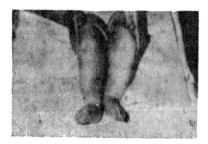

Figure 11–3

71. A 12-year-old girl complains of decreasing visual acuity and a slight feeling of discomfort in both eyes. Examination by an ophthalmologist reveals anterior uveitis. You suspect that the child may have

(A) leukemia
(B) toxoplasmosis
(C) toxocara infection
(D) hypoparathyroidism
(E) juvenile rheumatoid arthritis

72. A 12-year-old black male is evaluated for dry cough, dyspnea on effort, and fatigue of several months' duration. A chest roentgenogram reveals a bilateral diffuse interstitial infiltrate and bilateral hilar adenopathy. Physical examination reveals a clear chest but hepatosplenomegaly and generalized lymphadenopathy. You expect to find

(A) pancytopenia
(B) a positive tuberculin skin test
(C) a positive serum titer for *Borrelia burgdoferi*
(D) a decreased serum level of alpha-1-antitrypsin
(E) an elevated serum concentration of angiotensin-converting enzyme

73. Acute poststreptococcal glomerulonephritis in childhood

(A) is most common between 1 and 3 years of age
(B) usually follows the onset of a streptococcal infection by 2 to 3 days
(C) can result from either streptococcal pharyngitis or streptococcal impetigo
(D) is generally associated with transient hypercomplementemia
(E) usually presents as acute renal failure

74. The most consistent finding in lymphocytic thyroiditis (Hashimoto's thyroiditis) is

(A) enlargement of the thyroid gland
(B) hyperthyroidism
(C) hypothyroidism
(D) eosinophilia
(E) associated disturbances of the parathyroids

75. The most characteristic feature of the juvenile nasopharyngeal angiofibroma is

(A) its association with diabetes mellitus
(B) its predilection for pubescent females
(C) its tendency to bleed
(D) its lack of response to radiotherapy or chemotherapy
(E) the rapidity with which it metastasizes

76. The pulmonary function test most commonly used for home monitoring of a child with asthma is

(A) vital capacity
(B) functional residual capacity
(C) 1-second timed vital capacity (FEV_1)

(D) peak expiratory flow rate
(E) maximum midexpiratory flow rate

77. A 2-year-old child has had recurrent episodes of fever, cough, and pulmonary infiltrates on chest roentgenograms. Diagnostic evaluation reveals a normal sweat test, barium swallow, and serum immunoglobulins but a severe microcytic, hypochromic anemia. The child's diet is normal for age. Which of the following would be highest on your list of differential diagnoses?

(A) Cystic fibrosis
(B) Diffuse pulmonary hemangiomatosis
(C) Extramedullary pulmonary erythropoiesis
(D) Gastroesophageal reflux and hemorrhagic esophagitis
(E) Primary pulmonary hemosiderosis

78. An eczematoid rash may be seen in patients with

(A) leukemia
(B) Wiskott-Aldrich syndrome
(C) inflammatory bowel disease
(D) endocardial fibroelastosis
(E) Kawasaki's syndrome

79. A previously well 9-year-old boy develops an intensely pruritic rash consisting of roughly circular elevated lesions with pink edges and pale centers. Lesions are well circumscribed and range in size from 2 to 6 cm in diameter. The history is unremarkable, and physical examination is unrevealing except for the rash. Careful diagnostic workup probably will disclose

(A) a food allergy
(B) an occult malignancy
(C) a collagen vascular disease
(D) C_1-esterase inhibitor deficiency
(E) no specific cause for the rash

80. Most patients with XYY constitution are

(A) short
(B) homosexual
(C) behaviorally normal
(D) impulsive and antisocial
(E) severely mentally retarded

81. Precocious puberty secondary to a lesion of the central nervous system

(A) occurs only in boys
(B) is always isosexual
(C) is usually caused by a malignant hypothalamic tumor
(D) is associated with small gonads
(E) is usually incomplete

82. Precocious puberty has been noted in association with

    (A) hypoadrenalism
    (B) hypoparathyroidism
    (C) hyperparathyroidism
    (D) hypothyroidism
    (E) hyperthyroidism

83. Pseudohypoparathyroidism is associated with

    (A) short stature
    (B) renal failure
    (C) long, spindly fingers
    (D) generalized increased mineralization of bone
    (E) decreased serum levels of parathyroid hormone

84. The most consistent abnormality in Von Willebrand's disease is a

    (A) decreased platelet count
    (B) prolonged bleeding time
    (C) prolonged prothrombin time
    (D) prolonged partial thromboplastin time
    (E) decreased plasma level of factor XII

85. The most common cause of congenital hypothyroidism is

    (A) dysgenesis of the thyroid gland
    (B) a defect in thyroid synthesis
    (C) Hashimoto's thyroiditis
    (D) maternal ingestion of iodides
    (E) maternal iodine deficiency

86. Which of the following statements regarding cysticercosis is true?

    (A) Pancreatitis is common
    (B) Myocarditis is the most common manifestation
    (C) Infection generally results from ingestion of undercooked pork
    (D) In most cases there is meningitis with an intense eosinophilic pleocytosis of the CSF
    (E) In the United States it is most prevalent in the southwestern region and among Mexican immigrants

87. A 17-year-old boy with cystic fibrosis complains of a 5- to 10-lb weight loss over the past month unaccompanied by changes in his pulmonary or gastrointestinal symptoms. You suspect that he has developed

    (A) a bronchogenic carcinoma
    (B) an eating disorder
    (C) biliary cirrhosis
    (D) cor pulmonale
    (E) diabetes mellitus

88. The diagnosis of cystic fibrosis is usually confirmed by the finding of

    (A) elevated sweat chloride
    (B) decreased sweat chloride
    (C) elevated serum chloride
    (D) decreased serum chloride
    (E) elevated sweat and serum chloride

89. Which of the following statements regarding acute bacterial otitis media in childhood is correct?

    (A) Fever is common, but pain is rare
    (B) It is a common cause of deafness
    (C) Infection is almost invariably bilateral
    (D) The most frequent organism is *Staphylococcus aureus*
    (E) It usually can be treated successfully with antibiotics without tympanocentesis

90. An inguinal hernia in a 2-month-old girl

    (A) may contain an ovary
    (B) is usually a direct hernia
    (C) does not require surgical repair
    (D) is a sign of pseudohermaphroditism
    (E) is generally associated with an imperforate anus

91. Which of the following would be expected in a 6-month-old child with a large ventricular septal defect?

    (A) cyanosis
    (B) an enlarged heart
    (C) a continuous cardiac murmur
    (D) decreased pulmonary vasculature on roentgenogram
    (E) evidence of predominantly right ventricular hypertrophy on ECG

Please note the use of a negative qualifier such as EXCEPT, LEAST, or NOT in each of the following questions (Questions 92 through 106).

92. Manifestations of hypoparathyroidism include all of the following EXCEPT

    (A) pseudotumor cerebri
    (B) tingling of the hands and feet
    (C) cataracts
    (D) delayed eruption of teeth
    (E) hypophosphatemia

93. Thrombocytopenia may be seen in patients with all of the following EXCEPT

    (A) giant hemangiomas
    (B) splenomegaly
    (C) congenital thrombasthenia
    (D) Wiscott-Aldrich syndrome
    (E) cyanotic congenital heart disease

94. Ehlers-Danlos syndrome is associated with all of the following EXCEPT

    (A) fragile skin that splits on slight trauma
    (B) hyperextensibility of the joints
    (C) slow wound healing
    (D) easy bruising
    (E) prolonged bleeding time

95. Which of the following statements regarding multiple cartilaginous exostoses is NOT true?

(A) It is inherited as an autosomal dominant disorder
(B) Malignant degeneration is a known but late and infrequent complication
(C) Lesions may present with pain from pressure or joint involvement
(D) Most lesions are evident at birth
(E) Lesions may occur in the vertebral bodies and ilium as well as in long bones

96. Which of the following would NOT be expected in an 8-year-old child with Cushing's syndrome?

(A) Acne and hypertrichosis
(B) Anemia
(C) Hypertension
(D) Obesity
(E) Short stature

97. The nephrotic syndrome in childhood may be seen in association with all of the following EXCEPT

(A) Marfan's syndrome
(B) lupus erythematosus
(C) congenital syphilis
(D) renal vein thrombosis
(E) gold therapy

98. Appropriate management of acute renal failure includes all of the following EXCEPT

(A) oral aluminum hydroxide gels
(B) replacement of urinary sodium losses with sodium lactate or bicarbonate
(C) restriction of water intake to 300 mL/m^2 per day plus urine output
(D) zero caloric intake
(E) zero potassium intake

99. Which of the following statements regarding children with constitutional growth delay is INCORRECT?

(A) They are small for their age
(B) They undergo puberty at the normal age
(C) Skeletal maturation is delayed
(D) They can anticipate eventual normal adult height
(E) Thyroid function is normal

100. All of the following are typical of scabies EXCEPT

(A) intense pruritus
(B) sparing of the hands and feet
(C) linear lesion ending in a black dot
(D) involvement of several members of the family
(E) papules that become excoriated and crusted

101. Which of the following is LEAST frequent with rotavirus infection?

(A) Fever
(B) Vomiting
(C) Coryza preceding the diarrhea
(D) Blood and mucus in the stool
(E) Diarrhea lasting more than 48 hours

102. Achondroplasia has been associated with all of the following EXCEPT

(A) dwarfism
(B) hydrocephalus
(C) cranial deformities
(D) long, slender fingers
(E) extremities disproportionately short in relation to head and trunk

103. Occult bacteremia refers to the finding of a positive blood culture in a child without an obvious focus for the bacteremia. Which of the following is NOT correct?

(A) It is most common in children between 6 and 24 months of age
(B) The most common organism is *S. pneumoniae*
(C) It is more common in patients with white blood cell counts of 15,000/mm^3 or more
(D) It is more common in children with temperatures equal to, or greater than, 40°C
(E) It is seen primarily in children of lower socioeconomic classes

104. Viral bronchiolitis is characterized by all of the following EXCEPT

(A) a decrease in functional residual capacity
(B) air trapping on the chest roentgenogram
(C) hypoxemia
(D) inflammation and partial occlusion of bronchioles
(E) wheezing and tachypnea

105. Hypoglycemia may be seen in association with all of the following EXCEPT

(A) aspirin poisoning
(B) ethyl alcohol ingestion
(C) hyperthyroidism
(D) hypopituitarism
(E) Reye's syndrome

106. Which of the following manifestations of sarcoidosis would be LEAST likely in a 12-year-old child with the disease?

(A) Abnormal chest roentgenogram
(B) Diabetes insipidus
(C) Hepatosplenomegaly
(D) Iridocyclitis
(E) Lymphadenopathy

DIRECTIONS: This part of the test consists of a series of cases followed by a group of related questions. For each question, study the case and select the ONE best answer to complete each statement that follows. [*Note: The student should try to complete all questions about a case before looking at the answers.*]

Questions 107 through 110

On the second day of treatment for pneumococcal meningitis, a 10-month-old child who had been alert is noted to be lethargic. Serum electrolytes reveal: Na 120 mEq/L; Cl 82 mEq/L; K 3.1 mEq/L; BUN 2 mg/dL.

107. The most likely cause of the lethargy and hypo-electrolytemia in this patient is

(A) acute hepatic failure
(B) acute renal failure
(C) congestive heart failure
(D) inappropriate secretion of ADH
(E) subdural effusions

108. The appropriate test to confirm this diagnosis would be

(A) chest roentgenogram
(B) measurement of serum and urine osmolality
(C) determination of serum creatinine
(D) measurement of hepatic enzymes
(E) CT scan of the head

109. One would also expect this patient to exhibit

(A) polyuria
(B) hypotension
(C) metabolic alkalosis
(D) high urine specific gravity
(E) high serum alkaline phosphatase

110. The most appropriate management of this problem would be

(A) administration of hypertonic (3%) saline
(B) restriction of fluid intake to about 50 to 70% of maintenance requirements
(C) restriction of sodium intake to about 10% of normal
(D) administration of a diuretic such as furosemide

Questions 111 through 113

A 12-year-old child is admitted because of the sudden onset of coma. The child had been well until about 6 hours prior to admission, when he began to complain of a headache. The headache became more severe, and the child lapsed into coma. Physical examination reveals a temperature of 38.2°C. The child is flaccid and comatose. The remainder of the physical examination is unremarkable. A lumbar puncture reveals grossly bloody spinal fluid. After centrifugation, the fluid appears xanthochromic. There are 3,000 RBCs and 7 WBCs per cubic millimeter. The protein concentration is 400 mg/dL, and the glucose is 62 mg/dL.

111. The most likely etiology of the coma is

(A) intraventricular hemorrhage
(B) subarachnoid hemorrhage
(C) aqueductal stenosis
(D) viral encephalitis
(E) subdural effusion

112. Which of the following underlying structural abnormalities would most likely have led to the above event or condition?

(A) Absence of the corpus callosum
(B) Porencephalic cyst
(C) Cerebral arteriovenous malformation
(D) Cerebral aneurysm
(E) Arnold-Chiari malformation

113. The most appropriate next step at this time would be to

(A) obtain a CT scan of the head
(B) repeat the lumbar puncture
(C) administer fresh frozen plasma
(D) perform an exchange transfusion
(E) initiate a transfusion of packed red blood cells

Questions 114 through 116

A 21-day-old male infant is admitted because of vomiting for 12 days. Birth weight was 2,925 g. The child had been normal at birth and did well for the first 9 days of life. He was initially begun on breast feeding only, but on the eighth day of life, supplemental feeding with a commercially prepared cow milk formula was added. Vomiting began on the 10th day of life and persisted despite discontinuation of the prepared formula. On the 21st day of life, the child was hospitalized. Diarrhea had never been present. Several days prior to admission, the stools had become hard and infrequent. On admission, the anterior fontanel is sunken, the mucous membranes are dry, and skin turgor is poor. The diaper is dry, and the mother cannot recall when the child last urinated. The child appears poorly nourished. Wt. 2,850 g, PR 152, RR 12, T 37.5°C. Pulses and color are good. A firm, 3-cm, olive-shaped mass is palpated deep, just to the right of the midepigastrium.

114. The most likely cause of the abdominal mass is

(A) adrenal hemorrhage
(B) intussusception
(C) neuroblastoma
(D) pancreatic pseudocyst
(E) pyloric stenosis

115. One would expect the initial laboratory data to reveal

(A) mixed metabolic and respiratory acidosis
(B) mixed metabolic and respiratory alkalosis
(C) normal acid-base status
(D) primary metabolic acidosis
(E) primary metabolic alkalosis

116. Which of the following intravenous solutions would be most appropriate as the initial hydrating fluid?

(A) 5% dextrose in water
(B) Normal saline
(C) 140 mEq/L of Na, 120 mEq/L of Cl, 20 mEq/L of bicarbonate
(D) 5% glucose, 40 mEq/L of Na, 40 mEq/L of K, 80 mEq/L of Cl
(E) 3% dextrose plus 140 mEq/L of Na, 115 mEq/L of Cl, 20 mEq/L of bicarbonate, and 5 mEq/L of K

Questions 117 through 119

A 4-month-old infant is seen because of fever, irritability, and swelling over the jaw. The fever and irritability had been present for about 3 days before the mother noted the swelling. Physical examination reveals an irritable child with bilateral diffuse swelling of the lower face. The swelling is deep and firm. A distinct mass cannot be delineated. The remainder of the physical examination is normal.

117. The most likely diagnosis is

(A) cervical lymphadenitis
(B) fibrous dysplasia of the jaw
(C) infantile cortical hyperostosis
(D) mumps
(E) osteomyelitis of the mandible

118. One would expect a roentgenogram of the mandible to show

(A) no abnormality
(B) radiolucent areas
(C) cortical destruction and resorption
(D) thickening of the bony cortex and subperiosteal new bone formation
(E) diffuse osteoporosis

119. One would also expect to find

(A) polycythemia
(B) an elevated erythrocyte sedimentation rate
(C) an elevated BUN and serum creatinine
(D) a positive blood culture
(E) presence of sickle hemoglobin

Questions 120 through 122

A 2-year-old child is hospitalized because of fever, cough, and hepatomegaly. The child lives in a poor, crowded home on a small farm. No one else at home is ill. Physical examination reveals a thin child with marked hepatomegaly. The spleen is not palpable, and all lymph nodes are within normal limits. There are mild bilateral rales and wheezes, minimal tachypnea, and retractions. The remainder of the examination is within normal limits. Chest x-ray reveals bilateral scattered densities. White blood cell count is 14,000/mm^3 with 36% eosinophils.

120. Which of the following would be most likely to establish the diagnosis in this patient?

(A) Bone marrow aspiration
(B) Stool examination
(C) Blood smear
(D) Liver biopsy
(E) Duodenal aspiration

121. The child most likely acquired the disease by

(A) eating poorly cooked pork
(B) eating dirt
(C) kissing a dog
(D) contact with a sick bird
(E) contact with a sick rodent

122. Which of the following is LEAST likely also to be found in this patient?

(A) Nephritis
(B) Hyperglobulinemia
(C) Elevated serum anti-A and/or anti-B isohemagglutinin titer
(D) A retinal lesion
(E) Myocarditis

Questions 123 through 125

A 4-month-old girl is admitted because of failure to thrive and persistent pneumonia. The child was well at birth but severe, recurrent diarrhea began at about 6 weeks of age. At 8 weeks the child developed pneumonia, which responded only poorly to antibiotic therapy. Recurrent monilial infection of the skin and oral mucosa had been a problem. Physical examination reveals a small, poorly nourished child with moderate respiratory distress. There are bilateral rales, oral thrush, and a monilial-appearing rash in the diaper area. The remainder of the examination is within normal limits. The total white blood cell count is 5,200/mm^3 with 87% polymorphonuclear cells, 12% lymphocytes, and 1% eosinophils. Serum immunoglobulin levels are: IgA not detectable; IgG 280 mg/dL; IgM <5 mg/dL.

123. Which of the following diagnoses best explains the clinical picture?

(A) Pediatric AIDS
(B) Wiskott-Aldrich syndrome
(C) Hereditary agammaglobulinemia
(D) Severe combined immunodeficiency
(E) Transient hypogammaglobulinemia of infancy

124. On further evaluation one would also expect to find

(A) increased numbers of plasma cells on bone marrow examination
(B) enlarged superficial lymph nodes
(C) absent thymic shadow on chest roentgenogram
(D) positive intradermal reaction to *Candida* antigen
(E) Western blot positive for HIV

125. Chest roentgenogram reveals bilateral patchy consolidations and diffuse granular densities with an almost ground-glass appearance to the lungs. The most likely cause of this x-ray picture is

(A) pneumococcal pneumonia
(B) *Pneumocystis carinii* pneumonia
(C) pulmonary hemorrhage
(D) pulmonary lymphangiectasia
(E) miliary tuberculosis

Questions 126 through 128

A 4-month-old boy had been well until 4 weeks prior to admission, when vomiting and poor appetite were noted. Psychomotor development had been normal. The child was being fed whole cow milk and strained foods. Stools were normal. On the morning of admission, the child had a generalized convulsion and was brought to the emergency room, where the seizure was controlled with intravenous medication. A second seizure occurred about 1 hour later and again responded to intravenous medication. Physical examination revealed a pale, listless infant, poorly nourished, but in no acute distress. The height was at the 25th percentile, the weight at the 3rd percentile, and the head circumference over the 97th percentile on a standard growth curve. The anterior fontanel was full but not bulging. There were no focal neurologic signs. T 38°C, RR 16, HR 110, BP 70 by flush. The remainder of the examination was within normal limits.

126. Which of the following diagnoses is most likely?

(A) Tuberculous meningitis
(B) Mastoiditis
(C) Subdural hematoma
(D) Congenital toxoplasmosis
(E) Pseudotumor cerebri

127. Roentgenograms of the skull reveal widened sutures but no other abnormality. The eyes are dilated with atropine, and the fundi examined carefully. Bilateral retinal hemorrhages are noted. The most likely diagnosis now is

(A) Tuberculous meningitis
(B) Mastoiditis
(C) Subdural hematoma
(D) Congenital toxoplasmosis
(E) Pseudotumor cerebri

128. The correct diagnosis could best be established by

(A) lumbar puncture
(B) electroencephalography
(C) CT scan of the head
(D) bone marrow examination
(E) conjunctival biopsy

DIRECTIONS (129 through 135): Each set of matching questions in this section consists of a list of 4 to 26 lettered options followed by several numbered items. For each numbered item select the ONE lettered option with which it is most closely associated. Each lettered option may be selected once, more than once, or not at all.

Questions 129 through 135

A. Acetylcysteine	N. Methylene blue
B. Atropine	O. Naloxone
C. Ammonium chloride	P. Nitroprusside
D. Calcium chloride	Q. Phenobarbital
E. Deferoxamine	R. Phenylephrine
F. Digoxin	S. Physostigmine
G. EDTA	T. Potassium chloride
H. Ethanol	U. Potassium citrate
I. Fresh frozen plasma	V. Propranolol
J. Furosemide	W. Sodium bicarbonate
K. Glucagon	X. Sodium chloride
L. Methionine	Y. Sodium nitrite
M. Methyldopa	Z. Whole blood

For each drug or poison, select the most specific and most important antidote.

129. Lead

130. Iron

131. Acetaminophen

132. Organophosphate

133. Cyanide

134. Ethylene glycol

135. Morphine

DIRECTIONS (Questions 136 through 162): Each group of items in this section consists of lettered headings followed by a set of numbered words or phrases. For each numbered word or phrase, select

A if the item is associated with (A) <u>only</u>,
B if the item is associated with (B) <u>only</u>,
C if the item is associated with <u>both</u> (A) <u>and</u> (B),
D if the item is associated with <u>neither</u> (A) <u>nor</u> (B).

Questions 136 through 141

(A) Acute glomerulonephritis
(B) Minimal-change nephrotic syndrome
(C) Both
(D) Neither

136. Elevated serum antistreptolysin O titer

137. Response to corticosteroids

138. Hematuria

139. Hypercellularity of glomeruli, swelling of basement membrane, and subepithelial deposits of "electron-dense" material

140. Pneumococcal peritonitis

141. Eventual chronic renal failure in more than 50% of cases

Questions 142 through 144

    (A) Cystic fibrosis
    (B) Idiopathic celiac disease (gluten-induced enteropathy)
    (C) Both
    (D) Neither

142. Steatorrhea

143. Hepatoma

144. Management includes a wheat-free diet

Questions 145 through 146

    (A) Turner's syndrome
    (B) Klinefelter's syndrome
    (C) Both
    (D) Neither

145. Short stature

146. Infertility

Questions 147 through 150

    (A) Coxa plana (Legg-Calvé-Perthes disease)
    (B) Slipped femoral epiphysis
    (C) Both
    (D) Neither

147. Most common at around the time of puberty

148. May be bilateral

149. More common in girls than in boys

150. Associated with precocious puberty

151. Surgical nailing the treatment of choice

Questions 152 through 155

    (A) Autosomal recessive
    (B) X-linked recessive
    (C) Both
    (D) Neither

152. Clinical disease rare in females

153. Both parents generally clinically normal

154. Transmission of abnormal gene from father to son

155. Affected persons marrying normal persons usually have clinically normal offspring

Questions 156 through 158

    (A) Myasthenia gravis
    (B) Duchenne muscular dystrophy
    (C) Both
    (D) Neither

156. Muscle fasciculations

157. Skeletal muscle weakness

158. Involvement of cardiac muscle

Questions 159 through 162

    (A) Hereditary spherocytosis
    (B) Sickle cell disease
    (C) Both
    (D) Neither

159. Positive Coombs's test

160. Neonatal hyperbilirubinemia

161. Reticulocytosis

162. Abnormal hemoglobin electrophoresis

Answers and Explanations

1. (E) Secretory otitis media (SOM), also called serous OM and nonsuppurative OM, is a condition of persistent fluid in the middle ear. Although it is characterized by the absence of fever and the lack of signs or evidence of inflammation of the tympanic membrane (TM), pathogenic bacteria can be recovered from the middle ear in up to a third of cases. It is a common finding in young children, usually following an episode of acute bacterial OM. Most cases resolve spontaneously, although often only after many months. The classic finding, on which diagnosis is based, is a thickened TM that does not vibrate with pneumotoscopy. *(Hoekelman:1419; Rudolph:939)*

2. (A) Multicystic kidney is one type of renal dysplasia, a group of disorders characterized by developmental abnormalities of kidney structure and differentiation. The entity is *not* related to polycystic kidney disease. Bilateral multicystic kidneys are rapidly fatal in the newborn period. The unilateral multicystic kidney usually presents in infancy as an abdominal mass. Hypertension has been noted but is rare. In unilateral cases, renal function is preserved by the opposite normal kidney. *(Rudolph:1256)*

3. (B) The term Fanconi's syndrome currently is used to indicate a complex dysfunction of the proximal tubules characterized by glycosuria, aminoaciduria, and phosphaturia. Blood glucose as well as urea and creatinine levels usually are normal. It may be seen as an isolated finding (primary Fanconi's syndrome) or secondary to disorders such as cystinosis or tyrosinemia. [*Note:* Fanconi's syndrome is not related to Fanconi's anemia, an autosomal recessive disorder characterized by pancytopenia and hypoplastic thumb and radius.] *(Rudolph:1282)*

4. (E) The defect in proximal renal tubular acidosis is renal loss of bicarbonate because of an abnormally low threshold. Serum chloride is elevated, and serum bicarbonate is low. Therefore, choices **(A)**, **(C)**, and **(D)** can be eliminated. A distinctive feature of these patients is their unimpaired ability to excrete adequate amounts of titratable acid and thereby lower urinary pH. The urine pH usually is

acid in these patients when the serum bicarbonate level is low. However, if they are given an infusion of bicarbonate to raise the serum level, urine pH will be alkaline during the infusion. *(Rudolph:1277–1278)*

5. (E) The presence of bilateral renal masses and a midline suprapubic mass (the distended bladder) in a newborn infant is congenital urethral or bladder neck obstruction until proven otherwise. Posterior urethral valves are an especially important cause of such obstruction in the male infant. Early diagnosis is critical, as the renal parenchyma eventually will be destroyed by the resultant hydronephrosis. *(Rudolph:1297)*

6. (A) An abdominal or flank mass is the most common presenting sign in children with Wilms's tumor. Often, the mass is discovered on routine examination or during examination for a minor illness. Occasionally, the parents will bring the child to the physician because they note an enlarging abdomen or feel the mass themselves. *(Rudolph:1199)*

7. (E) In patients with acute poststreptococcal glomerulonephritis, clinical findings generally clear before the laboratory abnormalities do. Hypertension and edema usually clear in days to weeks. Serum complement (C_3) levels return to normal by 1 to 2 months. Impaired urea or creatinine clearance may last 6 months or more, and microscopic hematuria may persist for more than a year before finally resolving. *(Rudolph:1262)*

8. (E) *Pseudomonas aeruginosa* is the most common cause of fatal bacterial septicemia in most series of children with leukemia. *E. coli* and *S. aureus* also are common. The other bacteria listed are infrequently the cause of fatal sepsis in these patients. *(Am J Dis Child 122:283–287,1971)*

9. (B) In most regards, chronic ambulatory peritoneal dialysis compares favorably to other methods of chronic dialysis. Growth, dietary restrictions, and electrolyte problems are about the same as with other dialysis programs. However, there is a high rate of peritonitis. *(Rudolph:1252)*

10. **(D)** Autosomal recessive congenital nephrotic syndrome (NS) is believed to result from a defect in the chemical structure of the basement membrane and is characterized pathologically by microcytic dilatation of the proximal tubules. Proteinuria and edema develop early, and death from renal failure in a few months is common. As might be anticipated from the etiology and pathology, there is no response to corticosteroids. This genetic form of congenital NS must be distinguished from congenital NS with causes such as syphilis or renal vein thrombosis. *(Rudolph:1273)*

11. **(B)** Most cases of minimal-change nephrotic syndrome begin between 2 and 5 years of age with a peak age of onset between 2 and 3 years of age. This is especially true for those cases associated with minimal-change morphology. Older children presenting with nephrotic syndrome are more likely to have an underlying chronic nephritis (eg, membranoproliferative glomerulonephritis, lupus nephritis) rather than minimal-change nephrotic syndrome. *(Rudolph:1268)*

12. **(E)** A low serum concentration of the C3 component of complement in a child with nephrotic syndrome almost always indicates the presence of membranoproliferative disease (assuming that the child does not have systemic lupus). Membranoproliferative glomerulonephritis is very unlikely either to respond to corticosteroids or to remit spontaneously. *(Rudolph:1268–1269)*

13. **(D)** Uneven ventilation occurs early in an attack of asthma and leads to ventilation-perfusion imbalance and hypoxemia. At this stage, the patient is still able to "blow-off" carbon dioxide via the least-obstructed regions of the lung, so the arterial PCO_2 is normal or low. Hypoxemia characteristically precedes hypercarbia. Only when obstruction is so generalized and severe that alveolar ventilation falls does the arterial PCO_2 rise. Thus, early in an attack of asthma, the arterial PCO_2 is apt to be normal or low; the PO_2 is always low. *(Rudolph:507)*

14. **(B)** Generalized or diffuse hyperinflation of the lungs, manifested by an increased anteroposterior diameter of the thorax and flattened diaphragms, is the earliest and most frequent roentgenographic abnormality in children with asthma. Infiltrations, atelectasis, and pneumomediastinum are seen occasionally during an acute attack. Bronchiectasis is a rare complication and would suggest the possibility of an underlying disorder such as cystic fibrosis, immunodeficiency, foreign body, or recurrent aspiration. *(N Engl J Med 309:336,1900,1983; Rudolph:507)*

15. **(B)** Achondroplasia is an autosomal dominant Mendelian disorder. Most cases, however, are sporadic, the result of new autosomal dominant mutations. The incidence is approximately 1 in 26,000 live births. *(Rudolph:398)*

16. **(D)** For reasons that still are not understood, the most common bacterial organisms infecting the lungs of children with cystic fibrosis are *Staphylococcus aureus* and *Pseudomonas aeruginosa*. This has not changed much in the past two decades despite major changes in our antibiotic armamentarium. *Pseudomonas* is particularly difficult to eradicate despite sensitivity in vitro to a variety of antibiotics. *(Rudolph:1531)*

17. **(A)** Cleft lip, with or without cleft palate, seems genetically distinct from the isolated cleft palate. A sibling born to a child with either a cleft lip or a cleft palate has an increased risk of the same but not the other lesion. If the cleft is part of a recognized malformation syndrome, the genetics of that syndrome apply. When either cleft lip or cleft palate occurs as an isolated finding, the etiology is believed to be multifactorial, and recurrence risks in siblings are based on empiric data rather than on Mendelian patterns. *(Rudolph:433)*

18. **(D)** In the congenital abnormality of anomalous origin of the left coronary artery, the aberrant left coronary artery arises from the pulmonary artery rather than from the aorta. This results in perfusion of the left ventricle by poorly oxygenated blood under low pressure. Myocardial ischemia can be severe. The presenting signs are irritability (presumably from cardiac pain) and congestive heart failure. Myocardial infarction is not uncommon. *(Rudolph:1363–1364)*

19. **(E)** The findings of cyanosis and blood that is chocolate brown and does not become red on exposure to air are indicative of methemoglobinemia. One cause of methemoglobinemia is exposure to well water that has been contaminated with nitrites. Carbon monoxide poisoning (automobile exhaust) results in carboxyhemoglobin, which binds oxygen so tightly that it cannot be released to the tissues. In this situation the blood would be bright red rather than dark brown. Fava beans are a cause of hemolysis in patients with G6PD deficiency but are not a cause of methemoglobinemia. *(Rudolph:808)*

20. **(B)** The principal symptom of serous otitis media is hearing loss. Many cases are asymptomatic and are detected by the appearance of the tympanic membrane on routine physical examination or by a routine hearing test. Although the role of infection is uncertain, the pathogenesis appears to be primarily eustachian tube dysfunction. Fluid obtained by myringotomy may be thin or glue-like and is sterile

in about two-thirds to three-quarters of cases. *(Rudolph:940)*

21. **(D)** Pica may be defined as ingestion of nonfood substances such as dirt and flakes of peeling paint. The latter is important as a potential source of lead poisoning. In some cases, pica may be a sign of an emotional or behavioral problem. *(Rudolph:106)*

22. **(C)** The primary lesion in acne is plugging of the duct of the sebaceous gland by dried or excessive sebum and keratin. The obstructed gland (comedo) eventually becomes inflamed. The relative roles of fatty acids, bacteria such as *Propionibacterium acnes* and *Staphylococcus epidermidis*, and the immunologic response in determining this inflammatory reaction are uncertain. [*Note:* The question asked for the *primary* lesion in acne. Infection of the gland, which is an important factor in many cases, is a *secondary* rather than a primary lesion.] *(Rudolph:918)*

23. **(B)** Although all the diseases listed can cause nasal obstruction and discharge, allergic rhinitis is by far the most common and the most likely in this child. Bilateral choanal atresia causes respiratory distress in the neonatal period; unilateral atresia causes persistent unilateral purulent discharge. Immunodeficiency is most likely to cause chronic sinusitis and purulent discharge. Cystic fibrosis is much less common than allergy, and a defect in the cribriform plate is extremely rare. *(Rudolph:503–504)*

24. **(D)** Atopic dermatitis (eczema) is characterized by exudation, pruritus, and lichenification. Involvement in infancy is common, although the distribution and other features may be somewhat different than in older children. The classical adult distribution with predilection for popliteal and antecubital areas usually is not seen in infancy. Involvement of the face is common. Most patients have *elevated* serum IgE levels and normal levels of the other immunoglobulins. *(Rudolph:884–885)*

25. **(B)** The copperhead is a member of the group of poisonous snakes known as pit vipers or *Crotalids*. This group also includes the rattlesnake and the cottonmouth (water moccasin). All members of the group share similar toxins, the effects of which include local tissue injury and necrosis, neurologic manifestations, generalized bleeding, and shock. The severity of the reaction is related to the amount of venom injected (size of snake) and the size of the victim. Local reactions are most common and are seen in almost all significant envenomations. Systemic reactions are less frequent and generally are seen only with severe envenomations. *(Rudolph:825–826)*

26. **(E)** The major concern for children with chronic serous otitis is that the associated conductive hearing loss will interfere with speech and language development during the critical early years of life. Although some authors have suggested that permanent hearing loss may develop from damage to the middle ear, this is uncommon and, in any event, would be conductive rather than nerve deafness. These children are not especially subject to pyogenic complications such as mastoiditis, meningitis, and perforation of the tympanic membrane. *(Rudolph:940)*

27. **(E)** The sudden onset of bilateral sensorineural deafness without apparent etiology is a tragic but well-recognized event in childhood. These children do not go on to develop signs of any systemic illness, and the cause of the deafness is believed to be a viral labyrinthitis with destruction of the cochlea. *(Adv Otorhinolaryngol 20:229–235,1973; Otolaryngol Head Neck Surg 89:137–141,1981)*

28. **(E)** Nasal polyps are uncommon in childhood. The two leading causes are allergy (allergic rhinitis) and cystic fibrosis. Although allergy is more common, any child with nasal polyps probably should have a sweat test, since allergic manifestations are not uncommon in children with cystic fibrosis. Certain rare benign (hemangioma, fibroma) and malignant (rhabdomyosarcoma, esthesioneuroblastoma) lesions can be mistaken for polyps. *(Rudolph:504,1527,1529)*

29. **(C)** Unlike the situation in older children and adults, in infants the most frequent target organ of alpha-1-antitrypsin deficiency is the liver. This may take the form of prolonged neonatal cholestasis and/or cirrhosis and portal hypertension. Obstructive lung disease may be seen in older children but is rare in infancy. *(Rudolph:1069–1070,1545)*

30. **(C)** Unlike the situation in adults, in *infants* and children less than 7 years of age, Cushing's syndrome is almost always caused by an adrenal cortical tumor, usually a carcinoma. Pituitary dysfunction or pituitary tumor as a cause of increased cortisol production is exceedingly rare in young children. When it does occur, it is more properly referred to as Cushing's *disease*. Even more rarely, the syndrome can result from ACTH produced by a nonpituitary tumor. *(Rudolph:1604)*

31. **(B)** The most common tumor to cause destruction of the anterior pituitary gland in childhood is the craniopharyngioma. Gliomas, germinomas, and hamartomas also can involve the pituitary gland in childhood. The chromophobe adenoma is the most common destructive lesion in adults but is rare in childhood. *(Rudolph:1576)*

32. **(C)** In patients with sickle cell disease the hemoglobin is generally between 7 and 10 g/dL, although it may drop considerably lower during an aplastic or a hyperhemolytic crisis. Hemoglobin values above 10

g/dL are uncommon in children with sickle cell disease except in young infants, in whom the presence of fetal hemoglobin protects against sickling. *(Hathaway:487)*

33. **(B)** Sickle cell disease rarely is manifest during the neonatal period, when fetal hemoglobin is protective against sickling. Most splenic sequestration crises occur during infancy and early childhood and are uncommon after the fourth or fifth birthday, by which time autosplenectomy from recurrent infarctions has occurred. In patients with sickle-C disease or sickle-thalassemia, however, the spleen may remain large, and sequestration crises can occur into the teens and adulthood. *(Rudolph:1125–1126)*

34. **(A)** The fall in oxygen saturation from the left atrium to the left ventricle indicates a right-to-left shunt at the ventricular level. The drop in pressure from the right ventricle to the pulmonary artery and the low pulmonary artery pressure indicate pulmonic stenosis rather than pulmonary hypertension. A simple ventricular septal defect (VSD) or a VSD plus aortic valve insufficiency would cause a left-to-right shunt. Eisenmenger's syndrome is a VSD with pulmonary hypertension and reversal of shunt. The catheterization data indicate pulmonary stenosis and a right-to-left shunt through a VSD, findings most compatible with the diagnosis of tetralogy of Fallot. *(Rudolph:1397)*

35. **(B)** This child probably has cyclic neutropenia, a defect in the production of granulocyte-macrophage colony-stimulating factor (GM-CSF). In these patients GM-CSF is produced in a cyclic rather than continuous manner. Episodes of neutropenia, often accompanied by fever, aphthous stomatitis, and cervical lymphadenitis recur at *regular* intervals, usually every 21 to 42 days. Few other conditions have such a remarkable periodicity. Schwachman-Diamond syndrome is the association of neutropenia with exocrine pancreatic insufficiency. Chédiak-Higashi syndrome is an autosomal recessive disorder characterized by morphologically abnormal neutrophils (as well as eventual pancytopenia), recurrent infections, partial albinism, and mental retardation. *(Rudolph:1143)*

36. **(B)** Although some cases of encopresis may be secondary to organic causes (spina bifida, Hirschsprung's disease), the majority are psychological or behavioral in nature. Even when the encopresis is secondary to fecal retention, the fecal retention itself usually is on a psychological basis. In contrast, the majority of cases of enuresis are primary and generally are not considered to represent an emotional or behavioral disorder. Rather, enuresis probably reflects a disturbance of bladder physiology or sleep mechanism. Some cases of secondary enuresis (enuresis in a child who previously had been dry), however, do result from emotional factors. Most functional headaches are not migraines. *(Rudolph:110–112)*

37. **(B)** Hysterical episodes simulating seizures rarely are associated with bodily injury, incontinence, or postictal sleep. The pseudoseizures frequently are triggered by bizarre stimuli, and the pattern of the seizure changes often. The patient actually is awake and aware of his or her surroundings and events and can recall them later. *(J Pediatr 94:153,1979; Rudolph:1770)*

38. **(B)** Pseudotumor cerebri is also referred to as benign intracranial hypertension. These patients do not develop seizures, coma, or herniation syndromes. The only recognized permanent deficit is decreased visual acuity secondary to long-standing papilledema. *(Rudolph:1747–1748)*

39. **(A)** Fever, purulent nasal discharge, and local tenderness in the region of a nasal sinus (in this case, the maxillary sinus) are characteristic of acute sinusitis. Retropharyngeal abscess presents with fever, dysphagia, and sometimes respiratory distress, usually in a younger child. In the absence of redness or swelling around the eye, periorbital cellulitis would be an unlikely diagnosis. *(Rudolph:948)*

40. **(B)** Pulmonary hypertension with cor pulmonale is an infrequent but important complication of chronic upper airway obstruction secondary to enlarged tonsils and adenoids in young children. These children appear to hypoventilate, especially when asleep. The hypoxemia that results from the hypoventilation causes pulmonary arteriolar vasoconstriction, and this, in turn, results in cor pulmonale. *(Rudolph:954, 1389)*

41. **(C)** Essentially all febrile seizures occur in children between 6 months and 5 years of age. Indeed, most authors incorporate this age range into the definition of febrile convulsions, although some broaden the definition to between 3 months and 6 years. The peak age clearly is between 6 months and 3 years. In one study, the mean age was 23 months. One should be very suspicious of the diagnosis of a febrile seizure in a child much younger than 6 months or older than 5 years. *(Hathaway:667; Pediatrics 61:720,1978)*

42. **(C)** The clinical picture described is extremely suggestive of a brain tumor. Head tilt in these cases can arise from several mechanisms, including cranial nerve involvement with acute strabismus and secondary compensation by tilting the head. Head tilt is particularly common with posterior fossa tumors. Although headache and vomiting can be seen with a brain abscess, head tilt is very unusual in this condition. *(Rudolph:1682,1733)*

43. (C) Hartnup's disease is an inborn error of transport of tryptophan and certain other amino acids. There is increased renal tubular loss of the involved amino acids. The disorder is associated with attacks of cerebellar ataxia, which resolve spontaneously but also can be reversed by the administration of nicotinic acid. None of the other conditions listed is associated with ataxia. *(Rudolph:316)*

44. (B) In children with cleft palate or submucosal cleft palate or short palate, the adenoidal tissue helps close off the nasopharynx during speech. Removal of the adenoids in such children may precipitate nasal speech and generally is contraindicated. All of the other choices listed actually have been suggested as *indications* for adenoidectomy, although the usefulness of adenoidectomy in recurrent or persistent otitis media is questionable. *(Rudolph:954)*

45. (C) The rash described is that of a contact dermatitis, most likely from poison ivy. The lesions are papules and vesicles and are intensely pruritic. Restriction of the rash to the legs also is characteristic of poison ivy. Although the rash of Henoch-Schönlein purpura is usually restricted to below the waist, it is purpuric rather than pruritic. *(Rudolph:888)*

46. (E) Many cases of intestinal malrotation (a congenital malformation of bowel orientation) are associated with adhesive bands (Ladd's bands) that run from the cecum to the left upper quadrant and can partially or completely obstruct the duodenum. Most cases of malrotation present with vomiting within the first few weeks of life, either because of Ladd's band or because of a midgut volvulus. A few remain asymptomatic. There is no recognized association with hypoglycemia or necrotizing enterocolitis. *(Rudolph:1032)*

47. (C) The classic radiologic finding in duodenal atresia is dilatation of the stomach and of the proximal duodenum—the so-called "double-bubble" sign. Although there is no gas beyond the atretic duodenum, there is gas in the stomach and proximal duodenum, so the abdomen is not totally gasless. *(Hathaway:543)*

48. (D) Ketotic hypoglycemia is a substrate-limited normoinsulinemic condition of young children. There appears to be a problem in mobilizing amino acids, such as alanine, for gluconeogenesis. Serum alanine levels are low. Symptoms tend to improve with age, and spontaneous remission usually occurs before 10 years of age. Most of these children are thin. Attacks may be induced by a high-fat, low-calorie diet. *(Rudolph:328)*

49. (B) The picture described is most suggestive of the X-linked recessive disorder of end-organ insensitivity to androgenic hormones (testicular feminization). Although the 20,22-desmolase deficiency does cause male pseudohermaphroditism, the associated adre-

nal insufficiency is quickly fatal in infancy unless diagnosed and treated. All other forms of congenital adrenal hyperplasia are virilizing rather than feminizing. True hermaphroditism is very rare and requires that both testicular and ovarian tissue be present. No evidence for this is presented in this case. *(Rudolph:1656–1657)*

50. (D) Bleeding into the skin and mucous membranes (petechiae, ecchymosis, and epistaxis) is the most common manifestation of platelet dysfunction. Hemarthrosis is seen frequently in hemophilia but is uncommon in platelet disorders. Gastrointestinal bleeding, as well as spontaneous hemorrhage into brain and other viscera, occurs but, fortunately, is infrequent. *(Rudolph:1159)*

51. (D) Annular pancreas is a congenital malformation in which the pancreas encircles the duodenum. The condition may be asymptomatic or may cause partial or complete duodenal obstruction. The most frequent presenting complaint is vomiting. *(Rudolph: 1002)*

52. (E) Breath-holding spells always terminate spontaneously and are never fatal; they have no known relationship to sudden infant death syndrome. Breath-holding attacks are common in early childhood, with a peak incidence between 12 and 18 months, and usually disappear by about 5 years of age. The exact mechanism or etiology is not known. Although many youngsters will hold their breath to the point of cyanosis and syncope or seizure, there is nothing to suggest that breath holding is a type of epilepsy. Rather, the syncope and seizure are secondary to cerebral hypoxia. *(Rudolph:739)*

53. (D) The major manifestation of pinworm (*Enterobius vermicularis*) infection is rectal or perirectal itching. Mild infestations often are asymptomatic. Occasionally, the worms, which leave the rectum at night to lay their eggs in the perineal area, may wander into the vagina, causing pain and/or itching. A relationship to appendicitis has been suggested but is dubious. *(Rudolph:721)*

54. (D) Although all the conditions listed as possible answers are associated with bullous lesions, epidermolysis bullosa (EB) is the best fit and should be highest on the differential diagnosis. There are at least 15 known forms of EB, varying in severity and age of presentation. Many present in the newborn period, with lesions mostly at areas of friction or trauma, as described in this patient. Both drug-induced toxic epidermal necrolysis (rare in neonates) and staphylococcal scalded-skin syndrome (common in neonates) are associated with more generalized erythema and lesions than described in this patient. Neither the lesions of bullous impetigo nor the lesions of congenital syphilis are related to areas of trauma; the latter have a special predilection for the palms and soles. *(Rudolph:612,619,906–909)*

55. **(C)** Juvenile polyps are most commonly found in the rectum. These are hamartomas with inflammatory infiltration. They are not adenomatous polyps and are neither malignant nor premalignant. They generally present in the first 5 years of life with the passage of red blood streaking on the stool. *(Pediatr Clin North Am 32:1259–1260,1985; Rudolph:1029–1030)*

56. **(A)** The child described probably has a gastric trichobezoar (hair ball). It sounds as if she has trichotillomania, the habit of pulling out scalp hairs and swallowing them. Often, the hairs fail to pass from the stomach and form a mass, which causes pain and vomiting. The mass frequently is quite large and may be palpable on physical examination. *(Hoekelman:818)*

57. **(C)** Although advances in surgical care and the availability of antibiotics have reduced the overall mortality from appendicitis in the first 2 years of life to less than 1% (mortality rate in the neonatal period is still very high), the majority of cases are perforated by the time of diagnosis. There is no relationship to Meckel's diverticulum or hemangioma of the appendix, although some cases in young infants are related to colonic obstruction from Hirshsprung's disease. Fever is common. Surgical intervention is required in all cases of appendicitis regardless of age. *(Rudolph:1036; Hathaway:550)*

58. **(E)** Umbilical hernias are quite common, especially in premature and in black infants. Although there is an increased incidence of umbilical hernias in infants with a variety of syndromes (eg, Beckwith-Wiedmann) and diseases (eg, hypothyroidism), the great majority occur in otherwise normal infants. Most resolve spontaneously, and no therapy is required except for the rare case that incarcerates. An abdominal ultrasound examination should be done *only* if there is clinical evidence of an abdominal mass or ascites. Strapping or taping is ineffective and irritating and should not be advised. *(Hoekelman:1548; Hathaway:553)*

59. **(B)** Chylous ascites is characterized by a high concentration of lipids in the ascitic fluid. Most cases in infancy are caused by congenital malformation of lymph channels; occasional cases result from obstruction of the thoracic duct, tumor, inflammation, or intestinal obstruction. Loss of albumin, gammaglobulin, and lymphocytes in the ascitic fluid leads to depletion of these elements from the blood. The prognosis is guarded, even with treatment. Spontaneous resolution has been reported but is the exception rather than the rule. *(Hathaway:548–549)*

60. **(C)** The clinical picture described, including the pleural effusion, is typical of acute pancreatitis. Al-

though tuberculosis could explain the pleural effusion, it doesn't explain the acute abdomen. *C. difficile* can be a cause of severe pseudomembranous colitis but is not associated with an acute abdomen and doesn't explain the pleural effusion. *(Rudolph: 1028, 1044–1045)*

61. **(D)** Although idiopathic scoliosis can present at any stage of growth, it is most commonly manifest during or shortly before adolescence. It is considerably more frequent in girls than in boys. These children are mentally and intellectually normal. The condition is never painful and is usually detected on routine physical examination. *(Rudolph:1950–1951)*

62. **(E)** Thrombosis of the portal vein is the leading cause of portal hypertension in children *without evidence of cirrhosis*. In most cases, the thrombosis occurred in the neonatal period. Hepatic *function* is normal, and the children usually present years later with varices. Although obstruction of the portal vein by tumor could explain the clinical picture in this case, such an occurrence is exceedingly rare in childhood. Intrahepatic biliary atresia leads to biliary cirrhosis in the first year of life; the child would be jaundiced. *(Pediatr Clin North Am 32:1255–1258,1985; J Pediatr 103:696–702,1983; Rudolph:998)*

63. **(C)** Chronic cough, clubbing, and rectal prolapse should immediately suggest cystic fibrosis. All three of these findings are common in this disorder. None of the other disorders would explain all of the symptoms listed. Whipworms (rather than pinworms) can cause rectal prolapse but would not cause cough or clubbing, as there is no systemic or pulmonary phase of this parasite. Agammaglobulinemia can be associated with chronic pneumonia and bronchiectasis, and therefore cough and clubbing, but is not associated with rectal prolapse. *(Rudolph:1528–1529)*

64. **(B)** The minute structures attached to the hairs are most likely nits, the eggs of the scalp louse (pediculosis capitis). The safest and most effective treatment of scalp lice is the topical application of a 1% permethrin cream rinse. Griseofulvin is useful for certain fungal infections such as tinea capitis but is not effective against pediculosis. Tetracycline orally or topically is ineffective against lice. *(Hoekelman:1306–1307; Hathaway:280)*

65. **(B)** Chemical pneumonitis is the most common clinical manifestation of poisoning with hydrocarbons such as kerosene and may result from the aspiration of even minute amounts. Central nervous system changes are less common but can be seen, especially with large doses. Hepatic involvement is generally not a problem. Peripheral neuritis and aplastic anemia do not occur. *(Rudolph:804–805)*

66. **(B)** Congenital hypothyroidism may be associated with prolonged neonatal hyperbilirubinemia, either

unconjugated or mixed. The unconjugated hyperbilirubinemia is caused by impaired hepatic glucuronidation of bilirubin and by enhanced enterohepatic circulation of bilirubin secondary to decreased intestinal motility. The mechanism of the mixed hyperbilirubinemia is uncertain. Hypothyroidism also can be associated with anemia and impaired renal function, but these are mild. *(Hathaway:81)*

67. (B) Laryngomalacia is a condition of excessive compliance, or softness, of the cartilage of the larynx. It is presumed to be a problem of maturation rather than a congenital abnormality and is the most common cause of persistent inspiratory stridor in the young infant. Symptoms usually begin in the first month of life, are worse with agitation and in the supine position, and eventually resolve, usually by a year or so. Foreign body aspiration is an important cause of persistent stridor in the older infant and toddler but would be very unusual at this age. *(Rudolph:957; Hoekelman:1080)*

68. (B) Hypercalciuria has been found in a very significant number of children with otherwise unexplained gross or microscopic hematuria. In most cases, the hematuria is not associated with renal stones or precedes the formation of stones by many years. The serum level of calcium is normal in these patients. *(N Engl J Med 310:1345–1348,1984; J Pediatr 99:712–715, 716–719,1983; Rudolph:1242)*

69. (B) The chest roentgenogram reveals air trapping of the left lung with a shift of the heart and mediastinum to the right. This is most suggestive of a foreign body in the left mainstem bronchus. In the case of infantile lobar emphysema, the findings would be present in the first few months of life and would not cause the sudden onset of wheezing at 4 years of age. Also, in this condition, one lobe rather than an entire lung would be overdistended. Asthma is associated with bilateral, rather than unilateral, air trapping. *(Am J Dis Child 141:259–262,1987; Rudolph:1519)*

70. (B) The unequal leg length and asymmetry of the inguinal (anterior) and thigh (posterior) skin creases are indicative of severe congenital dislocation of the hip. Neither tibial torsion nor equinovarus deformity affect leg length or inguinal skin creases. Arthrogryposis is associated with severe contractures. *(Rudolph:1929–1931)*

71. (E) Any child with uveitis involving primarily the *anterior* structures of the eye should be suspected of having juvenile rheumatoid arthritis (JRA). This association is strongest in girls with the pauciarticular form of JRA, especially those who are antinuclear antibody positive. Toxoplasmosis and toxocara are more likely to be associated with *posterior* uveitis. Neither leukemia nor hypoparathyroidism is associated with uveitis. *(Rudolph:1906–1907)*

72. (E) This child most likely has sarcoidosis, and many patients with this disease have an elevated serum level of angiotensin-converting enzyme (ACE). Although not all patients with sarcoid have an elevated serum level of ACE, elevated levels are so infrequent in other conditions that it is a useful diagnostic test. Tuberculosis is the only other listed condition that might be considered for this youngster. However, the diffuse interstitial infiltrates (rather than a nodular or miliary picture) are not characteristic of tuberculosis, and the hilar adenopathy in tuberculosis is usually unilateral rather than bilateral. *(Rudolph:1542)*

73. (C) Acute glomerulonephritis (AGN) is most common between ages 5 and 10 years. It usually follows a streptococcal infection, either pharyngeal or skin, by 1 to 2 weeks rather than a few days. It is quite clear from renal biopsy studies that have included asymptomatic family members of the index case that poststreptococcal AGN is asymptomatic in 50 to 85% of cases. The most common presenting complaints are hematuria and/or edema. Acute renal failure occurs in only a small percentage of cases. Poststreptococcal AGN usually is associated with a *decreased* serum complement level. *(Rudolph:1260–1261)*

74. (A) Lymphocytic thyroiditis (Hashimoto's thyroiditis) is an autoimmune disorder, and circulating antithyroid antibodies can be demonstrated in most patients. However, other autoimmune disorders, including diabetes mellitus, adrenal insufficiency, hypoparathyroidism, and pernicious anemia, occur in only a *minority* of patients. The thyroid gland is *invariably enlarged*, often irregularly so. Most patients are euthyroid, some are hypothyroid, and a few are hyperthyroid. *(Rudolph:1634)*

75. (C) The juvenile nasopharyngeal angiofibroma is a *benign* lesion of the nasopharynx, presenting most frequently in *prepubescent males*. These tumors bleed easily and profusely. The most common mode of presentation is massive epistaxis. *(Hathaway:347; Am J Dis Child 135:535–537,1981)*

76. (D) The peak expiratory flow rate is easily measured with relatively inexpensive equipment designed for home use. All the other tests listed require more elaborate and more expensive equipment. Self-monitoring of peak expiratory flow by children has proved to be a very useful tool in adjusting medication and deciding when to seek medical attention. *(Rudolph:507)*

77. (E) Primary pulmonary hemosiderosis is an uncommon disease of unknown origin characterized by repeated pulmonary hemorrhages. The clinical picture of recurrent episodes of fever, cough, and radiographic infiltrates is frequently misinterpreted as recurrent pneumonia, especially in infants and young children who do not expectorate and in whom hemoptysis may go undetected. The first clue often is a severe iron deficiency anemia. Some of these infants or children have improvement in pulmonary manifestations when cow milk is eliminated from their diet. Diffuse pulmonary hemangiomatosis and extramedullary pulmonary erythropoiesis are nonentities. *(Rudolph:1543)*

78. **(B)** Most eczematoid rashes in childhood usually represent atopic dermatitis, either as an isolated disorder or in association with allergic diseases. Eczema also is seen in association with certain systemic disorders such as Wiskott-Aldrich syndrome and phenylketonuria but has no special association with leukemia, inflammatory bowel disease, endocardial fibroelastosis, or Kawasaki's syndrome. *(Rudolph:512,884–885,906)*

79. **(E)** The rash described in this question sounds like urticaria, for which there are many causes. Although allergy to foods, drugs, or chemicals is high on the list, in most cases no specific cause can be found. A few cases result from infections such as hepatitis virus or group A *Streptococcus*. A very few cases are caused by collagen vascular disease or malignancy. Hereditary deficiency of C_1-esterase inhibitor (extremely rare) is usually associated with angioedema rather than urticaria. *(Rudolph:516–517)*

80. **(C)** The XYY karyotype is relatively common, occurring in about 1 in 1,000 males. Patients with this karyotype generally are tall. It is debatable whether or not the XYY karyotype is associated with an increased risk of impulsivity, antisocial behavior, and psychopathic personality, but whether or not this is true, *most* XYY individuals are behaviorally normal, although IQ and language development tend to be low normal. *(Rudolph:1662)*

81. **(B)** Precocious puberty secondary to a central nervous system lesion is always isosexual, since it results from the release of gonadotropins. For the same reason, the gonads are large and mature early. Either males or females can be affected. Hamartomas of the hypothalamic region are the most common lesion. Neurofibromatosis, hydrocephalus, and tumors are other examples of diseases or lesions that can cause central precocious puberty. In many cases, a discrete lesion or cause cannot be identified. *(Rudolph: 1671–1673)*

82. **(D)** Precocious puberty has not been noted in association with hyperthyroidism but has been seen in association with *hypo*thyroidism. Precocious puberty also has been associated with gonadotropin-producing tumors such as hepatoblastomas and choriocarcinomas. It is not seen with hypoadrenalism or parathyroid disorders. *(Rudolph:1636,1672,1674)*

83. **(A)** The abnormality in pseudohypoparathyroidism is a defect in end-organ (kidney and bone) response to parathyroid hormone. Serum levels of parathyroid hormone are normal or elevated. Short stature and skeletal abnormalities, including demineralization, are common. Fingers are short and broad (brachymetacarpals). *(Rudolph:1647–1648)*

84. **(B)** Also called pseudohemophilia, Von Willebrand's disease is characterized by a prolonged bleeding time. There is a *variable* deficiency or molecular abnormality of factor VIII, giving a rise to *variably* abnormal PTT. The platelet count, factor XII level, and prothrombin time are all normal. *(Rudolph:1164–1165)*

85. **(A)** Dysgenesis (aplasia, dysplasia, hypoplasia) of the thyroid gland is the most common cause of congenital hypothyroidism. Inborn metabolic errors of thyroid synthesis are much less frequent. Maternal ingestion of iodides (as in expectorants) is a recognized cause of neonatal hypothyroidism but is rare today. *(Rudolph:1628–1629)*

86. **(E)** Cysticercosis is a condition of generalized tissue invasion by the larva of *T. solium* and results from the ingestion of *T. solium eggs* that have contaminated food or cooking utensils. Eating undercooked infected pork results in ingestion of an encysted worm, which causes an intestinal tapeworm infestation, not cysticercosis. Rarely, autoinoculation by the fecal-oral route may be the mechanism of infection in a patient with an intestinal *T. solium* tapeworm. Cysticercosis is endemic in Mexico. In the United States it is seen primarily in areas with large Latin American immigrant populations. The central nervous system is the most common target organ, and seizures are probably the most frequent presenting complaint. Meningeal involvement with abnormal cerebrospinal fluid findings occurs in fewer than half the cases of cysticercosis, and even in these cases, eosinophilia of the cerebrospinal fluid usually is not marked. [*Note:* Attention to terms such as "generally" and "in most cases" is important.] (Pediatr Clin North Am *32:953–966,1985; Rudolph:736–737*)

87. **(E)** Diabetes mellitus is a common development in the adolescent and older patient with cystic fibrosis. It results from pancreatic fibrosis and beta-cell destruction. It behaves like maturity onset diabetes, with little tendency to ketoacidosis. Diabetes should always be considered when an older child with cystic fibrosis loses weight. *(Rudolph:1528–1529)*

88. **(A)** Elevated sweat chloride concentration is an almost universal finding in patients with cystic fibrosis (CF). Serum electrolytes, in contrast, are usually normal, although hyponatremia may occasionally develop *secondary* to the sweat abnormality. The sweat test is the diagnostic test for CF. Normal children have sweat chloride concentrations less than 40

mEq/L, whereas CF patients have concentrations greater than 60 mEq/L. *(Rudolph:1528–1530)*

89. **(E)** The bacteria most commonly involved in *acute* otitis media in childhood are *Streptococcus pneumoniae, Hemophilus influenzae,* and beta-hemolytic streptococci. *Staphylococcus aureus* is only an infrequent cause. Earache is common, as any pediatrician and many parents can attest. One or both ears may be involved. Drainage by tympanocentesis is seldom needed, since most cases respond to appropriate antibiotic therapy. Tympanocentesis is frequently necessary for *chronic serous* otitis media. *(Pediatrics 65:917,1980; Hoekelman:1417–1419)*

90. **(A)** Inguinal hernias are not at all rare in female infants, and the great majority of these infants are genetically female and otherwise normal. Such hernias may contain intestine or an ovary, either of which can incarcerate. Prompt surgical correction is indicated. Most inguinal hernias in infants, males or females, are indirect. *(Rudolph:1041–1042; Hathaway: 552–553)*

91. **(B)** Large ventricular septal defects (VSD) usually are associated with left deviation of the electrical axis and evidence of left ventricular hypertrophy on electrocardiogram, although signs of combined ventricular hypertrophy are not uncommon. An enlarged heart is common, but the pulmonary vasculature is increased, not decreased. The murmur of a VSD is systolic rather than continuous. With large left-to-right shunts and a high pulmonary flow, there also may be a middiastolic rumble but still *not* a continuous murmur. *(Rudolph:1365–1366)*

92. **(E)** Pseudotumor cerebri (headache, vomiting, and papilledema) may be seen in association with hypoparathyroidism. Stiffness and tingling of the extremities may precede frank tetany or carpopedal spasms. Teeth erupt late and irregularly. Cataracts occur, usually late. Hypocalcemia and *hyper*phosphatemia are characteristic. *(Rudolph:1647)*

93. **(C)** Thrombocytopenia occurs in all of the conditions listed except thrombasthenia. In cases of splenomegaly and giant hemangiomas, the thrombocytopenia is secondary to platelet sequestration or trapping. In Wiscott-Aldrich syndrome, an X-linked immunodeficiency disorder, the platelets are intrinsically abnormal and have a shortened survival time. The mechanism of the thrombocytopenia occasionally seen in children with cyanotic congenital heart disease is unclear, but increased peripheral destruction seems to be a factor. Congenital thrombasthenia (Glanzmann's disease) is an autosomal recessive disorder of platelet *function* associated with normal numbers and morphology of platelets. *(Rudolph:1159–1161)*

94. **(E)** Ehlers-Danlos (EDS) syndrome is a group of disorders involving genetic abnormalities of collagen and other supporting tissues. All tests of hemostatic function are normal in patients with EDS. There is no generalized bleeding tendency, although prolonged bleeding may occasionally be seen as a result of gaping wounds. Hyperextensibility of the joints, easy rupture of skin, easy bruising, and poor wound healing are characteristic of this disorder. Nine varieties of EDS have been described. Not all features are found in every type. *(Rudolph:413–415)*

95. **(D)** In the disorder of multiple cartilaginous exostoses, fragments of cartilage become separated from the epiphyseal line and are incorporated in the shaft of the bone, where they continue to proliferate. The exostoses usually are not evident clinically or radiographically at birth but appear after 2 or 3 years of age. Tubular bones, ribs, vertebral bodies, scapulae, and iliac crests may be involved. The disorder follows an autosomal dominant pattern of inheritance. *(Rudolph:404–405)*

96. **(B)** Obesity, mainly central in distribution, and growth retardation (short stature) generally are the primary features of Cushing's syndrome (hyperfunction of the adrenal cortex) in childhood. Acne, hypertrichosis, hypertension, and striae are other common findings. Anemia is not a feature of Cushing's syndrome. Indeed, cortisone stimulates the bone marrow with resultant polycythemia. *(Rudolph:1487–1489)*

97. **(A)** Diseases associated with the nephrotic syndrome (NS) in childhood include systemic lupus erythematosus, congenital syphilis, and renal vein thrombosis. Medications that can cause nephrotic syndrome include tridione, penicillamine, and gold salts. Most cases of NS, however, are secondary to primary renal disorders such as minimal-change disease or membranoproliferative glomerulonephritis. Marfan's syndrome is not associated with renal involvement. [*Note:* To answer this question, the examinee must be certain *either* that Marfan's syndrome is not associated with NS or that all the other items listed are.] *(Rudolph:1267)*

98. **(D)** Appropriate management of acute renal failure includes fluid restriction to insensible loss (usually 300 mL/m^2) plus urine output. Urinary sodium loss should be replaced, preferably with sodium lactate or sodium bicarbonate to minimize metabolic acidosis. Since hyperkalemia is one of the major threats to life in acute renal failure, all potassium intake generally should be avoided. Tissue catabolism, with release of intracellular potassium and metabolic acids, can be minimized by the administration of at least 400 calories/m^2 that are free of potassium. The intake of protein must be restricted, although administration of a balanced mixture of amino acids may sometimes be helpful. Oral aluminum hydroxide to

decrease absorption of phosphate is necessary in many cases to prevent hyperphosphatemia and hypocalcemia. Although not needed in all cases, it certainly is an *appropriate* part of therapy. *(Rudolph:1246–1247)*

99. **(B)** Children with constitutional growth delay have no endocrine disease but lag behind their peers in both growth and physiologic maturation. Such children are small for their age. Bone age also is delayed and therefore is commensurate with height. *Puberty is delayed*, and, consequently, growth continues for a longer than normal period of time, resulting in an ultimate adult height that is normal. *(Rudolph:235; J Pediatr 92:697–704,1978)*

100. **(B)** Scabies is characterized by intense pruritus that starts 2 to 3 weeks after the onset of infection and is presumed to be caused by hypersensitivity to the mite, its eggs, or its feces. The typical lesion is a papule that becomes excoriated and crusted. The hands and feet often are the sites of earliest and most intense involvement, especially in patients beyond infancy. The classical lesion is a burrow, a linear eruption ending in a black dot (the buried insect), but often this is obscured by the excoriations of scratching. Involvement of other family members in addition to the patient is common. *(Pediatr Clin North Am 32:989–995,1985; Hoekelman:1307)*

101. **(D)** Rotavirus is the agent most frequently recovered from the stool of infants and young children with viral gastroenteritis. Fever and vomiting are common. Coryza and other upper respiratory symptoms occasionally precede the gastrointestinal symptoms. Blood or mucus in the stool is very infrequent, as is the finding of fecal leukocytes on microscopic examination of a stool specimen. *(Rudolph:670–671)*

102. **(D)** The selective disturbance of skeletal growth in achondroplasia results in disproportionately short extremities. In the extremities the proximal bones are further disproportionately shortened in relation to the distal bones. The fingers, however, are short and stubby. Hydrocephalus is seen occasionally, possibly related to a small foramen magnum. Overall height, of course, is markedly decreased. These patients characteristically have a relatively large head, bulging forehead, and depressed nasal bridge. *(Rudolph:398–399)*

103. **(E)** Occult bacteremia, a positive blood culture in a febrile child who appears well enough to be treated as an outpatient, is recognized as an important problem. It is most common in children between 6 and 24 months of age with temperatures of 40°C or greater and white blood cell counts of 15,000/mm³ or greater, although these features cannot be used to accurately identify each individual patient who will have a positive blood culture. *S. pneumoniae* accounts for the majority of cases, with *H. influenzae, N. meningitides*, and *Salmonella* species accounting for most of the remaining cases. The problem is equally prevalent in middle-income private patients and in lower-socioeconomic-level clinic patients. *(J Pediatr 109:1–8, 1986)*

104. **(A)** Viral bronchiolitis is an acute infectious disease characterized by inflammatory occlusion of small airways. Wheezing, tachypnea, and hypoxemia are common. Hyperaeration is evident on chest roentgenograph. The air trapping results in an *increased* functional residual capacity. *(Rudolph:1520–1521)*

105. **(C)** Hypoglycemia has been noted occasionally in children with hypothyroidism, but not with hyperthyroidism. Both panhypopituitarism and isolated growth hormone deficiency have been associated with hypoglycemia. A significant percentage of children with Reye's syndrome, especially those less than 2 years of age, are hypoglycemic. Hypoglycemia is a recognized complication of poisoning with ethyl alcohol and with aspirin, much more frequently in children than in adults. *(Rudolph:327–330)*

106. **(B)** Pituitary involvement, with resultant diabetes insipidus, is a very rare manifestation of sarcoidosis in children. Lymphadenopathy, hepatosplenomegaly, and ophthalmologic findings are much more common. Abnormal chest roentgenograms are present in most patients except those in the first few years of life. *(Rudolph:1542)*

107. **(D)** The syndrome of inappropriate secretion of antidiuretic hormone (SIADH) is a common complication of a variety of central nervous system problems, including bacterial meningitis. Usually the SIADH resolves as the meningitis is treated, even if a subdural effusion is present. *(Rudolph:561,1581–1582)*

108. **(B)** Theoretically, the syndrome of inappropriate ADH secretion would be most accurately diagnosed by measurement of serum ADH levels. However, an assay for antidiuretic hormone is not readily available. Therefore, the diagnosis usually is confirmed by demonstrating a low urine output and inappropriate high urine osmolality in the presence of low serum osmolality. *(Rudolph:561,1581–1582)*

109. **(D)** Patients with inappropriate secretion of ADH have a decreased urine output and are hypervolemic. They are neither hypotensive nor alkalotic. The urine specific gravity is high. As a matter of fact, high urine specific gravity is one of the criteria for the diagnosis of SIADH. *(Rudolph:561,1581–1582)*

110. **(B)** Therapy of inappropriate ADH secretion consists primarily of fluid restriction and, of course, treatment of the underlying condition, in this case, bacterial meningitis. Attempts to correct the hyponatre-

mia by administration of sodium usually result in more retention of water and further hypervolemia and edema. Intravenous administration of hypertonic saline would be indicated only if the hyponatremia were life threatening. Maintenance amounts of sodium should be administered. Diuretics are not very effective in this condition. *(Rudolph:561,1581–1582)*

111. (B) The cerebrospinal fluid findings, especially the xanthochromic appearance after centrifugation, indicate an intracranial hemorrhage. The bleeding is primarily subarachnoid, or, at least, there has been extension of the bleeding into the subarachnoid space. Intraventricular hemorrhage is uncommon except in the small, premature infant. Fever is seen in patients with intracranial hemorrhage. *(Rudolph:1753)*

112. (C) Of the abnormalities listed, only cerebral arteriovenous malformation (AVM) and aneurysm predispose to hemorrhagic disasters. In children, cerebral AVMs are the most common cause of spontaneous intracranial hemorrhage. Unlike the situation in adults, intracranial hemorrhage in children is rarely from a ruptured aneurysm. *(Rudolph:1753)*

113. (A) The most appropriate management at this time would be to perform a CT scan, followed, *if necessary*, by arteriography. It would not have been unreasonable to have performed the CT prior to the lumbar puncture. It is a question of judgment of the likelihood of meningitis in this child with only a slight fever. There is no need to repeat the lumbar puncture at this time. Intracranial hemorrhage rarely is associated with volume depletion or the need for transfusion. In the absence of evidence of a bleeding disorder, there is no indication for administration of fresh frozen plasma. *(Rudolph:1753)*

114. (E) The clinical picture described, including the olive-shaped mass, are almost pathognomonic for infantile hypertrophic pyloric stenosis. Intussusception is rare in the neonatal period and is unlikely to cause vomiting for 12 days without signs of obstruction or other intraabdominal catastrophe. The mass associated with neuroblastoma or adrenal hemorrhage is more lateral (or in the flank), and vomiting is not especially frequent with either of these two conditions. *(Rudolph:1001)*

115. (E) Most infants with hypertrophic pyloric stenosis develop a metabolic alkalosis secondary to the loss of hydrogen ion in the vomitus, which in this condition is essentially pure gastric secretion. Metabolic alkalosis occurs so regularly in this disorder that it often is used as a diagnostic feature. *(Rudolph:1001)*

116. (B) The physical findings suggest that the child is moderately dehydrated. Glucose and water alone is never the appropriate hydrating or maintenance so-

lution for an infant or a child. Bicarbonate should be withheld from this child, who is not described as appearing clinically acidotic and who is very likely to have a metabolic alkalosis secondary to the prolonged vomiting. Indeed, the respiratory rate of 12 is rather slow for an infant of this age and could be explained on the basis of respiratory compensation for a metabolic alkalosis. Although the child might be *hypo*kalemic secondary to prolonged alkalosis, there also is the possibility of *hyper*kalemia secondary to dehydration and prerenal azotemia. Normal saline is the most appropriate initial rehydrating fluid. *(Rudolph:1001)*

117. (C) The clinical picture and the age of the patient are typical for infantile cortical hyperostosis (Caffey's disease), a rare inflammatory disease of bone of unknown etiology. The swelling in mumps is generally higher, in the preauricular region, and the examiner usually can outline the swollen parotid gland. Mumps is rather uncommon in the first 6 months of life. The mandible is an uncommon site for osteomyelitis, and one would expect unilateral rather than bilateral findings. Fibrous dysplasia is not associated with systemic signs and usually begins in childhood rather than infancy. Acute cervical lymphadenitis usually is unilateral and presents as a mass rather than as diffuse swelling. *(Rudolph:409)*

118. (D) The typical radiographic abnormalities found in patients with infantile cortical hyperostosis are cortical thickening and subperiosteal new bone formation. There are no osteoporotic or radiolucent changes. *(Rudolph:409)*

119. (B) A markedly elevated erythrocyte sedimentation rate is characteristic of this condition. Anemia, leukocytosis, and elevated serum *alkaline* phosphatase are frequent. The blood culture is negative, renal function is normal, and the disease is not associated with sickle cell disease. *(Rudolph:409)*

120. (D) This child most likely has visceral larva migrans (VLM), which in this country usually is caused by *Toxocara canis* or *Toxocara cati*, the dog and cat ascarids, respectively. Diagnosis can be established by biopsy of an involved organ such as lung or liver. Since the human is an unnatural host, the parasite does not complete its life cycle, and ova or worms do not appear in the stool or in duodenal fluid. The diagnosis cannot be established by examination of the bone marrow or a blood smear. Serologic tests are helpful. Most patients, if not blood type AB, have markedly elevated anti-A and/or anti-B isohemagglutinin antibody titers. Often the diagnosis is made on the basis of the clinical, hematologic, and serologic data without liver biopsy. [*Note:* The question asked which of the listed procedures would be most likely to establish the diagnosis, not whether or not the procedure was necessary or indicated.] *(Rudolph:719)*

121. (B) *Toxocara canis* infection usually is acquired by eating soil contaminated by dog stool. The *T. canis* eggs that are passed in the dog's stool are not directly infective, but in the soil the eggs develop into infective ova containing second-stage larvae. Infection, therefore, is probably not acquired by direct contact with the animal but only by contact with infected soil, usually as a result of geophagy. *(Rudolph:719)*

122. (A) Nephritis is not a usual part of the clinical picture of visceral larva migrans. Neurologic involvement, ophthalmic (retinal) lesion, and myocarditis are well-recognized complications. As mentioned above, an elevated serum concentration of anti-A and/or anti-B isohemagglutinin titers, as well as total immunoglobulin level, is common. *(Rudolph:719)*

123. (D) The most likely diagnosis is severe combined immunodeficiency syndrome (SCIDS). Both Wiskott-Aldrich syndrome and hereditary agammaglobulinemia are X-linked recessive conditions and, therefore, are unlikely in this female child. Most 3-month-old infants have low but detectable levels of IgA and IgM (normal range for 3-month-old: 3 to 90 and 115 to 120 mg/dL, respectively). The IgG is maternal. Patients with AIDS usually have elevated levels of immunoglobulins. Also, infants with AIDS are usually not this sick this early; infants with SCIDS often are. Patients with transient hypogammaglobulinemia of infancy usually are not as sick as this patient, and infection generally does not start as early as 6 weeks. Of the diagnoses listed, only SCIDS explains all the findings including lymphopenia. *(Rudolph: 463–464; Hathaway:1102)*

124. (C) Severe combined immunodeficiency is associated with an absence or paucity of plasma cells in the bone marrow, absence or paucity of superficial lymphoid tissue, and an absent thymic shadow on chest roentgenogram. Cutaneous reactivity to various common antigens is absent. In an immunologically normal child with *Candida* infection, one would expect to find a positive reaction to intradermal testing with *Candida* antigen. In a child with severe combined immunodeficiency, there is global anergy, and all skin tests are nonreactive. *(Rudolph:463–464)*

125. (B) The roentgenographic picture described is typical of *Pneumocystis carinii* infection, to which these infants are unduly susceptible. Viruses such as cytomegalovirus could produce a similar picture, but this is not listed as a choice. Lymphangiectasia is a congenital lesion of the lung, unrelated to immunologic disorders. Neither pneumococcal pneumonia nor pulmonary hemorrhage is likely to be so protracted or indolent. Miliary tuberculosis is a possibility but

usually does not produce such extensive bilateral disease or a ground-glass appearance radiographically. It also is uncommon in patients this young. *(Rudolph:463–464)*

126. (C) Of the conditions listed, subdural hematoma is the most likely and would best explain all the clinical findings. Tuberculous meningitis can cause obstructive hydrocephalus and a large head, but one would expect fever, and cranial nerve abnormalities usually are evident on physical examination. Mastoiditis is generally associated with fever and, by itself, would not explain the neurologic findings. Pseudotumor cerebri is relatively benign and is not associated with convulsions. All three conditions—tuberculous meningitis, mastoiditis, and pseudotumor—are uncommon in the first few months of life. With congenital toxoplasmosis one would expect more chronic findings and delayed psychomotor development. *(Rudolph:1706–1707,1760)*

127. (C) Retinal hemorrhages may be found in up to 40% of cases of subdural hematoma and usually are indicative of a shaking injury as a form of child abuse. The forceful shaking of the infant creates shearing forces in the brain and retina, resulting in bleeding in both organs. In congenital toxoplasmosis one finds a chorioretinitis rather than hemorrhage. *(Rudolph:1706–1707,1760)*

128. (C) The diagnosis of subdural hematoma usually can be easily and definitively established by CT scan of the head. The electroencephalogram might be suggestive of cortical damage or a lesion or might be normal but would not be diagnostic. Examination of cerebrospinal fluid is apt to be unrewarding. Occasionally, one may find an elevated protein concentration, especially as a consequence of associated subarachnoid hemorrhage, but, again, this would not be diagnostic. Lumbar puncture in a patient with increased intracranial pressure is not without risk. In this child, it would be preferable to obtain the CT scan before a lumbar puncture. *(Rudolph:1706–1707,1760)*

129. (G) EDTA is the chelation agent of choice for children with significantly elevated blood lead levels. Children with blood lead levels of 25 mg/dL or greater should undergo chelation therapy with $CaNa_2$-EDTA. In cases of very high blood levels (>70 mg/dL) or overt encephalopathy, the EDTA should be preceded by a dose of BAL. Chelation with oral *meso*-1,3-dimercaptosuccinic acid (DMSA) appears promising and eventually may replace EDTA, especially for patients with only moderately elevated blood lead levels. *(Rudolph:808; Hathaway:947–948; J Pediatr 113:751–757,1988)*

130. (E) Children with either acute iron poisoning or

chronic iron overload from repeated transfusions should be treated with the iron-chelating agent deferoxamine. For acute ingestion, the drug usually is administered intravenously. *(Rudolph:806; Hathaway:946–947)*

131. (A) If treatment is begun within 24 hours of ingestion, acetylcysteine may prevent hepatic injury from acetaminophen ingestion. Acetaminophen itself is not hepatotoxic, but some of its metabolites are. These hepatotoxic metabolites ordinarily are inactivated by glutathione as soon as they are formed. Large overdoses of acetaminophen deplete the liver's stores of glutathione, permitting the toxic metabolite to accumulate. Acetylcysteine replenishes hepatic glutathione, protecting the liver from the toxic byproducts of acetaminophen metabolism. *(Rudolph: 788–789; Hathaway: 934–935)*

132. (B) Atropine is an important part of the treatment of organophosphate poisoning. Although it has little effect on the central nervous system effects of organophosphate, atropine will control respiratory secretions and other cholinergic effects. Pralidoxime, a cholinesterase-regenerating oxime, may be needed to reverse muscle weakness. *(Rudolph:814–815; Hathaway:946)*

133. (Y) Cyanide binds to intracellular iron in the cytochrome system, interfering with aerobic metabolism. Amyl nitrite by inhalation (pearls) or sodium nitrite solution (3%) intravenously will reverse the intracellular effects of cyanide by oxidizing hemoglobin to methemoglobin, which then binds cyanide tightly. Administration of sodium thiosulfate hastens conversion of cyanide to the less toxic thiocyanate. *(Rudolph:800–801; Hathaway:932)*

134. (H) Ethylene glycol is the primary component of antifreeze. Organic acids formed by metabolism of ethylene glycol are more toxic than the parent compound and are responsible for most of the major toxicity. Ethanol, an effective antidote, works by competing for the enzyme alcohol dehydrogenase, which catalyzes the first step in the metabolism of ethylene glycol. The same enzyme initiates the metabolic pathway for methanol and isopropyl alcohol, and therefore, ethanol is also useful in treating poisoning with these substances. *(Rudolph:802–803)*

135. (O) Naloxone is a competitive antagonist to the opiates, including morphine. The drug is best administered intravenously. The usual dose is 0.03 mg/kg, but a second larger dose (0.1 mg/kg) may be given if there is no response. Naloxone is not itself a depressant and is a very safe drug. *(Rudolph:813; Hathaway: 949)*

136. (A) Most cases of acute glomerulonephritis are poststreptococcal, and some evidence of an antecedent streptococcal infection, such as an elevated anti-

streptolysin 0 titer, usually can be found in these patients. No such relationship exists for minimal-change nephrotic syndrome. *(Rudolph:1260–1261)*

137. (B) Most cases of minimal-change nephrotic syndrome respond to corticosteroids. Poststreptococcal acute glomerulonephritis does not respond to corticosteroids. *(Rudolph:1261–1262,1269)*

138. (C) Hematuria is present in most cases of poststreptococcal acute glomerulonephritis, and dark urine is the presenting complaint in many cases. Hematuria, usually microscopic, is present in 20 to 50% of cases of minimal-change nephrotic syndrome. [*Note:* Even though hematuria is present in fewer than half of the cases of minimal-change disease, it still is *associated* with this condition. The finding of microscopic hematuria would not rule against minimal-change nephrotic syndrome.] *(Rudolph:1260–1261,1268)*

139. (A) Hypercellularity of glomeruli, swelling of basement membrane, and subepithelial deposits of "electron-dense" material are the classical microscopic and electron microscopic changes of poststreptococcal acute glomerulonephritis. In contrast, as the name implies, minimal-change nephrotic syndrome is characterized by minimal changes on light microscopy. Examination by the electron microscope, however, reveals fusion of foot processes. *(Rudolph:1260–1261,1267)*

140. (B) Patients with nephrotic syndrome and ascites are at increased risk of peritonitis. In untreated cases, pneumococcus is the major etiologic organism. In patients receiving adrenocorticosteroids, other organisms are more common. *(Rudolph:1269)*

141. (D) Both poststreptococcal acute glomerulonephritis and minimal-change nephrotic syndrome have an excellent prognosis. Most cases of acute glomerulonephritis, especially poststreptococcal glomerulonephritis, end in complete remission. Probably fewer than 10% of cases progress to chronic renal disease. More than half of the cases of minimal-change nephrotic syndrome respond well to treatment with prednisone and have few or no relapses. Even those with frequent relapses (about 40% of cases) usually do not progress to chronic renal failure, although proteinuria and edema may be a continuing problem. *(Rudolph:1262,1269–1270)*

142. (C) Fat malabsorption and steatorrhea are present in both cystic fibrosis and celiac disease. In the former it results primarily from pancreatic insufficiency. In the latter condition it is secondary to villous atrophy. *(Rudolph:1017,1043,1528)*

143. (D) Neither cystic fibrosis nor celiac disease has any association with hepatoma. There is an increased incidence of lymphoma and esophageal cancer in adult patients with celiac disease. This may relate more to associated HLA typing and immunologic mechanism than to the celiac disease itself. *(Rudolph:1017,1043, 1528)*

144. **(B)** A wheat-free diet is indicated in patients with celiac disease, which is a gluten-induced enteropathy. Gluten is a protein found only in wheat. Patients with cystic fibrosis are quite capable of handling dietary gluten and do not require a wheat-free diet. *(Rudolph:1017)*

145. **(A)** Turner's syndrome is the syndrome of gonadal (ovarian) dysgenesis and an XO karyotype. These patients are phenotypic females. They are characteristically *short* and stocky with broad chest and short neck. Webbed neck, coarctation of the aorta, cubitus valgus, and short fourth metacarpal are other common features. Klinefelter's syndrome is the syndrome of gonadal (seminiferous tubule) dysgenesis and an XXY karyotype. These patients are phenotypic males and tend to be *tall* and eunuchoid with small testes. Behavioral problems and mental retardation are common. *(Rudolph:1658–1662)*

146. **(C)** Hypogonadism and infertility are present in both Turner's syndrome and Klinefelter's syndrome. *(Rudolph:1658–1662)*

147. **(B)** Coxa plana, or Legg-Calvé-Perthes disease, is a condition of avascular necrosis of the femoral head and is most common between 4 and 10 years of age. Slipped femoral epiphysis is a condition of slippage of the femoral shaft relative to the femoral head at the epiphyseal plate and is most common in the teen years. Slipped femoral epiphysis is rarely seen before the age of 10 years. *(Rudolph:1941–1944)*

148. **(C)** Although both coxa plana and slipped femoral epiphysis usually are unilateral, bilateral involvement can occur in either condition. Bilateral disease is seen in up to 20% of patients with slipped femoral epiphysis. Bilateral involvement also occurs in children with coxa plana, although less frequently than in slipped femoral epiphysis. *(Rudolph:1941–1944)*

149. **(D)** Both coxa plana and slipped femoral epiphysis are more common in boys than in girls. Coxa plana is six times more common in boys than girls, whereas slipped femoral epiphysis is only slightly more common in boys than girls. *(Rudolph:1941–1944)*

150. **(D)** Neither coxa plana nor slipped femoral epiphysis has been associated with precocious puberty. *(Rudolph:1941–1944)*

151. **(B)** Surgical intervention, with nailing of the femoral shaft to the femoral head, is the treatment of choice for slipped femoral epiphysis. Legg-Calvé-Perthes disease (coxa plana) usually is self-limited and responds to conservative management with bed rest, traction, or casting. The blood supply to the femoral head reestablishes itself, and the necrotic tissue is replaced by healthy bone. When surgery is required for severe cases, arthrotomy or osteotomy is performed; nailing is unnecessary. *(Rudolph:1941–1944)*

152. **(B)** In cases of X-linked recessive disease, the female is generally heterozygous and clinically unaffected. If the abnormal gene is itself very common, then affected (homozygous) females will exist, but much less frequently than affected males. In the case of autosomal recessive disorders, males and females are affected equally. *(Rudolph:265–269)*

153. **(C)** In recessive disorders (autosomal or X-linked), both parents generally are clinically normal. In the case of an autosomal recessive disease, both parents are carriers but phenotypically normal. In X-linked recessive disorders, the mother is a carrier and the father is genetically normal. Both parents, therefore, are clinically (phenotypically) normal. *(Rudolph:265–269)*

154. **(A)** In the case of an X-linked gene, the father cannot transmit the abnormal (X) gene to a son. The father must contribute the Y, not the X gene, if the offspring is to be a male. In autosomal recessive disorders, both parents must contribute an aberrant gene in order for the child to be clinically affected. *(Rudolph:265–269)*

155. **(C)** Children born to a union between a person with a recessive disease and a (phenotypically) normal person will be clinically unaffected. In the case of an X-linked disorder (for example, hemophilia), the affected male can transmit either the normal Y gene, in which case the child is a genetically and clinically normal male, or the X gene, in which case the child is a female carrier. In the case of an autosomal recessive disorder such as cystic fibrosis, the carrier state or gene frequency in the Caucasian population is approximately 1 in 20. Since the *affected* individual is homozygous, he or she must contribute the CF gene. The normal mate has only a 1 in 20 chance of being a carrier and, *if* a carrier, has only a 50% chance of passing the CF gene. Therefore, only 1 in 40 children would be expected to have the disease. *(Rudolph:265–269)*

156. **(D)** Muscle fasciculations are indicative of anterior horn cell disease and are not seen in disorders of the distal motor unit. Myasthenia is a disease of the neuromuscular synapse. Muscular dystrophy is a primary degenerative muscle disease. Neither disease involves the anterior horn cell, and neither is associated with fasciculations. *(Rudolph:1799–1804)*

157. (C) Both myasthenia gravis and muscular dystrophy are associated with skeletal muscle weakness. In the case of myasthenia, the onset of weakness can be either sudden or gradual. In the case of muscular dystrophy, the onset is gradual, often insidious. *(Rudolph:1799–1804)*

158. (B) Children with Duchenne muscular dystrophy often have some cardiac involvement demonstrated on electrocardiogram. Clinically evident cardiomyopathy is well recognized, albeit infrequent. In contrast, cardiac muscle is spared in myasthenia gravis. *(Rudolph:1799–1804)*

159. (D) A positive Coombs's test is a reflection of circulating antibodies directed against the erythrocytes and may be seen in *acquired* spherocytosis associated with autoimmune hemolytic anemia. However, neither *hereditary* spherocytosis nor sickle cell disease involves autoantibodies, and therefore, the Coombs's test is negative in both conditions. *(Rudolph:1123–1127,1132–1134)*

160. (A) Hereditary spherocytosis frequently presents in the newborn period with hyperbilirubinemia severe enough to require treatment with phototherapy or even exchange transfusion. Symptoms of sickle cell anemia, in contrast, do not become apparent until levels of fetal hemoglobin, which inhibits sickling, have decreased, usually no sooner than a few months of age. *(Rudolph: 1123–1127,1132–1134)*

161. (C) Both spherocytosis and sickle cell anemia are associated with hemolytic anemia. Reticulocytosis, therefore, is common in both conditions. In some patients with spherocytosis, hemolysis may be mild, and reticulocytosis may be the only evident abnormality. *(Rudolph:1123–1127,1132–1134)*

162. (B) The basic defect in sickle cell disease is the genetically encoded production of sickle hemoglobin, an abnormal hemoglobin that can be demonstrated on hemoglobin electrophoresis. Hereditary spherocytosis involves a defect in the red blood cell membrane; the hemoglobin in this disorder is normal. *(Rudolph:1123–1127,1132–1134)*

BIBLIOGRAPHY

Alvarez F, Bernard O, Brunelle F, et al. Portal obstruction in children. *J Pediatr.* 1983;103:696–702.

Brown JW, Voge M. Cysticercosis. A modern day plague. *Pediatr Clin North Am.* 1985;32:953–966.

Esclamado RM, Richardson MA. Laryngotracheal foreign bodies in children. A comparison with bronchial foreign bodies. *Am J Dis Child.* 1987;141:259–262.

Gershel JC, Goldman HS, Stein RE, et al. The usefulness of chest radiographs in first asthma attacks. *N Engl J Med.* 1983;309:336–339.

Graziano JH, Lolancono NJ, Meyer P. Dose-response study of oral 2,3-dimercaptosuccinic acid in children with elevated blood lead concentrations. *J Pediatr.* 1981;113:751–757.

Gurevitch AW. Scabies and lice. *Pediatr Clin North Am.* 1985;32:989–995.

Hathaway WE, Groothius JR, Hay WW, et al. *Current Pediatric Diagnosis & Treatment.* 10th ed. Norwalk, Conn: Appleton & Lange; 1991.

Hoekelman RA, Friedman SB, Nelson NM, et al. *Primary Pediatric Care.* 2nd ed. St. Louis, Mo: Mosby Year Book; 1992.

Hughes WT. Fatal infections in childhood leukemia. *Am J Dis Child.* 1971;122:283–287.

Kalia A, Travis LB, Brouhard BH. The association of idiopathic hypercalciuria and asymptomatic gross hematuria in children. *J Pediatr.* 1983;99:716–719.

Massab HF. The role of viruses in sudden deafness. *Adv Otorhinolaryngol.* 1973;20:229–235.

McLellan D, Giebink GS. Perspectives on occult bacteremia in children. *J Pediatr.* 1986;109:1–8.

Nelson KB, Ellenberg JH. Prognosis in children with febrile seizures. *Pediatrics.* 1978;61:720–727.

Oldham KT, Lobe TE. Gastrointestinal hemorrhage in children. *Pediatr Clin North Am.* 1985;32:1247–1263.

Paradise JL. Otitis media in infants and children. *Pediatrics.* 1980;65:917–943.

Rimoin DL, Horton WA. Short stature. Part II. *J Pediatr.* 1978;92:697–704.

Roy S, Stapelton B, Noe HN. Hematuria preceding renal calculus formation in children with hypercalciuria. *J Pediatr.* 1983;99:712–715.

Rudolph AM, Hoffman JIE, Rudolph CD. *Pediatrics.* 19th ed. Norwalk, Conn: Appleton & Lange; 1991.

Scheider S, Rice DR. Neurologic manifestations of childhood hysteria. *J Pediatr.* 1979;94:153–156.

Sessions RB, Zarin DP, Bryan RN. Juvenile nasopharyngeal angiofibroma. *Am J Dis Child.* 1981;135:535–537.

Stapleton FB, Roy S III, Noe NH, et al. Hypercalciuria in children with hematuria. *N Eng J Med.* 1984;310:1345–1348.

Practice Test Subspecialty List

ALLERGY AND IMMUNOLOGY

78, 79, 123, 124, 125

CARDIOLOGY

18, 34, 91

DERMATOLOGY

22, 24, 45, 54, 64, 100

ENDOCRINOLOGY

30, 31, 48, 49, 66, 74, 81, 82, 83, 85, 87, 92, 96, 99, 105, 145, 146

GASTROENTEROLOGY

29, 51, 55, 56, 59, 60, 62, 63, 114, 115, 116, 142, 143, 144

GENERAL PEDIATRICS

117, 118, 119

GENETICS

15, 17, 80, 94, 102, 152, 153, 154, 155

HEMATOLOGY AND ONCOLOGY

6, 8, 32, 33, 35, 50, 84, 93, 159, 160, 161, 162

INFECTIOUS DISEASES

39, 53, 86, 89, 101, 103, 107, 108, 109, 110, 120, 121, 122

NEUROLOGY

38, 41, 42, 43, 52, 111, 112, 113, 126, 127, 128, 156, 157, 158

ORTHOPEDICS

61, 70, 95, 147, 148, 149, 150

OTOLARYNGOLOGY

1, 20, 23, 26, 27, 28, 44, 75

POISONING (TOXICOLOGY)

19, 21, 25, 65, 129, 130, 131, 132, 133, 134, 135

PSYCHOSOCIAL PEDIATRICS

36, 37

PULMONARY

12, 14, 16, 40, 67, 69, 72, 88, 76, 77, 104, 106

RENAL

2, 3, 4, 5, 7, 9, 10, 11, 12, 68, 73, 97, 98, 136, 137, 138, 139, 140, 141

RHEUMATOLOGY

71

SURGERY

46, 47, 57, 58, 90

Index

The numbers following each entry indicate the corresponding chapter and question numbers.

ABO incompatibility disease, 3–19
Abetalipoproteinemia, 7–29
Abuse, child, 5–5, 5–6, 5–25, 5–28, 5–40, 9–53
Accidents, 5–35
Acetaminophen
  poisoning, 5–2
    use of acetylcystein in, 11–131
  toxicity of, 8–66
Achondroplasia
  features of, 11–102
  increased intracranial pressure in, 9–56
  mode of inheritance in, 11–15
Acidosis, with diarrhea and dehydration, 7–14
Acne, 11–22
  neonatal, 3–64
  pustular, 8–34
Acyclovir, oral, 8–5
Adenoidectomy, submucosal cleft palate as contraindication to, 11–44
Adenoids, hypertrophy of, causing cor pulmonale, 11–40
Adenosine deaminase deficiency, 6–125
Adolescence
  definition of, 2–50
  psychological problems in, 2–51
Adrenal hyperplasia, congenital, 1–22, 2–94, 3–73, 10–107, 10–108, 10–109, 10–110
Agammaglobulinemia, hereditary, 6–122
Albinism, association with tyrosinase deficiency, 7–46
Alkaline phosphatase, serum levels of, 2–9
Alkalosis
  metabolic, 7–36
  with pyloric stenosis, 9–123
Allopurinol, 8–31
Alpha–1–antitrypsin deficiency, 11–29
Alveoli, pulmonary, number at birth, 2–55
Amino acids, essential, 4–23
Amphetamines, abuse of, 5–45
Ampicillin
  bacterial resistance to, 8–42
  rash with, 8–41
Amyl nitrate, abuse of, 5–44

Anemia
  in endocarditis, 9–120
  in newborn, 3–96
  iron deficiency, 9–33, 9–88
    prematurity as factor in, 3–81
    relation to cow milk intake, 4–19
  megaloblastic, 9–54
Aniridia, association with Wilms' tumor, 9–13
Annular pancreas, 11–51
Aperts syndrome, 9–15
Appendicitis, in less than 2-year-old, 11–57
Arbovirus, mosquitoes as vectors in, 6–12
Arteriovenous malformation, 3–50, 9–68
Ascaris lumbricoides
  intestinal obstruction with, 6–48
  pulmonary involvement with, 6–49
Ascites, chylous, 11–59
Aspirin
  contraindication in children with bleeding problems, 9–131
  disturbance of hemostasis with, 5–50
  poisoning, 5–23, 5–24, 5–47
Asthma
  arterial blood gases in, 11–13
  management of acute attack, 10–6, 10–7, 10–8, 10–9, 10–10
  monitoring of peak expiratory flow in, 11–76
  roentgenographic abnormality in, 11–14
Ataxia
  acute cerebella, 9–11
  in Hartnup disease, 11–43
Atopic dermatitis, 11–24
Atrial septal defect, 9–52, 9–113, 10–76, 10–77, 10–78, 10–79, 10–80
Atropine, use in organophosphate poisoning, 11–132
Automobile safety, 5–34
Autosomal recessive disorders, 11–153, 11–154, 11–155

Bacteremia, occult, 11–103
Bacterial endocarditis, antibiotic prophylaxis against, 8–12
Bed, resistance to, 2–14

Bile, in vomitus, 9–122
Biliary atresia, 1–35, 3–95
Bilirubin
    excretion of, in utero, 3–13
    production from hemoglobin, 2–14
    unconjugated, albumin binding of, 3–21
Bladder control, age of attainment, 2–72
Blindness, detection of, 2–82
Blood count, normal in 2-year-old, 9–86
Blood pressure
    measurement of, 9–2
    normal value at 2 years, 2–23
Blood transfusions, use in hemolytic anemia, 8–11
Body proportions, 2–36, 2–66
Body water, total, change with age, 2–11
Bonding, maternal-infant, 2–32
Bone age, 2–33
Botulism, infantile, 1–14
Brain abscess, association with cyanotic congenital heart disease, 9–28
Brain tumors, 9–24
    head tilt in, 11–42
Breast abscess, in newborn, 3–1
Breath-holding spells, 11–52
Bronchiolitis
    viral, 1–2, 11–104
    wheezing with, 6–15
Bronchopulmonary dysplasia, 3–33
Bronze baby syndrome, 10–84

Caffey disease, 11–117, 11–118, 11–119
Calcium, requirement for, 4–14
Carbohydrate, as source of calories, 4–26
Cefoxitin, effect against anaerobes, 8–79
Ceftazidime, effect against Pseudomonas, 8–78
Celiac disease, 9–5
    use of wheat-free diet in, 11–144
Cellulitis, periorbital, 9–66
Cephalhematoma, 3–55
Cephalosporins
    effect against E. coli, 8–81
    lack of effect against Listeria, 8–80
    second generation, 8–77
Cerebral palsy, 9–9, 9–10
Cerebrospinal fluid, protein concentration of, in neonate, 2–24
Child abuse. See Abuse, child
Chlamydia psittaci, 6–95
Chlamydia trachomatis, 6–98
Cholesterol, elevated serum level of, 7–28
Chorea
    Huntington, 9–94, 9–96
    rheumatic, 9–16, 10–111, 10–112, 10–113, 10–114, 10–115, 10–116
        treatment of, 8–30
Chronic granulomatous disease, 6–19
Circumcision
    arguments for, 1–17
    indications for, 1–18
Cleft palate, 11–17
    submucosal, 11–44
Clubfoot deformity, 3–59
Coarctation of the aorta, 9–77
Cocaine, 5–43
    cerebral infarction in neonate due to maternal use of, 1–5
Coccidiomycosis, 6–83

Condyloma accuminatum, 1–31
Congenital adrenal hyperplasia, see adrenal hyperplasia, congenital
Congenital heart disease, cyanotic, 3–45
    management of neonate with, 10–68, 10–69, 10–70, 10–71, 10–72
Convulsions. See Seizures
Coombs' test, 11–159
Cor pulmonale, from chronic upper airway obstruction, 11–40
Coronary artery, anomalous origin of, 11–18
Corticosteroids, side effects of, 8–68
Cortisone, dexamethasone equivalent of, 8–24
Craniopharyngioma, 9–4, 11–31
    growth curve in, 2–42
Craniosynostosis, 9–15
Cranium, at birth, relative size of, 2–34
Cri du chat syndrome, 3–109
Crigler-Najjar syndrome, 1–36
Cushing syndrome, 1–96, 11–30, 11–96
Cyanide poisoning, 11–133
Cyanosis
    causes of, 3–98
    peripheral, normal in newborn, 3–44
Cyclophosphamide, hemorrhagic cystitis with, 8–29
Cystic fibrosis, 11–63
    diabetes in, 11–87
    genetics of, 1–1
    meconium ileus in, 9–91
    pancreatic insufficiency in, 9–26
    pulmonary involvement in, 11–16
    sweat test in, 11–88
Cystic hygroma, 9–34
Cysticercosis, 11–86
Cytomegalovirus
    congenital, 1–7, 3–3, 3–4, 3–47
    mononucleosis picture with, 6–42

DPT vaccine, use of, 6–9
Deafness, sudden onset, 11–27
Death rate, pediatric, 9–1
Deferoxamine (desferrioxamine), use in iron poisoning, 5–1, 8–54
Dehydration
    fluid management in, 7–12, 10–17, 10–18, 10–19, 10–20, 10–21
    secondary to diarrhea, acidosis in, 7–14
Denver Developmental Screening Test, 2–67
Dermatomyositis, 9–27
Development, 2–19
    of 1-month-old, 2–2
    of 3-month-old, 2–71
    of 4-month-old, 2–4
    of 6-month-old, 2–5
    of 7-month-old, 2–92
    of 14-month-old, 2–90
    of 1-year-old, 2–73
    of 3-year-old, 2–83, 2–84
    of 4-year-old, 2–13
    of 5-year-old, 2–15, 2–85
    of 6-year-old, 2–16, 2–74
Developmental screening tests, categories in, 2–70
Dexamethasone, cortisone equivalent of, 8–24
DiGeorge syndrome, 3–46
Diabetes insipidus, nephrogenic, 8–7
Diabetes mellitus, 7–41
    excessive insulin dosage in, 8–50
    insulin requirement in, with bed rest, 8–6
    in cystic fibrosis, 11–87

monitoring home control in, 7–42
onset in children, 7–22
polyuria in, 7–16
Diabetic ketoacidosis
dosage of insulin in, 8–58
serum osmolality in, 7–21
Dialysis, continuous ambulatory peritoneal, 11–9
Diamond Blackfan syndrome, 9–42
Diaphragmatic paralysis, associated with brachial plexus palsy, 3–53
Diazoxide, 8–25
Diencephalic syndrome, 9–14
Digoxin, dosage in premature infant, 8–48
Diphenhydramine, dosage of, 8–23
Diphtheria
neurologic complications of, 6–62
treatment of, 8–49
Diuretics
effect on blood pressure, 8–84
use in congestive heart failure, 8–82
Doriden, abuse of, 5–42
Double aortic arch, 9–114
Down's syndrome, 3–108
association with duodenal atresia, 9–124
in newborn, informing parents of, 2–7
Drowning, 5–32
Drug abuse, 5–39
Ductus arteriosus, patent, 9–43
Duodenal atresia, 9–121, 11–47
Dysautonomia, familial, 9–55

EDTA, use in lead poisoning, 11–129
Echolalia, normal, 2–30
Eczema, 11–24. *See also* Atopic dermatitis
Ehlers-Danlos syndrome, 11–94
Electrocardiogram, 2–22, 9–106, 9–107, 9–108, 9–109
Emesis, induced, use in poisoning, 5–29
Encephalocele, 3–83
Encopresis, 11–36
Endocardial fibroelastosis, 9–45
Endocarditis, bacterial, 9–21
Entamoeba histolytica, 8–59
Enterobius vermicularis, 6–92
Epiglottitis, acute, 8–14
Epstein-Barr virus, as cause of mononucleosis, 6–63
Erythema nodosum, 1–23
Erythema toxicum, 3–31
eosinophils in, 3–70
Erythroblastopenia, transient, 9–47
Ethosuximide, use in absence seizures, 8–18
Ethylene glycol, poisoning, 11–134
Exostosis, multiple cartilaginous, 11–95

Failure to thrive
evaluation of infant with, 10–49, 10–50, 10–51, 10–52, 10–53, 10–54
nonorganic causes of, 1–19
Fanconi's syndrome, 11–3
Fasciculations, muscle, 11–156
Fat necrosis, subcutaneous, in newborn, 3–79
Fat
as percentage of body weight, related to age, 2–12
as source of calories, 4–27, 4–28
content of milk, 4–10

Feeding, infant
fluid requirements for, 4–6
introduction of solids in, 4–1, 4–2
low birth weight, 3–29
use of commercial formula in, 1–15
Femoral epiphysis, slipped, 8–63, 10–87, 10–88, 10–89, 11–147, 11–151
Fetal heart rate monitoring, 3–93
Fetal hemoglobin, 2–20
Fetus, weight of at 28 weeks, 3–27
Fluids, requirement for, 7–1, 7–2, 7–3, 7–4, 7–5, 7–6, 7–7, 7–8, 7–9, 7–34, 7–35
Fluoride, 8–64
Folic acid, deficiency, 4–16
Fontanel, anterior
age of closure, 2–39
at birth, 2–38
Food poisoning, staphylococcal, 6–27
Foreign body
pulmonary, 11–69
swallowed, 8–3
Fracture, epiphyseal, 5–22
Friedreich ataxia, 9–94, 9–95, 9–97
Fructose intolerance, hereditary, 7–39
Fruit juice, source of calories in, 4–30
Fundoplication, use in treatment of GER, 8–16
Furosemide, toxicities of, 8–85

G-6-P-D deficiency, see glucose–6-phosphate dehydrogenase deficiency
Galactokinase deficiency, 7–19
Galactosemia, 7–20, 7–23, 10–55, 10–56, 10–57
Gastroesophageal reflux, surgical treatment of, 8–16
Gaucher's disease, 7–30
Gender identity, during infancy, 2–76
Gentamicin, dose in neonate, 8–44
Gesell schedules, use in 1-year-old, 2–79
Gestation, 40-weeks, signs of 3–28
Glaucoma, congenital, 3–42
Glomeruli, renal, number at birth, 2–56
Glomerulonephritis
acute, 10–1, 10–2, 10–3, 10–4, 10–5, 11–136, 11–139
poststreptococcal, 11–7, 11–73
Glucose-6-phosphate dehydrogenase deficiency, 7–38, 9–65, 10–101, 10–102, 10–103, 10–104, 10–105, 10–106
Glutethimide, overdose with, 5–20
Glycogen storage disease, 7–18, 7–27, 7–43
Gonococcal ophthalmia neonatorum, 3–7
Grasp reflex, in newborn, 3–30
Grasp response, voluntary, 2–18
Griseofulvin, 8–60
Group B streptococcus, as cause of neonatal meningitis, 3–77
Growth delay, constitutional, 11–99
Growth hormone, deficiency of, 2–43
Growth, pattern of during childhood, 2–40
Guillain-Barré syndrome, 10–43, 10–44, 10–45, 10–46, 10–47, 10–48
Gynecomastia, physiologic, 2–45

HIV, clinical features of, 6–78
congenital, EB virus infection with, 6–65
Hallucinogenic drugs, 5–16, 5–17
Hartnup disease, ataxia in, 11–43
Head circumference
at birth, 2–63
growth of, 2–64, 2–65

Head injury, 5–3
Heart failure, causes of, 9–115
Height. *See also* Length
  annual increase during school-age years, 2–62
Hemangioma, capillary, 3–68
Hematuria, 11–138
  due to hypercalciuria, 11–68
  microscopic, chronic, 1–24
Hemiparesis, detection of, 2–81
Hemoglobin
  fetal, 3–82
  normal value at 1 year, 2–53
Hemolytic disease of the newborn, 3–20
Hemophilia, 9–126, 9–128
  treatment of, 8–1, 8–51
Hemophilus influenzae B, immunization against, 1–12
  prophylaxis with rifampin, 6–61
Hemosiderosis, primary pulmonary, 11–77
Henoch-Schönlein purpura, 1–26, 9–40
Hepatitis A, preicteric, 1–11
Hepatitis B, chronic infection with, 6–56
  preicteric, 6–55
Hepatitis, viral, 6–117, 6–118, 6–119, 6–120, 6–121
  acute, 10–22, 10–23, 10–24, 10–25
  fulminant, 6–54
Hepatoblastoma, 8–36, 9–69
Hepatoma, 11–143
Hernia
  inguinal, in female, 11–90
  umbilical, 11–58
Heroin, 5–36, 5–38
Herpangina
  causes of, 6–60
  clinical findings in, 6–59
Herpes simplex
  meningoencephalitis, 6–53
  ophthalmolitis, 6–64
Hip, congenital dislocation of, 11–70
Hirschsprung's disease, 9–46, 9–93
Histoplasmosis, 6–2
Hodgkin disease, 9–50, 9–80
Homocystinuria, 7–17, 7–44
Honey, association with infantile botulism, 1–14
Hospitalization
  of infant, psychological trauma of, 2–47
  of toddler, psychological trauma of, 2–48
Huntington chorea. *See* Chorea, Huntington
Hurler syndrome, 1–29
Hyperbilirubinemia, neonatal
  management of 3–111, 3–112, 3–113, 3–114, 3–115, 3–116,
    10–61, 10–62, 10–63, 10–66, 10–67, 10–81, 10–82, 10–83,
    10–84, 10–85, 10–86
  neurologic damage from, 3–101
  physiologic, 1–34, 3–88, 3–105
Hypercalciuria, hematuria with, 11–68
Hypernatremia, treatment of, 7–13
Hyperostosis, cortical, infantile. *See* Caffey disease
Hyperthermia, malignant, 9–19
Hypocalcemia, 6–123
  in newborn, 3–52, 3–71
Hypoglycemia, 7–37
  conditions associated with, 11–105
  in newborn, 3–58
  ketotic, 11–48
  secondary to drugs, 5–46
Hypoparathyroidism, 11–92

Hypothyroidism
  congenital, 11–66, 11–85
  neonatal, epiphyseal dysgenesis in, 3–75

Immunization
  DPT, 6–128
    convulsion following, 10–97, 10–98, 10–99, 10–100
  H. influenzae, 6–133
  measles, 6–130
    used of killed vaccine, 6–132
  polio, 6–129
  rubella, 6–131
Immunodeficiency, 6–124, 6–126, 6–127, 9–98
  severe combined, 11–123, 11–124, 11–125
Immunoglobulins, serum, 6–3, 6–66, 6–99, 6–100, 6–101, 6–102,
  6–103
Incontinentia pigmenti, 3–80
Infant of diabetic mother, 3–103
Inflammatory bowel disease, 8–53
Inhalants, abuse of, 5–19, 5–37
Injection, intramuscular, sites for, 8–39
Injury prevention, 5–11
  child's judgement in, 5–27
Insulin
  NPH, 8–76
  use in children, 1–10
  effect of bed rest on requirement for, 8–6
  lente, 8–72
  regular, 8–75
  semilente, 8–74
  ultralente, 8–73
Intelligence (IQ), measurement of, 2–31
Intrauterine transfusion
  complications of, 3–16
  indication for, 2–15
Intraventricular hemorrhage, 3–43
Intussusception, 9–25, 10–26, 10–27, 10–28, 10–29
Ipecac, contraindication to use of, 5–31
Iron deficiency anemia. *See* Anemia
Iron poisoning, 5–33, 8–54, 11–130
Isoniazid, 8–27

Kawasaki syndrome, 9–79
Kernicterus
  early signs of, 3–18
  relation to serum level of bilirubin, 3–17
Kerosene, ingestion of, 11–65
Klinefelter's syndrome, 1–8
  infertility in, 11–146

LSD, 5–18
Lactase deficiency, intestinal, 9–38
Langerhan's cell histiocytosis, 9–71, 10–90, 10–91, 10–92, 10–
  93
Language development, in 14-month-old, 2–6
Laryngomalacia, 11–67
Latency, 2–78
Laugh, social, 2–87
Lead
  lack of nutritional value, 4–22
  poisoning, 5–7
    screening for, 5–8
    signs of, 5–9

use of EDTA in, 11–129
Learning disorder, 2–3
Lecithin-sphingomyelin ratio, in amniotic fluid, 3–32
Legg-Perthe disease, 11–148, 11–149
Length
    gain during first year of life, 2–60
    gain during second year of life, 2–61
Letterer-Siwe disease. *See* Langerhan's cell histiocytosis
Leukemia, 9–62, 9–89
    CNS, involvement in, 9–63
    treatment of, 8–32, 8–70
Lice, scalp, treatment of, 11–64
Listeria monocytogenes
    meningitis due to, 6–45
    neonatal infection with, 3–6
Lordosis, normal in toddler, 2–49
Low birth weight, 3–24, 3–25, 3–89
Lupus erythematosus, systemic, prognosis, 9–73
Lyme disease, 1–25
Lymphoid hyperplasia, in childhood, 2–54
Lymphoma, non-Hodgkin, 9–61

Malignancy, conditions associated with increased risk of, 9–83
Malrotation, intestinal, 11–46
Maple syrup urine disease, 7–24, 7–47, 8–61
Marfan's syndrome, 2–95
Marijuana, 5–15, 5–41
Massive infantile spasms. *See* Seizures
Maternal-infant interaction, 2–29
McCune-Albright syndrome, 9–41
Measles, 6–85, 6–86, 6–87, 6–88, 6–109, 6–110, 6–111, 6–112, 6–113, 6–115
    complications of, 6–69
    immunization against, 6–116
    mortality, in undeveloped countries, 6–7
    rash of, 6–50
    use of immunoglobulin in unimmunized contacts of, 6–46
    vaccine, age of first dose, 6–8
Meconium
    aspiration syndrome, 1–9, 3–2
    failure to pass, 3–78
Medulloblastoma, 9–84
Menarche, relation to Tanner stage, 2–68
Meningitis
    empiric antibiotic treatment of, 8–38
    neonatal, 3–5
    beyond the newborn period, 6–52
    H. influenzae, 6–61
    Listeria monocytogenes, 6–45
    meningococcal, treatment of, 8–46
    pneumococcal, SIADH secretion in, 11–107, 11–108, 11–109, 11–110
    subdural effusions with, 6–41
    symptoms of, 6–39
    tuberculous, 6–11
Methadone, ingestion of, 8–28
Methanol, poisoning with, 8–21
Methemoglobinemia, due to well water, 11–19
Methyl alcohol, poisoning, 5–1
Methylphenidate, 8–4
Milk, composition of, 4–25
Minimal change disease, as cause of nephrotic syndrome, 1–3
Molluscum contagiosum, 1–30
Mononucleosis, 10–11, 10–12, 10–13, 10–14, 10–15, 10–16

cytomegalovirus as cause of, 6–42
    clinical features of, 6–72
    clinical picture of, 1–6
    Epstein-Barr virus as cause of, 6–63
Morphine, poisoning, use of naloxone in, 11–135
Mortality, neonatal, 3–22, 3–23, 3–26
Mosquitoes, as vectors in arbovirus infection, 6–12
Muscular dystrophy, Duchenne, 11–158
Multicystic kidney, 11–2
Mumps, 10–94, 10–95, 10–96
    aseptic meningitis with, 6–38
Murmur, of atrial septal defect, 9–52
Murmurs, new, in endocarditis, 9–116
Muscle mass, growth of, 2–41
Myasthenia gravis, 11–157
    newborn of mother with, 3–57
Mycobacteria, atypical, 6–16
Mycoplasma pneumonia, 8–13
    neurologic complications with, 6–14

Naloxone, use of, 8–67
Nasal polyps, 11–28
Nasopharyngeal angiofibroma, juvenile, 11–75
Necator americanus, 6–89
Necrotizing enterocolitis, 3–67
Neisseria gonorrhea
    extragenital complications of, 6–51
    immunity to, 6–58
    infection in prepubertal girls, 6–25
    pelvic inflammatory disease secondary to, 6–84
    urethritis, in male, 6–26, 8–65
Neisseria meningitidis
    meningitis, treatment of, 8–46
    rifampin as prophylaxis for, 6–43
    shock with, 6–40
Nephrotic syndrome
    age of onset, 11–11
    conditions associated with, 11–97
    congenital, 11–10
    pneumococcal peritonitis in, 11–140
    response to corticosteroids in, 11–137
    serum complement in, 11–12
Neuroblastoma, 9–12, 9–35, 9–36
Neuromotor development, pattern of, 2–1
Neutropenia, cyclic, 11–35
Niacin, deficiency of, 4–31, 4–32
Nitrite, poisoning with, 8–22
Nodules, subcutaneous, in rheumatic fever, 9–117
Nucleated red blood cells, in newborn, 3–119

Oedipal years, 2–77
Ophthalmia neonatorum, gonococcal, 3–7
Organicacidemia, presentation in neonatal period, 3–56
Organophosphate poisoning, 5–14
    use of atropine in, 11–132
Osmolality, serum
    in diabetic ketoacidosis, 7–21
    normal, 7–15
Osteogenesis imperfecta, 7–31
Otitis externa, 9–37
Otitis media
    bacterial, acute, 11–89
    serous, chronic, 8–35, 11–1, 11–20, 11–26
Ovulation, relation to menarche, 2–52

Pancreatic enzymes, use in cystic fibrosis, 8–52
Pancreatic insufficiency, 9–26
Pancreatitis, acute, 11–60
Pancytopenia, acquired, 9–90
Pasteurella multocida, 6–94
Peak expiratory flow, monitoring in asthma, 11–76
Penicillin, oral, 8–43
Periorbital cellulitis, 11–39
Pertussis, 6–96, 10–33, 10–34, 10–35
    blood count in, 6–36
    choice of antibiotic for, 8–45
    clinical course of, 6–35
    susceptibility of newborns to, 3–10
Petechiae, in endocarditis, 9–118
Phenobarbital, newborn of mother abusing, 3–76
Phenothiazine poisoning, 5–10
Phenylketonuria, 7–45
    screening for, 7–25
    treatment of, 7–26
Phenytoin, gingival hyperplasia with, 1–4
Pica, 11–21
Pierre Robin syndrome, 3–60
Pinworms, 11–53
Pityriasis rosea, 1–32, 1–33
Platelet disorders, manifestations of, 11–50
Poison ivy dermatitis, 11–45
Poisoning, 5–48, 5–49
    organophosphate, 1–21
Polio, immunization against, 6–10
Polycystic kidney disease, 9–133, 9–134, 9–135, 9–136
Polycythemia, neonatal, 3–99
Polyps, intestinal, juvenile, 11–55
Pompe's disease, 7–27
Porphyria, congenital, 7–51
Portal vein, thrombosis of, 11–62
Posterior urethral valves, 11–5
Potassium
    requirement for, 7–11
    serum value in newborn, 3–91
Prader-Willi syndrome, 9–75
Pralidoxime, use in organophosphate poisoning, 8–55
Precocious puberty, 11–150
    associated with hypothyroidism, 11–82
    secondary to CNS lesion, 11–81
Prednisone, alternate day dosage, 8–10
Prochlorperazine poisoning, 5–10
Propranolol, use in SVT, 8–19
Propylthiouracil, 8–9
Protein, recommended daily intake, 4–11, 4–12
Pseudocholinesterase deficiency, 8–33
Pseudohypoparathyroidism, 11–83
Pseudotumor cerebri, 9–59, 11–38
Puberty, delayed, ultimate height in, 2–44
Pulmonary venous drainage, anomalous, 9–22
Pustulosis, neonatal, 3–8
Pyloric stenosis, hypertrophic, 11–114, 11–115, 11–116
    alkalosis with, 7–36
    surgical treatment of, 9–125
Pyridoxine, use in neonatal convulsions, 3–61
Pyruvate kinase deficiency, 7–32

Q fever, spread of, 6–68
QT interval, syndrome of prolongation of, 8–15

Rabies, 6–105, 6–106, 6–107
Radial head, subluxation of, 5–21
Renal agenesis, 3–72
Renal failure
    acute, 11–98
    chronic, 8–71, 11–141
Renal function, in infant, 2–57
Renal tubular acidosis, 11–4
Renal vein thrombosis, in newborn, 3–94
Respiratory distress syndrome
    absence of wheezing in, 3–92
    acidosis in, 3–34
    hypoxia in, 3–41
    prematurity as etiologic factor in, 3–35
    roentgenographic findings in, 3–37
    signs of, 3–36
    surfactant in, 3–40
    use of continuous airway pressure in, 3–38
Respiratory rate, normal in 1-year-old, 2–21
Reticulocyte count, in newborn, 3–118
Retinoblastoma, 1–20, 9–39
Retinopathy of prematurity, 3–39
Rheumatic fever
    arthritis in, 9–18
    chorea in, 9–16, 9–32
    Jones criteria for, 9–70
    prevention of recurrences of, 9–30
Rheumatoid arthritis, juvenile, 9–58
    uveitis, in, 11–71
    serum rheumatoid factor in, 9–29
Rhinitis, allergic, 11–23
Rifampin, use for prophylaxis with *N. meningitidis*, 6–43
Riley-Day syndrome, 9–55
Rocky Mountain spotted fever, 6–34, 10–36, 10–37, 10–38
Roseola, 6–57
Rotavirus, 11–101
Rubella
    arthritis with, 6–114
    congenital, 3–100, 6–5
    consequences of maternal infection, 6–71
    immunization against, 6–116
    infection in young children, 6–82

Salicylate. *See* Aspirin
Salmonella infection, 6–18
Sarcoidosis, 11–106
    angiotensin-converting enzyme in, 11–72
Scabies, 11–100
Scalded skin syndrome. *See* Toxic epidermal necrolysis
Scarlet fever, 6–29, 6–30, 6–73, 6–74
Scoliosis, idiopathic, 11–61
Seizures, 9–99, 9–103, 9–104
    absence, 8–18, 9–101, 9–105
    febrile, 8–8, 10–58, 10–59, 10–60, 11–41
    following DPT immunization, 10–97
    grand mal, 9–100, 9–102
    hysterical, pseudo, 11–37
    massive infantile spasms, 9–48, 9–49, 9–51
    neonatal, 3–63
    partial complex, 9–17
Sepsis
    gram negative, 9–129
    in child with leukemia, 11–8

Septostomy, atrial, balloon, 9–23
Shaken infant syndrome, 5–25
Shellfish poisoning, 5–12
Shigella infection, 6–21
Short stature, familial, 2–69
Sickle cell disease, 9–64, 9–87
    abnormal hemoglobin electrophoresis in, 11–162
    dactylitis in, 9–31
    hemoglobin level in, 11–32
    reticulocytosis in, 11–161
    splenic sequestration in, 11–33
Sit without assistance, age of attainment, 2–88
Skim milk
    dangers of use of in infant feeding, 4–24
    source of calories in, 4–29
Skin, red coloration of in newborn, 3–65
Sleep, position for infants, 1–13
Small for gestational age infant, definition of, 1–16
Small for gestational age infants, 3–102
Smallpox, vaccination for, 6–6
Smile, social, 2–86
Snake bite, copperhead, 11–25
Sodium, daily requirement, 7–10
Soy-protein formula, use in infant feeding, 4–21
Spasms, infantile. *See* Seizures
Spasmus nutans, 9–60
Speech, at 4 years, 2–28
Spherocytosis, hereditary, neonatal hyperbilirubinemia with, 11–160
Spider, brown recluse, bite of, 5–30
Spinal muscle atrophy, infantile, 9–8, 9–57
Spirillum minus, 6–93
Spironolactone, potassium sparing effect of, 8–83
Spleen
    congenital absence of, 9–81
    rupture of, 5–26
Splenectomy, indication for, 8–69, 9–130
Splenic sequestration, in sickle cell disease, 11–33
Stairs, ability to walk up, age of attainment, 2–91
Staphylococcus
    pneumonia due to, 6–32
    toxins associated with, 6–75
Steatorrhea, 11–142
Streptococcus pneumoniae, pneumonia with, 6–31
Streptococcus
    group A, infection in children less than 1 year, 6–28
    group B, infection, early onset, 6–44
Strongyloides stercoralis, 6–4
Sturge-Weber Syndrome, 1–28
Subarachnoid hemorrhage, management of child with, 11–111, 11–112, 11–113
Subdural effusion, with bacterial meningitis, 6–41
Subdural hematoma, 9–3, 11–126, 11–127, 11–128
    in newborn, 3–90
Sudden infant death syndrome, 9–72
    association with prone sleep position, 1–13
Suicidal behavior, during adolescence, 2–75
Suicide, 5–4
Sweat test, in cystic fibrosis, 11–88
Sweating, in infant, as sign of heart failure, 3–51
Synostosis, sagittal, premature, 3–62
Syphilis
    congenital, 3–87, 6–22, 6–23, 6–24, 10–30, 10–31, 10–32, 11–54
    primary, treatment of, 8–40

Tablespoon, volume of, 8–37
Tachycardia, supraventricular, 9–20
Tanner stage 3 sexual development, 2–17
Tay-Sachs disease, 9–6, 10–39, 10–40, 10–41, 10–42
Teeth
    deciduous, 2–25, 2–26
    permanent, first, 2–27
Television, amount of time spent viewing, 2–46
Temper tantrums, 2–8
Testicle, undescended, 8–2
Testicular feminization syndrome, 11–49
Tetanus, 6–108
    neonatal, 3–12, 6–33
    trismus with, 6–104
Tetany, neonatal, 3–66
Tetracycline, dental discoloration with, 8–62
Tetralogy of Fallot, 8–17, 9–44, 9–76, 9–78, 9–111, 11–34
Thrombocytopenia absent radii syndrome, 3–85
Thrombocytopenia
    causes of, 9–82
    diseases associated with, 11–93
    idiopathic, 9–85, 9–127, 9–132, 10–73, 10–74, 10–75
        use of intravenous immunoglobulin in, 8–47
    in neonate, 3–117
Thrush, in newborn, 3–11, 3–48
Thymus
    appearance on chest roentgenogram, 3–84
    involution during undernutrition, 4–13
Thyroiditis, lymphocytic (Hashimoto), 11–74
Thyrotoxicosis, neonatal, 3–74
Toddler, developmental thrust of, 2–10
Tonic neck reflex, age at which present, 2–93
Tourett syndrome, 1–27
Toxic epidermal necrolysis, 3–9, 3–69
Toxic shock syndrome, staphylococcal, 6–1
Toxocara canis. *See* Visceral larva migrans
Toxoplasmosis
    acquired, 6–77
    congenital, 6–76
Transposition of the great arteries, 9–23, 9–112
Tremors, in neonate, 3–104
Trichobezoar, 11–56
Trichuris trichiuria, 6–91
Trisomy 13, 3–107
Trisomy 18, 3–106
Tuberculin test, positive, management of 8–26
Tuberculosis
    meningitis in, 6–11
    miliary, 6–13
    pleural effusion in, 6–81
    primary pulmonary, 6–17, 6–67, 6–79, 6–80
    use of isoniazid in, 8–27
Turner's syndrome, 3–110
    infertility in, 11–146
    short stature in, 11–145
Typhoid fever, 6–20, 6–37

Undernutrition, effects of, 4–4
Urea cycle defects
    genetic, 7–48, 7–50
    hyperammonemia in, 7–49
Urethral obstruction, 11–5
Urinary tract infection, neonatal, 3–86
Urticaria, 11–79
Uveitis, in juvenile rheumatoid arthritis, 11–71

Varicella
  clinical features of, 6–70
  neonatal, 3–9
Vegan diet, 4–17
Ventricular septal defect, 9–74, 9–110, 11–91
Vesicoureteral reflux, treatment of, 8–56
Visceral larva migrans, 6–47, 6–90, 11–120, 11–121, 11–122
Vitamin A, 4–3
Vitamin B$_{12}$, deficiency, 4–15
Vitamin C, deficiency of, 4–33, 4–34
Vitamin D, 4–8, 4–9
Vitamin E, 4–18
Vitamin K
  content in milk, 4–7
  use in newborns, 4–5
Vitamins, fat soluble, 4–20
Volvulus, midgut, association with malrotation, 9–92
Vomiting, in first day of life, causes of, 3–97
Vomitus, bile-stained, 9–122
Von Willebrand's disease, 11–84

Waferin, poisoning with, 8–20
Walk without assistance, age of attainment, 2–89
Wechsler Intelligence Scale, 2–80
Weight gain
  during first 3 months of life, 2–37
  during first year of life, 2–58
  during second year of life, 2–59
Weight loss, immediate neonatal, 2–35
Werdnig-Hoffman disease. *See* Spinal muscular atrophy
Wheezing, due to aspirated foreign body, 11–69
Wilms' tumor, 11–6
  aniridia with, 9–13
  cure rate in, 8–57
Wilson's disease, 7–33, 9–7, 9–67
Wilson-Mikity syndrome, 3–49
Wiskott-Aldrich syndrome, rash in, 11–78

X-linked recessive disorders, 11–152
XYY chromosomal constitution, 11–80

NAME _____

ADDRESS _____

Street

_____

City   State   Zip

DIRECTIONS

MAKE ERASURES COMPLETE

Mark your social security number from top to bottom in the appropriate boxes on the right. Refer to the section " HOW TO TAKE THE PRACTICE TEST" in the introduction to the book for more information. PLEASE USE NO. 2 PENCIL ONLY.

SOCIAL SECURITY NUMBER

| 0 1 2 3 4 5 6 7 8 9 |
| 0 1 2 3 4 5 6 7 8 9 |
| 0 1 2 3 4 5 6 7 8 9 |
| 0 1 2 3 4 5 6 7 8 9 |
| 0 1 2 3 4 5 6 7 8 9 |
| 0 1 2 3 4 5 6 7 8 9 |
| 0 1 2 3 4 5 6 7 8 9 |
| 0 1 2 3 4 5 6 7 8 9 |
| 0 1 2 3 4 5 6 7 8 9 |

1 Ⓐ Ⓑ Ⓒ Ⓓ Ⓔ
2 Ⓐ Ⓑ Ⓒ Ⓓ Ⓔ
3 Ⓐ Ⓑ Ⓒ Ⓓ Ⓔ
4 Ⓐ Ⓑ Ⓒ Ⓓ Ⓔ
5 Ⓐ Ⓑ Ⓒ Ⓓ Ⓔ
6 Ⓐ Ⓑ Ⓒ Ⓓ Ⓔ
7 Ⓐ Ⓑ Ⓒ Ⓓ Ⓔ
8 Ⓐ Ⓑ Ⓒ Ⓓ Ⓔ
9 Ⓐ Ⓑ Ⓒ Ⓓ Ⓔ
10 Ⓐ Ⓑ Ⓒ Ⓓ Ⓔ
11 Ⓐ Ⓑ Ⓒ Ⓓ Ⓔ
12 Ⓐ Ⓑ Ⓒ Ⓓ Ⓔ
13 Ⓐ Ⓑ Ⓒ Ⓓ Ⓔ
14 Ⓐ Ⓑ Ⓒ Ⓓ Ⓔ
15 Ⓐ Ⓑ Ⓒ Ⓓ Ⓔ
16 Ⓐ Ⓑ Ⓒ Ⓓ Ⓔ
17 Ⓐ Ⓑ Ⓒ Ⓓ Ⓔ
18 Ⓐ Ⓑ Ⓒ Ⓓ Ⓔ
19 Ⓐ Ⓑ Ⓒ Ⓓ Ⓔ
20 Ⓐ Ⓑ Ⓒ Ⓓ Ⓔ
21 Ⓐ Ⓑ Ⓒ Ⓓ Ⓔ
22 Ⓐ Ⓑ Ⓒ Ⓓ Ⓔ
23 Ⓐ Ⓑ Ⓒ Ⓓ Ⓔ
24 Ⓐ Ⓑ Ⓒ Ⓓ Ⓔ
25 Ⓐ Ⓑ Ⓒ Ⓓ Ⓔ

26 Ⓐ Ⓑ Ⓒ Ⓓ Ⓔ
27 Ⓐ Ⓑ Ⓒ Ⓓ Ⓔ
28 Ⓐ Ⓑ Ⓒ Ⓓ Ⓔ
29 Ⓐ Ⓑ Ⓒ Ⓓ Ⓔ
30 Ⓐ Ⓑ Ⓒ Ⓓ Ⓔ
31 Ⓐ Ⓑ Ⓒ Ⓓ Ⓔ
32 Ⓐ Ⓑ Ⓒ Ⓓ Ⓔ
33 Ⓐ Ⓑ Ⓒ Ⓓ Ⓔ
34 Ⓐ Ⓑ Ⓒ Ⓓ Ⓔ
35 Ⓐ Ⓑ Ⓒ Ⓓ Ⓔ
36 Ⓐ Ⓑ Ⓒ Ⓓ Ⓔ
37 Ⓐ Ⓑ Ⓒ Ⓓ Ⓔ
38 Ⓐ Ⓑ Ⓒ Ⓓ Ⓔ
39 Ⓐ Ⓑ Ⓒ Ⓓ Ⓔ
40 Ⓐ Ⓑ Ⓒ Ⓓ Ⓔ
41 Ⓐ Ⓑ Ⓒ Ⓓ Ⓔ
42 Ⓐ Ⓑ Ⓒ Ⓓ Ⓔ
43 Ⓐ Ⓑ Ⓒ Ⓓ Ⓔ
44 Ⓐ Ⓑ Ⓒ Ⓓ Ⓔ
45 Ⓐ Ⓑ Ⓒ Ⓓ Ⓔ
46 Ⓐ Ⓑ Ⓒ Ⓓ Ⓔ
47 Ⓐ Ⓑ Ⓒ Ⓓ Ⓔ
48 Ⓐ Ⓑ Ⓒ Ⓓ Ⓔ
49 Ⓐ Ⓑ Ⓒ Ⓓ Ⓔ
50 Ⓐ Ⓑ Ⓒ Ⓓ Ⓔ

51 Ⓐ Ⓑ Ⓒ Ⓓ Ⓔ
52 Ⓐ Ⓑ Ⓒ Ⓓ Ⓔ
53 Ⓐ Ⓑ Ⓒ Ⓓ Ⓔ
54 Ⓐ Ⓑ Ⓒ Ⓓ Ⓔ
55 Ⓐ Ⓑ Ⓒ Ⓓ Ⓔ
56 Ⓐ Ⓑ Ⓒ Ⓓ Ⓔ
57 Ⓐ Ⓑ Ⓒ Ⓓ Ⓔ
58 Ⓐ Ⓑ Ⓒ Ⓓ Ⓔ
59 Ⓐ Ⓑ Ⓒ Ⓓ Ⓔ
60 Ⓐ Ⓑ Ⓒ Ⓓ Ⓔ
61 Ⓐ Ⓑ Ⓒ Ⓓ Ⓔ
62 Ⓐ Ⓑ Ⓒ Ⓓ Ⓔ
63 Ⓐ Ⓑ Ⓒ Ⓓ Ⓔ
64 Ⓐ Ⓑ Ⓒ Ⓓ Ⓔ
65 Ⓐ Ⓑ Ⓒ Ⓓ Ⓔ
66 Ⓐ Ⓑ Ⓒ Ⓓ Ⓔ
67 Ⓐ Ⓑ Ⓒ Ⓓ Ⓔ
68 Ⓐ Ⓑ Ⓒ Ⓓ Ⓔ
69 Ⓐ Ⓑ Ⓒ Ⓓ Ⓔ
70 Ⓐ Ⓑ Ⓒ Ⓓ Ⓔ
71 Ⓐ Ⓑ Ⓒ Ⓓ Ⓔ
72 Ⓐ Ⓑ Ⓒ Ⓓ Ⓔ
73 Ⓐ Ⓑ Ⓒ Ⓓ Ⓔ
74 Ⓐ Ⓑ Ⓒ Ⓓ Ⓔ
75 Ⓐ Ⓑ Ⓒ Ⓓ Ⓔ

76 Ⓐ Ⓑ Ⓒ Ⓓ Ⓔ
77 Ⓐ Ⓑ Ⓒ Ⓓ Ⓔ
78 Ⓐ Ⓑ Ⓒ Ⓓ Ⓔ
79 Ⓐ Ⓑ Ⓒ Ⓓ Ⓔ
80 Ⓐ Ⓑ Ⓒ Ⓓ Ⓔ
81 Ⓐ Ⓑ Ⓒ Ⓓ Ⓔ
82 Ⓐ Ⓑ Ⓒ Ⓓ Ⓔ
83 Ⓐ Ⓑ Ⓒ Ⓓ Ⓔ
84 Ⓐ Ⓑ Ⓒ Ⓓ Ⓔ
85 Ⓐ Ⓑ Ⓒ Ⓓ Ⓔ
86 Ⓐ Ⓑ Ⓒ Ⓓ Ⓔ
87 Ⓐ Ⓑ Ⓒ Ⓓ Ⓔ
88 Ⓐ Ⓑ Ⓒ Ⓓ Ⓔ
89 Ⓐ Ⓑ Ⓒ Ⓓ Ⓔ
90 Ⓐ Ⓑ Ⓒ Ⓓ Ⓔ
91 Ⓐ Ⓑ Ⓒ Ⓓ Ⓔ
92 Ⓐ Ⓑ Ⓒ Ⓓ Ⓔ
93 Ⓐ Ⓑ Ⓒ Ⓓ Ⓔ
94 Ⓐ Ⓑ Ⓒ Ⓓ Ⓔ
95 Ⓐ Ⓑ Ⓒ Ⓓ Ⓔ
96 Ⓐ Ⓑ Ⓒ Ⓓ Ⓔ
97 Ⓐ Ⓑ Ⓒ Ⓓ Ⓔ
98 Ⓐ Ⓑ Ⓒ Ⓓ Ⓔ
99 Ⓐ Ⓑ Ⓒ Ⓓ Ⓔ
100 Ⓐ Ⓑ Ⓒ Ⓓ Ⓔ

101 Ⓐ Ⓑ Ⓒ Ⓓ Ⓔ

102 Ⓐ Ⓑ Ⓒ Ⓓ Ⓔ

103 Ⓐ Ⓑ Ⓒ Ⓓ Ⓔ

104 Ⓐ Ⓑ Ⓒ Ⓓ Ⓔ

105 Ⓐ Ⓑ Ⓒ Ⓓ Ⓔ

106 Ⓐ Ⓑ Ⓒ Ⓓ Ⓔ

107 Ⓐ Ⓑ Ⓒ Ⓓ Ⓔ

108 Ⓐ Ⓑ Ⓒ Ⓓ Ⓔ

109 Ⓐ Ⓑ Ⓒ Ⓓ Ⓔ

110 Ⓐ Ⓑ Ⓒ Ⓓ Ⓔ

111 Ⓐ Ⓑ Ⓒ Ⓓ Ⓔ

112 Ⓐ Ⓑ Ⓒ Ⓓ Ⓔ

113 Ⓐ Ⓑ Ⓒ Ⓓ Ⓔ

114 Ⓐ Ⓑ Ⓒ Ⓓ Ⓔ

115 Ⓐ Ⓑ Ⓒ Ⓓ Ⓔ

116 Ⓐ Ⓑ Ⓒ Ⓓ Ⓔ

117 Ⓐ Ⓑ Ⓒ Ⓓ Ⓔ

118 Ⓐ Ⓑ Ⓒ Ⓓ Ⓔ

119 Ⓐ Ⓑ Ⓒ Ⓓ Ⓔ

120 Ⓐ Ⓑ Ⓒ Ⓓ Ⓔ

121 Ⓐ Ⓑ Ⓒ Ⓓ Ⓔ

122 Ⓐ Ⓑ Ⓒ Ⓓ Ⓔ

123 Ⓐ Ⓑ Ⓒ Ⓓ Ⓔ

124 Ⓐ Ⓑ Ⓒ Ⓓ Ⓔ

125 Ⓐ Ⓑ Ⓒ Ⓓ Ⓔ

126 Ⓐ Ⓑ Ⓒ Ⓓ Ⓔ

127 Ⓐ Ⓑ Ⓒ Ⓓ Ⓔ

128 Ⓐ Ⓑ Ⓒ Ⓓ Ⓔ

129 Ⓐ Ⓑ Ⓒ Ⓓ Ⓔ Ⓕ Ⓖ Ⓗ Ⓘ Ⓙ Ⓚ Ⓛ Ⓜ
　　Ⓝ Ⓞ Ⓟ Ⓠ Ⓡ Ⓢ Ⓣ Ⓤ Ⓥ Ⓦ Ⓧ Ⓨ Ⓩ

130 Ⓐ Ⓑ Ⓒ Ⓓ Ⓔ Ⓕ Ⓖ Ⓗ Ⓘ Ⓙ Ⓚ Ⓛ Ⓜ
　　Ⓝ Ⓞ Ⓟ Ⓠ Ⓡ Ⓢ Ⓣ Ⓤ Ⓥ Ⓦ Ⓧ Ⓨ Ⓩ

131 Ⓐ Ⓑ Ⓒ Ⓓ Ⓔ Ⓕ Ⓖ Ⓗ Ⓘ Ⓙ Ⓚ Ⓛ Ⓜ
　　Ⓝ Ⓞ Ⓟ Ⓠ Ⓡ Ⓢ Ⓣ Ⓤ Ⓥ Ⓦ Ⓧ Ⓨ Ⓩ

132 Ⓐ Ⓑ Ⓒ Ⓓ Ⓔ Ⓕ Ⓖ Ⓗ Ⓘ Ⓙ Ⓚ Ⓛ Ⓜ
　　Ⓝ Ⓞ Ⓟ Ⓠ Ⓡ Ⓢ Ⓣ Ⓤ Ⓥ Ⓦ Ⓧ Ⓨ Ⓩ

133 Ⓐ Ⓑ Ⓒ Ⓓ Ⓔ Ⓕ Ⓖ Ⓗ Ⓘ Ⓙ Ⓚ Ⓛ Ⓜ
　　Ⓝ Ⓞ Ⓟ Ⓠ Ⓡ Ⓢ Ⓣ Ⓤ Ⓥ Ⓦ Ⓧ Ⓨ Ⓩ

134 Ⓐ Ⓑ Ⓒ Ⓓ Ⓔ Ⓕ Ⓖ Ⓗ Ⓘ Ⓙ Ⓚ Ⓛ Ⓜ
　　Ⓝ Ⓞ Ⓟ Ⓠ Ⓡ Ⓢ Ⓣ Ⓤ Ⓥ Ⓦ Ⓧ Ⓨ Ⓩ

135 Ⓐ Ⓑ Ⓒ Ⓓ Ⓔ Ⓕ Ⓖ Ⓗ Ⓘ Ⓙ Ⓚ Ⓛ Ⓜ
　　Ⓝ Ⓞ Ⓟ Ⓠ Ⓡ Ⓢ Ⓣ Ⓤ Ⓥ Ⓦ Ⓧ Ⓨ Ⓩ

136 Ⓐ Ⓑ Ⓒ Ⓓ

137 Ⓐ Ⓑ Ⓒ Ⓓ

138 Ⓐ Ⓑ Ⓒ Ⓓ

139 Ⓐ Ⓑ Ⓒ Ⓓ

140 Ⓐ Ⓑ Ⓒ Ⓓ

141 Ⓐ Ⓑ Ⓒ Ⓓ

142 Ⓐ Ⓑ Ⓒ Ⓓ

143 Ⓐ Ⓑ Ⓒ Ⓓ

144 Ⓐ Ⓑ Ⓒ Ⓓ

145 Ⓐ Ⓑ Ⓒ Ⓓ

146 Ⓐ Ⓑ Ⓒ Ⓓ

147 Ⓐ Ⓑ Ⓒ Ⓓ

148 Ⓐ Ⓑ Ⓒ Ⓓ

149 Ⓐ Ⓑ Ⓒ Ⓓ

150 Ⓐ Ⓑ Ⓒ Ⓓ

151 Ⓐ Ⓑ Ⓒ Ⓓ

152 Ⓐ Ⓑ Ⓒ Ⓓ

153 Ⓐ Ⓑ Ⓒ Ⓓ

154 Ⓐ Ⓑ Ⓒ Ⓓ

155 Ⓐ Ⓑ Ⓒ Ⓓ

156 Ⓐ Ⓑ Ⓒ Ⓓ

157 Ⓐ Ⓑ Ⓒ Ⓓ

158. Ⓐ Ⓑ Ⓒ Ⓓ

159 Ⓐ Ⓑ Ⓒ Ⓓ

160 Ⓐ Ⓑ Ⓒ Ⓓ

161 Ⓐ Ⓑ Ⓒ Ⓓ

162 Ⓐ Ⓑ Ⓒ Ⓓ